The neurologists

10794842

MANCHESTER
1824

Manchester University Press

The neurologists

A history of a medical specialty in modern Britain, c. 1789–2000

Stephen T. Casper

Manchester University Press

Published by Manchester University Press
Altrincham Street, Manchester M1 7JA, UK
www.manchesteruniversitypress.co.uk

British Library Cataloguing-in-Publication Data is available

Library of Congress Cataloging-in-Publication Data is available

ISBN 978 0 7190 9981 6 *paperback*

First published by Manchester University Press in hardback 2014

This edition first published 2015

Printed by Lightning Source

For the Association of British Neurologists

Contents

List of tables and figures *page* ix
Foreword by Robert Y. Moore xi
Preface xv

Introduction: from physician to neurologist 1
1 Physicians in neurological societies; neurologists in general medical societies 29
2 The First World War and the transformation of neurology 59
3 Neurology in interwar Britain 97
4 Neurology and state medicine 122
5 The integrative legacy of contemporary specialists in neurology 153

Notes 179
Select bibliography 237
Index 264

Tables and figures

Tables

1 Proposers for Fellowship in the Royal Society 49

2 Positions of prestige in British medicine occupied by members of the Neurological Society 53

Figures

1 Numbers of members held in common with the Neurological Society 51

Foreword

Medicine has a long history as both a practical enterprise and a scientific discipline. By the middle of the nineteenth century, the field of medicine was divided broadly, but not exclusively, into internal medicine and surgery. During the last half of that century, specialisation emerged within internal medicine as physicians recognised new diseases and developed tools for increasingly accurate diagnosis, the necessary prelude to assignment of therapy. In this book, Stephen T. Casper, an American trained at the Wellcome Centre for the History of Medicine at University College London, turns our attention to the origins and early history of the medical discipline of neurology in the United Kingdom from the mid-nineteenth to the mid-twentieth century. This period is particularly interesting and important in the history of modern neurology because it was then that British neurology began to lead the rest of the world. The forces that drove this ascent to excellence are evident. Industrialisation, already well underway in the United Kingdom, forced rural manpower to move to urban areas for work. Of all urban areas in the United Kingdom, London grew the most. A concentration of population resulted not only in an increased incidence of contagious diseases such as tuberculosis but also in an increased concentration of diseases with a relatively low prevalence, a characteristic of most neurological diseases other than epilepsy (the incidence of cerebrovascular disease, currently the most common neurological disease in industrialised countries, was relatively low, reflecting the short life expectancy of the period). A general recognition of the need for physicians who had specialised interest and experience in neurological diseases had not developed but was stimulated, as often happens, from an unexpected source.

In 1859, the National Hospital for Diseases of the Nervous System, the first hospital dedicated to neurologic diseases, was established. This occurred not out of an evident medical need but from the foresight and enthusiasm of a layperson, Miss Julia Chandler.[1] That a need did exist is established not only in the success of the National Hospital but by the founding of two additional hospitals, the Maida Vale (1867) and West End (1878) hospitals. The first National Hospital physicians included Jabez Ramskill, an early student of epilepsy, and Charles Eduardo Brown-Séquard, describer of the syndrome of spinal cord hemisection, and John Hughlings Jackson. Brown-Séquard was born on the island of Mauritius, then a British possession; hence, he was British by birth. He was also a relentless and peripatetic proselytiser for himself and neurology, crossing the seas to become a professor at Harvard and to succeed Claude Bernard as professor at the College de France. Aside from his syndrome – the manifestations of hemisection of the spinal cord – Brown-Séquard contributed little of lasting value, but did serve to turn a young Jackson towards neurology. Jackson became recognised as one of the founders of British neurology and, in the assessment of many, was the greatest thinker in the history of neurology. Gordon Holmes writes:'Jackson's work does not simply belong to the history of neurology. It remains today a live and vitalising force in the thought of all who seek depth as well as width of knowledge in the fields of neurophysiology and clinical neurology, and who wish to understand more than the reading of instruments of precision can tell them.'[2] The rest, as the saying goes, is history. It is, of course, the history Professor Casper relates for us.

An unforeseen factor that impelled the development of neurology was its complexity. Neurology is now known to deal with more than 700 inherited diseases and a further host of vascular, trauma, degeneration, immune abnormalities, metabolic disorders, neoplasia, and others as the fundamental aetiology.[3] Unlike other medical specialists, neurologists receive only modest assistance from the laboratory, physiology or imaging. Their ability to diagnose and treat neurological illness is much dependent on history and neurological examination.

To conclude these comments, I can envisage the potential reader perusing the shelf of 'new arrivals' in a bookshop. Interested in neurology and history, she picks up this book. The dust cover is attractive but, like all sceptics, she proceeds further to peruse the contents list to determine if the book is at all 'up her alley'. This assured, she goes on to the Foreword to assess its promise for enlightenment and pleasure. If this is you, my reader, let me give you my wholehearted endorsement of this book. It contains the story of a critical period in the evolution of modern neurology during a crucial time and in the country that led the advance. It is well written, forceful yet nuanced, engaging and stimulating, and above all, informative.

Robert Y Moore, MD, PhD, MD (Hon)
Love Family Professor Emeritus of Neurology
University of Pittsburgh

Preface

Neurology, like history, is a fascinating subject. And like history, nothing about neurology is simple. Throughout all of my research, one observation in particular has always struck me as noteworthy about neurology. While many physicians and scientists have engaged with the history of their fields, I think there are few academic disciplines or clinical specialties where that is so especially the case as it is for neurology. Why this is the case forms one of the major preoccupations of this study. The tentative answer to be found in the subsequent pages is that the professional identity of past neurologists has traditionally been grounded in a set of spirited, integrative dispositions and appreciations. The implications of such an outlook has been that historically the identity of a neurologist ultimately derived of a mixture of the actions of those scientists, physicians, and philosophers who first took as their object the mind, brain, and nervous system.

Yet the story does not really end there, because even as neurologists began retrospectively reconstructing past identities, another cultural formation began transforming the nature of scientific and medical work in Europe, North America, and beyond. It was not wholly inevitable that divisions of labour began to transform the factories and plantations of the modern world. It was still less inevitable that the middle classes should have acquired similarly divided characteristics; nevertheless, the professions, academic disciplines, and clinical specialties emerged in a world that saw in classification and social segmentation the virtue of progress.

Few ideas capture so clearly that world's optimism than the idiom of *specialisation*. As a phenomenon, specialisation, especially as it appeared in the writing of Herbert Spencer, came to appear an atavism of our Neolithic past and a natural law of the growth of knowledge and technological progress. Yet the idea of *specialisation* first came into this world to describe linguistic phenomenon; it moved from there readily into the evolutionary discourses of the pre- and then post-Darwinian worlds, and from there it aided and abetted a new organic conception of society that would in time become the favourite metaphorical trope of functionalist sociology. In this sense, *specialisation* was an idea peculiar to modernity; it would become an idea that lost much of its lustre (although not its reality) in the Digital Age.

The neurologists thus found themselves products of specialisation even as those figures who created that identity found virtues in a style of science and medicine that was the opposite of the word. At times, specialisation became such a force in the construction of their professional identity that it threatened their professional existence with still greater internal divisions. How the neurologists managed to keep their integrative outlook may help us to understand specialisation with a little more clarity. It also helps us to understand precisely why history beckons to so many neurologists. And perhaps, too, their story can shed light on a new phenomenon that began occurring in the last decades of the twentieth century – the rise of a culture that ascribed ever greater importance to the brain.

Such a narrative would not have been possible without the support of many people over the years. This study began as a doctoral dissertation at the Wellcome Trust Centre for the History of Medicine at University College London. Without the support of others in my cohort – Nandini Bhattacharya, Candice Guillet-Delisle, and Liew Kai Khiun – I very much doubt that I should have come as far as I did with this study. Similarly, I am indebted to Janet Browne, Roger Cooter, Anne Hardy, Rhodri Hayward, Christopher Lawrence, Helga Satzinger, and Andrew Wear. Each in a variety of ways inspired and encouraged me, and they made the London Centre the rich environment it was for those of us lucky enough to have briefly travelled through it. There, I also benefited from the expertise of Bruce Moran, Kiheung Kim, Katrina Gatley, Akinobu Takabayashi, and Richard Barnett.

Along the way, a number of others offered me assistance in this project. To them I can only give here too brief acknowledgement. John C. Burnham has been an amazing colleague on this journey. From him, I have learnt what it means to be passionate about history and the history of medicine.

Finally, I wish to pay a special tribute to L. Stephen Jacyna. His scholarship and his mentorship have been of singular importance to me; I have benefitted greatly from his advice, guidance and encouragement over the years.

Many thanks also to Max Stadler, Delia Gavrus, Katja Guenther, Fabio de Sio and Frank Stahnisch. Equally, I owe much to a University of Minnesota cohort, especially John Eyler, Jole Shackelford, Jennifer Gunn, Sally Kohlstedt, and Jacob Steere-Williams. Similarly, Matthew Stanley, Jesse Ballenger, Kenton Kroker, Russell Johnson, Piers J. Hale, Sheila Weiss, Laura Ettinger, Daniel Bradburd, Christopher Robinson, Steve Sturdy, Marjorie Lorch, Stanley Finger, Paul Foley, Tobias Rees, and the late Harry Marks all helped along the way.

A number of neurologists aided me throughout this project. Michael O'Brien was of special importance, both as a source of knowledge for this study and as a second supervisor to an unlikely student of the history of British neurology. The late Ian McDonald shared a number of wonderful stories about British neurology with me. So, too did Alistair Compston, William Goody, Lord Walton, Sir Roger Bannister, Michael Jefferson, Pauline Monro, David Shaw, and Christopher Gardner-Thorpe. Much of this project was supported by a generous fellowship from the Association of British Neurologists. I am grateful to them for an opportunity that launched me into a career as an historian of medicine and especially for the independence they gave me in exploring the history of British neurology.

Although they are too numerous to list here by name, I would also like to thank all of those who opened up their archives to me. I would especially like to mention the descendants of Edwin Bramwell and the descendants of W. Russell Brain. Both families gave me very privileged access to documents that as yet remain beyond the public record. I would also like to express gratitude to everyone at Manchester University Press.

Finally, I would like to express my appreciation to all of those who heroically read or almost read complete versions of this manuscript. My parents, my wife, John C. Burnham, Ellen Dwyer, Delia Gavrus, L. Stephen Jacyna, and two anonymous reviewers at Manchester University Press.

Introduction: from physician to neurologist

Writing to the Moncrieff-Arnott Professor of Clinical Medicine at Edinburgh University, the American surgeon Harvey Cushing asked Edwin Bramwell: 'Have there ever been any professors of neurology anywhere in Great Britain?' It was September 1934. Cushing was preparing an address for the opening celebration of the newly endowed Montreal Neurological Institute on the necessity for common unity between neurologists, neurosurgeons, and psychiatrists.[1]

'Is it', Cushing continued, 'that professors of medicine took an interest in neurology and were loath to give it up to the specialists? Would your father [Byrom Bramwell], for example, have cared to have a neurological unit and give up his general work to the infirmary? And would you have been glad to do the same?' It was curious, Cushing reflected, that although by the close of the nineteenth century there had been professors of mental and nervous diseases in America, the first professorship in neurology had been founded in Philadelphia only in 1903.[2]

In his reply, Edwin Bramwell wrote: 'There has never been, so far as I am aware, a Professor of Neurology in Great Britain.' He then added:

> My father had wider interests in various departments of medicine, and he would I know have been loath to give up his general work in the infirmary and take over a neurological unit. I too would be very sorry now, at any rate, to confine myself to purely neurological Hospital material. I always recall a remark of [William] Gowers, who by the way, was at one time Professor of Clinical Medicine at University College [London], 'a neurologist must be a specialist, but he cannot be an extremist.'[3]

This remarkable exchange between Harvey Cushing, a founder of modern neurosurgery, and Edwin Bramwell, a neurologist and son of a founder of modern neurology, frames the larger question this study explores across two centuries of British medical history. Why, despite often-alleged origins in antiquity, did neurology in Britain endeavour for so long to become a formally recognised specialty within general medicine?[4]

To answer this question, it is necessary to follow a complicated story, one involving individuals, institutions, and ideas all located in the complex, shifting social and cultural ferment of nineteenth- and twentieth-century Britain. Over that two-century period physicians and scientists found themselves, often reluctantly, occupying a new role as members of an ever-more specialist and ever-more medical enterprise called neurology. That story of their reluctance not only describes the by now well-worn tale of medical resistance to the advance of specialisation; significantly, it also calls attention to the fact that in Britain neurology was considered a socially preeminent and general form of scientific and medical knowledge. To define neurology as a specialty was therefore to engage in an act approaching contradiction. Neurologists, even after they had become specialists, sought and found ways to circumvent the ideals of specialisation and to continue thinking broadly about the medicine and science of the brain, nerves, and mind. Indeed, it was this propensity to think expansively that would eventually underpin and legitimate the popular rise of neurologically inclined culture in the late twentieth-century.[5]

In the early nineteenth century, neurology was broadly defined and included scientific and clinical knowledge of the mind, brain, and nervous system. Although that definition would narrow over the next two centuries, the world that nineteenth century British 'neurologists' inhabited aspired to medical generalism, gentlemanly science, and universalism. It would thus only be after the mid-twentieth century and with the emergence of neuroscience that neurology would come to be defined solely by its clinical orientation and that its practitioners would be called, one and all, 'the neurologists'.

Any number of histories of neurology, neuroscience, clinical practice, and of medicine and science offer an entrance into this story.[6] At the same time a sophisticated historical and sociological literature devoted to analysing the specialisation of medicine has made clear the many pitfalls and traps that loom beyond.[7] Such scholarship provides this account with a map for reconstructing the story through the eyes of the individuals involved, their contemporaries (particularly other physicians), and the already mature profession of medicine in Britain.[8] What therefore will become clear by the close of this journey is that the emergence of neurology was not predicated upon the hard work of a few brilliant, like-minded individuals alone. Rather, and surprisingly so, it was through a commitment to general medicine – one held by physicians of all stripes and intentions – that neurology became a demarcated area of clinical practice.

The story of British neurology thus sheds light on the wider history of general medicine in modern-era Britain; it is a story that enlarges upon historian Christopher Lawrence's pioneering identification of a patrician mindset in the habits of the consultant class of medical professionals in modern era Britain.[9] But there is more besides, for it was in this period that modernity in its many guises appeared. It was a time of steam travel, mass democracy movements, wars, new forms of communication, international banking, and imperialism. In consequence, the story of neurology is also a transnational one, for the practices and knowledge in science and medicine began to circulate rapidly through an epistolary economy comprising professional journals, translated books, conferences, and international philanthropy.[10]

The science and medicine of the nervous system in modern Britain

In the history of medicine and science, the brain, nerves, and nervous diseases have long been topics of interest.[11] This book accordingly builds on many excellent studies of the medical and scientific fields associated with those organs and diseases.[12] In the specific case of British neurology there are several useful edited volumes, many empirically rich biographical and autobiographical works, and numerous rigorous intellectual histories which have supported this book's general reconceptualisation.[13] In addition, there are books focusing on neurology in North America and Europe,[14] as well as several recent revisionist works examining the role of culture and society in shaping public and scientific conceptions of the nerves. These works have made clear that those physicians and scientists in Britain (and elsewhere) had long recognised that a proportion of the sick and infirm across the ages suffered from diseases or injuries of the nervous system.[15] It was obvious in the nineteenth century that even before there was anything akin to a recognisable medical profession, people had observed and feared the signs of these fatal or permanently disabling disorders. The experiences and treatment of, for example, paralysis, epilepsy, blindness, weakness, tremors, and even madness had left behind extensive historical documents, even from as distant a past as antiquity.

In the case of Britain, many physicians and scientists were steeped in a tradition of classical education. It had been obligatory for them to read Latin and Greek. Most were therefore aware that early philosophers like Plato and Aristotle had identified and articulated the relationship between the organs of the nerves and intellect.[16] The contributions of such figures as Hippocrates, Galen, and Avicenna to the doctrine of the nerves were also known in nineteenth-century Britain.[17] Indeed, at the beginning of that century, the discoveries of the ancients remained strongly authoritative. The prominence of that authority would erode only slowly with the advent of a modern medicine that increasingly challenged the authority of bygone epochs.[18]

One of the ways in which British physicians and scientists were able to question and transcend the authority of the past was through the invention of a somewhat romantic style of history in the Enlightenment tradition that argued for the positive development of the progress of knowledge.[19] This mode of historical understanding, which drew upon the contributions of such nineteenth-century luminaries as William Whewell, August Comte, and Herbert Spencer, infused much historical writing with teleological motifs and sometimes added a dimension that came to be described famously in the twentieth century as the Whig tradition in the history of science.[20] Such a tradition appeared, for instance, in 1902, when scientist and physician David Ferrier opened his Harveian Oration at the Royal College of Physicians with the observation that 'since the time of Harvey ... neurology had consisted largely in speculations as to the seat of the rational soul.'[21] It was this tradition that at once recognised and aggrandised the contributions of past scientists and physicians while simultaneously creating a lasting foundation for transcending classical authority for neurology.[22]

By the close of the nineteenth century, British physicians and scientists had developed a notion of how progress in the study of the brain, spine, and nerves had been achieved. For them, figures in the Renaissance had drawn upon the works of the Greek and Arabic traditions and created lasting theses about the functions of those organs.[23] These figures had also made pioneering inquiries into the relationship between the nervous organs, mind and heart, which became tenants not just of medicine but also philosophy and religion. Through the anatomy of Andreas Vesalius and Thomas Willis, the philosophy of René Descartes, and the physiology of Jean François Fernel, so their story of discovery went, early modern humoral medicine and science had fashioned a rational nomenclature that sought, as it did in all areas of natural philosophy, an ever-more refined categorisation of the anatomy, physiology, and diseases of the nerves.[24] It was this Whig tradition that appeared in the first histories of neurology that were written by British, American, and French medical historians (many of whom were practising clinicians).[25]

What has often gone unrecognised about this tradition was that even as it cast the history of the mind, nerves, and brain into a very long history, those modern fields – anatomy, physiology, neurology, psychiatry, and psychology – that most benefited from this long narrative had only just begun acquiring their modern professional stature in the nineteenth century. It was this paradox that was captured by the correspondence between Harvey Cushing and Edwin Bramwell.[26]

This seeming paradox is perhaps most easily explored through the history of the word 'neurology', which has curious and largely British origins. Thomas Willis coined the word in his *Cerebri Anatome*, which first appeared in 1664.[27] Yet, despite these seventeenth-century origins, for all practical purposes few figures used the word over the next two centuries in medical or lay literature.[28] It appeared rarely in medical texts and notices of medical lectures in the eighteenth century. By the time the phrenologists had begun extolling their theories at the end of the eighteenth century, the word seems to have passed into a wider medical parlance that had acquired something of a popular (some might suggest quackish) mystique.[29] The word was certainly uncommon in the nineteenth-century medical literature before 1850. It was first used in the *Lancet* in an 1859 article that reported on the lectures of a John Coghill, entitled: 'On the Structure and Relations of the Nervous System at the Periphery, Including the Neurology of the Organs of Special Sense'.[30] The word's first appearance in the *British Medical Journal* was somewhat later. In an 1861 letter, Thomas Pope questioned the therapeutic action of mercury in disease and wondered whether his contemporaries could infer 'that muscle, abstractedly, is capable of motion or sensation?' The answer, he cautioned in that journal's earliest usage, was that 'neurology says no.'[31] George Beard, a North American and one of the earliest self-described neurologists *and* medical electrologists, observed in 1874 that 'neurology' then was 'an old though not much used term'.[32]

As might be expected from this brief account, historians have noted that there is little evidence indicating that 'neurology' was understood uniformly across generations and locales.[33] It is perhaps equally important to note that the conceptual foundations of neurology and its history as a specialty diverge. As the story recounted in the subsequent chapters will make clear, the formal specialty of neurology in Britain had its origins in late nineteenth-century Victorian medicine and acquired a specialised form that is recognisable to our contemporary sensibilities only in the interwar period of the twentieth century.[34]

The construction of the nervous system and its diseases in Britain

The medicine of the early modern European world was dominated by humoral constitutionalism.[35] Illness, a single phenomenon visited by God or ill-fortune upon the sick, occurred when the humours of the body became imbalanced, demanding a traditional medical attention that sought to re-establish their equilibrium. By the turn of the nineteenth century, however, this medical order – one derived from the authoritative doctrines of the ancients – showed evidence of its decline in the face of numerous challenges to its credibility. On one side were discoveries of general value in natural philosophy that revealed that the received wisdom of the ancients was often and unquestionably in error. This fact, compounded by an emergent Enlightenment culture fascinated with collecting, categorising, and cataloguing all aspects of the natural world, revealed as well that there was potentially more in God's creation than literal biblical tradition explained. At the same time, the advent of new political philosophies central to the emergence of the liberal industrial order created a new individualist political and economic culture, which simultaneously also engendered a new medicine of individuals.[36] Although endowed differently by the Creator, individuals were nevertheless equally made up of the same malleable stuff – i.e. the flesh, bones, nerves and sinews of infinitely perfectible man. Medical and scientific knowledge of the body, in consequence, became ever-less focused on humours and constitutions, and ever-more focused on understanding the uniform characteristics of human anatomy, pathology, and disease.[37]

Paris, one seat of these new practices, saw its post-Revolution reformed hospitals and universities espouse an ethos determined to 'distinguish and separate' the natural world.[38] 'When the brain dies, the animal life dies, for the functions of this life, either directly or indirectly, have their seat in the brain,' wrote French anatomist Marie François Xavier Bichat in his *Physiological Researches on Life and Death*, no doubt thinking of all of 'the bodies of persons who had been guillotined' while simultaneously ushering in his theory of bodily tissues, the common practice among medical men of mortuary pathology, and a new style of medical examination of patients' bodies informed by statistics and microscopy.[39] 'Symptoms so different, and all comprehended under the general title of insanity, required, on my part, much study and discrimination,' wrote Philippe Pinel in his famous 1801 *Treatise on Insanity*, a text filled with 'cautious and repeated examinations into the condition of individuals' and which announced a new moral calculus for the asylum in post-Revolutionary France.[40] In this way, proponents of natural philosophy and the modern political ideologies, as well as figures in the new French Republic's bureaucracies, nurtured and stimulated the spread of clinical specialties and academic disciplines, and they thus dictated the new terms under which physicians 'consoled and classified' their patients.[41]

Circumstances across the English Channel were removed from the more drastic changes felt in Revolutionary and Napoleonic France.[42] The diploma systems of the various Royal Colleges continued to determine professional status in medicine and surgery in the major metropolitan areas, while in the more provincial regions general practitioners and their apprentices provided medical services to the rural needy.[43] At the same time, physicians and scientists felt the influence of trends on the Continent, especially those who trained in that then-hotbed of dissent and radicalism (also the venerable seat of British medicine), Edinburgh. Reform was in the air. In 1815 the Apothecaries Act standardised and regulated the practices of apothecaries. The Anatomy Act of 1832 modernised the medical curriculum,[44] and the 1858 Medical Act placed medical school degrees and the diplomas of the Royal Colleges on an ostensibly more or less equal footing. The Act also unified medicine and surgery for the first time through the creation of a Medical Directory that contained the names of all practitioners with the legal right to practise medicine. It also formalised the increasing antipathy to medical specialisation in Britain. Quite simply, the register's authors did not acknowledge specific specialties. Thus, even as specialist hospitals and medical specialists appeared more and more as a fixture of Britain's reforming medical culture, reformers within that same medical culture resisted efforts by some medical practitioners to cultivate the specialist's mystique.[45] They were reluctant to endorse efforts by colleagues to create new specialist departments in the general hospitals or to introduce specialised courses to the medical curriculum. A consultant in medicine had to have general abilities.[46] Specialisation, by contrast, hinted at narrowness, mediocrity, and perhaps quackery.

In one limited sense, however, specialists with interests in the nervous system had been around for at least as long as oculists had been treating diseases of the eyes.[47] Moreover, philosophical and medical interest in the nervous system was piqued from the seventeenth century onwards, famously so in the eighteenth-century work of George Cheyne (1671–1743), who had published his *The English Malady* in 1733. There he combined a mechanistic discussion of the nerve 'tubes' and their 'elastic properties' with broader condemnation of English decadence, which he supposed blameworthy for numerous nervous complaints.[48] Such medical theories and philosophical speculations were becoming increasingly influential in proto-psychological discussions and medical discourses on the nervous system. At the same time, at least in Edinburgh, the common understanding of the nervous system shifted from the Cartesian mechanism to a wider-ranging vitalism.[49] The nerves thus acquired rich philosophical connotations in Georgian and subsequently Victorian Britain even as they remained a shifting anatomical and physiological concept.[50] In consequence, physicians over the next two centuries unwittingly followed Cheyne's pattern by routinely situating the causes of nervous conditions in observable parallels in social and cultural phenomena around which public appreciations or anxieties had coalesced.[51]

Enlightenment constructions of the anatomy and function of the brain, nerves, and reflexes were also contingent upon their social and cultural contexts: by the nineteenth century the brain had acquired its centrality as the organ of bodily and cognitive control and the seat of madness.[52] Since the classical period, scholars, natural philosophers, and physicians had held that the nerves formed a series of connected tubes distributed across the body. Those tubes arose from the brain.

The brain secreted an ethereal fluid that flowed through the nerves. The nerves, involved in sensation and motion, facilitated the movement of this fluid, which they called the animal spirits – the prime agent, some believed, for the soul.[53]

Others, less motivated by theological commitments, sought material or mechanical explanations.[54] The discovery of static electricity in the eighteenth century, and subsequent observations about its effect on the bodies of animals, inspired Luigi Galvani and Alessandro Volta to wonder whether animals contained an intrinsic source of electricity. Volta argued that an extrinsic fluid connected the body with the environment. Galvani, by contrast, held that the body generated its own supply.[55] Their controversy, unresolved by the start of the nineteenth century, became complicated further by the spread of what some deemed quack medical therapies that relied upon electricity or pseudo-science.[56] The backdrop for their controversy was the early nineteenth-century public acclaim for the various traders in the medical marketplace who sold cures and claims about animal magnetism, physiognomy, phrenology, and mesmerism.[57] One such figure, perhaps representative of those movements, was a Mr Spencer T. Hall who advertised a series of lectures in the *Liverpool Mercury* on: 'his experiments in Mesmric Sonambulism and Somniloquence, Phreno-Mesmerism, Neurology, Musical Exstacy' in 1846.[58]

The psychology of the early nineteenth century left some with less philosophical and spectacular inclinations exasperated. In his 1811 essay on the anatomy of the brain, Charles Bell (1774–1842) complained in the opening paragraphs, 'The want of any consistent history of the Brain and Nerves, and the dull unmeaning manner which is in use of demonstrating the brain, may authorise any novelty in the manner of treating the subject.' He then added: 'I have found some of my friends so mistaken in their conception of the object of the demonstrations which I have delivered in my lectures, that I wish to vindicate myself at all hazards. They would have it that I am in search of the seat of the soul; but I wish only to investigate the structure of the brain.'[59] In many respects, this was a new secular programme for the anatomy of the brain and nerves – a view that had led to Bell's much-contested discoveries of the motor functions of the anterior roots of the spinal cord and claims that parts of the brain had distinct functions.[60]

The anatomical and physiological approach that characterised Bell's work became typical of all areas of hospital practice.[61] Physicians and surgeons, many of them having served as army and naval surgeons in the Napoleonic Wars, slowly became accustomed to elaborating the old anatomy and physiology through the new techniques of mortuary pathology. They came also to reconceive disease theories and the application of science to diagnostic medicine. If the sick sometimes had different symptoms, the new pathologists noted that specific diseases resided within particular 'tissues'.[62] By the mid-nineteenth century, the work of Matthias Schlieden (1804–81), Theodor Schwann (1810–82), Rudolf Virchow (1821–1902), and others had shifted the site of disease pathology from tissues to cells, the discrete unit of physiological function.[63]

Did the nervous system comprise these discrete units? No one was sure at the beginning of the nineteenth century. Charles Bell had noted that 'papilla' on the tongue could detect one stimulus alone – taste or pressure.[64] Such a functional observation combined with Marshall Hall's study of excitatory-motor reflexes, and Robert Bentley Todd and William Bowman's histological observations of nerve tissues, as elaborated in their *Physiological Anatomy and Physiology of Man*, might have enhanced that view further, but definitive evidence would not be forthcoming until the close of the nineteenth century.[65] Even if this question had been resolved earlier, tracing nervous conditions back to the cells, especially those that manifested as mental disorders without apparent lesion, would have elicited controversy.[66] Few European or North American scientists or physicians involved themselves so directly in what amounted to philosophical speculations. As far as the mind was concerned, most adopted a psychophysical parallelism, especially following Thomas Laycock's 1840 publication on *Nervous Diseases of Women*, a work devoted to physiological psychology.[67]

Though theological or philosophical speculations were less influential in the scientific construction of the nervous system, culturally embedded judgements often were, and perhaps none more so in Britain than the 'British man's' sense of his superiority in the hierarchy of humanity.[68] Meanwhile the normative conventions of Victorian bourgeois society often dictated and determined interpretations of scientific knowledge. Scientists and physicians routinely incorporated metaphors as socially, morally, and philosophically ambiguous as 'inhibition' into their interpretation of the physiological functions of the nervous system. In effect, they naturalised the social values of Victorian Britain.[69] Still, people understood the definition of the

ferment in which their work was embedded. To modern historical sensibilities such pairings as phrenology and physiognomy, animal electricity and mesmerism, pathology and physiology, philosophy and psychology can begin to conjure the constructions of the nervous system that had dominated the scientific and cultural landscapes of Enlightenment and Victorian Britain. Many of the educated middle classes in the nineteenth century would, for example, have been familiar with Thomas Hobbes' *Leviathan* and may even have noted his attention to the function of the nerves in its opening chapters. 'For what is the *Heart*', Hobbes wrote, 'but a *Spring*; and the Nerves. but so many *Strings*'.[93] Equally for others Jean-Jacques Rousseau's identification of the body politic in his *Social Contract* with anatomical metaphor, and particularly his comparison of the body's heart with executive power and the body's brain with legislative power, would have summoned tropes extending back to Shakespeare's London.[94] In this manner, the nervous system had emerged in the Enlightenment and after as a locus of political rights, a progenitor of human instincts, the substance of irrational spirits, and the originator of will and language. Its many products included the passions, sensibility, and civilisation; its diseases included madness, hysteria, and even genius.[95]

The subject of the nerves, spine, brain, and mind thus invited a gentlemanly generality in the eighteenth century.[96] The same universality was true in the nineteenth century. It remained very much the case even at the close of the twentieth century. That a number of scientific disciplines and clinical specialties dealing with the nervous system emerged over that same period and in this context is therefore undeniable. Nevertheless, many involved in these fields often felt ambivalent about such specialist identities. While this was especially true for physicians and scientists in Britain, it was also characteristic of their counterparts in philosophy, science, and medicine across Europe and North America. Certainly, there were any number of figures in all of those places who endeavoured to claim the nervous system as their own, to define its limits, cultivate younger disciples, build schools of thought, found hospitals or university departments, and accord to themselves the status of pioneer. But such attempts were often short-lived, faddish, and denigrated by subsequent generations, as was clearly the fate for mesmerism and phrenology.[97]

It might seem self-evident that physicians and scientists with interests in the nervous system and its diseases would have been in conflict with the dominant generalist medical idioms of their day. Surely such interests were specialist by definition. Far from seeing themselves and their knowledge that way, Georgian and Victorian doctors and scientists with interests in the nervous system regarded their work as in keeping with the broadminded, inclusive value system of medicine and science. In so far as they were able, they sought to fashion the knowledge of the nervous system as a subject of supreme value to science and medicine and of universal value to humanity. They invested the pathology and physiology of the nervous system with insights of general scientific, medical, and humanistic value. They sought to create institutions that reflected these generalist commitments, and they memorialised and commemorated in obituaries habits in their forebears that conformed to these same social and culture appreciations. In this way, even as the specialist figure of the medical neurologist became ever more common in the halls of British medicine, the individuals who cultivated and fashioned the neurological identity continued to imbue it with the habits of philosophical breadth, scholastic catholicity, generalist medical acumen, and broad scientific learnedness.

Of course, such a self-fashioned identity as a 'Renaissance man' (or, more rarely, woman) of medicine and science does not readily lend itself to a straightforward history of either neurology or medical specialisation. It requires an acknowledgement that the social and intellectual conception of medical and scientific neurology was never constant. Moreover, the individuals themselves never adopted a programmatic, unified view of their work and subject.[98] Thus, the way physicians and scientists understood the science and medicine of the nerves metamorphosed several times over the course of the two centuries, approximately 1800–2000.[99] From intellectual worlds as far apart as phrenology and comparative zoology to more practical distances between, for example, rehabilitative electrical therapeutics and prophylactic vaccines, the science and medicine of neurology was constantly reforged.[100] Some influences were intrinsic to changes in the science and medicine but others were made in larger social, cultural and economic terms; war, economic depression, the advent of 'Big Science', and the growth of the modern welfare state were all forces the exacted change on the development of specialisation. It was larger structures and changes in the nature of British political economy and culture that ultimately led neurologists to adopt specialisation for themselves and to start moderating their claims that they had a universalistic outlook.

Such an assertion leads inevitably to a question of comparison. Was this unique to British neurology? Or was this the case for British ophthalmology, psychiatry, psychology, internal medicine, and surgery? The answer is somewhere in between. Of course, physicians and scientists working in all areas of clinical and scientific practice developed their own methods, technologies, and professional social and cultural commitments, even as these were influenced by historical changes.[101] Moreover, the advent of specialisation did not instantly transform the consciousness of individuals into specialist mentalities. These were generational processes and all of these fields developed within generational time. The evolving culture of general medicine constantly influenced each field in different ways. But, as this book shows, the science and medicine of the nerves was different from other fields. Neurology in Britain was as much a science as it was an area of clinical practice.[102] The analysis of the physiology of the brain, the anatomy of the spine, and production of behaviours, for instance, opened up numerous possibilities for laboratory and medical research and treatment.[103] The deficits created by nervous diseases often revealed as much as could be shown about the proper function of the nervous system in the human subject. And all of these facts meant that the question of the relationship between mind and brain was never distant in discussions of perception, sensation, madness, or the role of culture in the production of normative behaviour.[104] It was, in other words, somewhat easier for physicians and scientists with interests in the nervous system to maintain a generalist, universalistic, polymathic pose and to view with suspicion attempts to narrow their sphere of practice.

Such assertions bring the other set of questions to the fore. Was there something unique about medical specialisation in Britain and about the specialisation of neurology in particular? The answers to these questions are more difficult. Medical specialists in North America and Europe had been available since the early nineteenth century (perhaps even earlier). But it could be argued with some justification that medical historians have exaggerated both the frequency of clinical specialisation and the exclusivity with which physicians and surgeons adopted their specialties.

There were material advantages to being a specialist. But there were material advantages to being a competent generalist as well. It is not difficult to infer why so many clinicians stayed comfortably in that middle ground throughout the nineteenth century. In any case, it was only with the advent of dedicated departments in hospitals and universities in the twentieth century that the specialist became a more common medical figure. British resistance to specialisation can hardly be claimed to be unique – the tropes against specialisation abound almost everywhere in the Western world – but British physicians were perhaps singular in that they resisted longer than most of their international contemporaries.

Neurology itself may well have been different too. It should not escape attention that early physicians with interests in nervous diseases brought a broad outlook to their practice. It seems to have been a common feature of neurology that it attracted men and women who saw the entirety of human knowledge and culture as an intact record of the qualities and abilities of the human nervous system. Thus the stories historians have told about, for example, hysteria, neurasthenia, and depression direct us towards the broader point that this intense curiosity about human behaviour often slipped into normative judgement about normal and pathological behaviour. Such a slip would not have occurred without the broad construction of the knowledge of the human nervous system, and that broad construction was hardly unique to British physicians; indeed figures like the American Silas Weir Mitchell or the Frenchman Jean-Martin Charcot appear especially exemplary of the habit of mind.

Places and spaces: identity in the hospitals

The most vocal opponents of specialisation in the nineteenth and twentieth centuries were medical consultants. They often greeted specialisation, as well as most innovations in science and medical practice, with profound resistance.[105] This fact, historians Steve Sturdy and Roger Cooter have noted, appears rather strange because consultants were the practitioners most likely to work in the specialist hospitals.[106] As Rosemary Stevens observed, of the 195 physicians working in London general hospitals in 1899, only 31 did not hold positions in a specialist hospital.[107] Given this demographic fact, it is somewhat difficult to understand why physicians were so reluctant to endorse specialisation.

One explanation must be that the habits and dispositions of consultants made them perceive mediocrity in specialisation. After the 1858 Medical

Act, figures at the Royal College of Physicians London had acted quickly to re-establish their authority, introducing the Member of the Royal College of Physicians (MRCP), a higher diploma. The new diploma effectively reinforced an emergent class structure within medicine. It formalised the difference between consultants and general practitioners. Specialisation, however, implied that physicians could possess real expertise only in a limited area. Most of them would have objected to such a notion, a point further enforced by the higher diploma.

Firstly, they regarded the body as a united subject. The colour of the skin, the taste of urine, or a twitching of the eyes were all clues to an underlying condition.[108] In 1840, Thomas Laycock, a physician with interests in nervous diseases and promulgator of the notion that reflexes could be found at all levels of the nervous system, contemplated how conditions of the kidneys could sometimes induce 'cerebral disease, as coma, convulsions, and apoplexy'. This led him to remark that, although he was not anxious that 'we should become exclusively "water-doctors"...it could not but be beneficial to practice, if practitioners were to examine the morbid changes of the urine.'[109] Pathological examinations, like those advocated by Laycock, demonstrated that disease worked across the whole body. Johns Hughlings Jackson (1835–1911), Physician to the National Hospital for Epilepsy and Paralysis, observed:

> If anyone were to work on different sections of medical practice, so as merely to add isolated series of facts to one another, he would really make little progress in cultivating his own mind. Such a man would dwell with exaggeration – hurtful to his own organisation of medical knowledge – on amaurosis as a defect of sight, and too little on it as a defect of specialised part of universal sensation.[110]

The finest medical discoveries were those that worked on the whole body. The intrinsic worth of aseptic and antiseptic techniques, for instance, was their general applicability. William Hale-White retrospectively judged Joseph Lister's (1827–1912) prevention of suppuration remarkable precisely because it worked on a united body.[111] Specialised knowledge, even of the nervous system and its diseases, appeared irreconcilably narrow in contrast.

Secondly, there were more pragmatic grounds for resisting specialisation. On one hand, hospitals throughout Britain were in a perpetual state of financial crisis. Since their chief sources of income were benefactions and subscriptions, altering the arrangements of hospital wards by creating specialist departments would have incurred immediate rises in expenditure for which funds were unavailable.[112] They meant also increasing the size of the resident staff. The large wards Florence Nightingale (1820–1910) called for throughout her career offered not just hygienic advantages but financial ones as well. One night nurse could provide adequate care for a large ward but not for several specialised wards.[113] On the other hand, hospital administration and physicians alike worried that increasing specialised practice would also complicate medical teaching. Experience in the general wards, especially for students, they felt, should mirror the disorder encountered in general practice.[114]

Opposition to specialisation did not, however, prevent it from occurring. Specialists became early fixtures in British medicine. They (or more especially their patrons) established hospitals and private practices frequently and early. The founding of Moorfields Eye Hospital in 1804 was one of the earliest examples; by 1900, there were 128 specialist hospitals in England and Wales. While those hospitals in London were indeed 'centres of specialist teaching and research',[115] the clinical staff in those hospitals was nevertheless highly mobile.[116] Junior appointments in all hospitals were a means for young physicians to remain employed within the medical hierarchy until their election to the position of assistant physician or full physician within a larger hospital brought them the status to acquire an income from private practice.[117] Terms of appointment in any hospital could therefore be short. Moreover physicians often held many appointments, sometimes simultaneously, in different specialist and general hospitals throughout their careers. Such was the case for physicians with interests in nervous diseases who saw a career in general medicine as the best path to financial security and professional regard.

This required balance between an individual's obligation to his or her current employer and long-term career plans presented administrators of specialist hospitals with a dilemma; prospective employees came with divide loyalties. For example, when administrators at the National Hospital for Epilepsy and Paralysis in Queen Square hired its first Surgeon, a Mr Russell, they insisted that he resign from his appointments and obligations at other hospitals. This in fact he chose not to do, leading to his rather immediate dismissal. The Hospital Board then hired John Hughlings Jackson as assistant physician.[118] Because rising to the status of full physician aided the growth of a private practice and income, individuals' circumstances and their participation in specialist practice was often more by luck than planning.

If the identity of these physicians and scientists appears somewhat fluid now, it should nevertheless be obvious that physicians and scientists throughout this period experienced no crisis of identity *per se*. They worked wherever they found employment and opportunity, which after 1859 included specialist hospitals for epilepsy and paralysis.

A number of specialist hospitals for the treatment of epilepsy, paralysis and other nervous diseases sprang up in Britain in the mid-nineteenth century. Of these, the aforementioned National Hospital in Queen Square, London, has received the most extensive historical attention.[119] Although devoted to all conditions ostensibly neurological, it is clear that the original impetus of the hospital's founders, as revealed by their letters, was not to establish a new specialty of medicine but rather to provide a less stigmatising environment than the asylum for patients suffering from diseases differing from insanity.[120] Thus the eventual seat of London neurology began not as a dream of a group of like-minded medics, but rather it was the realisation of Victorian families concerned to place ailing patients in an allegedly better hospital environment.

Less is known about the origins of other hospitals for the treatment of nervous conditions in London and whether the same motivation underpinned their foundation. There is a sense, however, that both the Maida Vale Hospital and West End Hospital were the pet projects of less reputable doctors. Another reason may be that the physicians at the National tended to claim that they sent patients suffering from mental diseases elsewhere, whereas their competitors treated mental and nervous patients alike. To be sure, both Maida Vale and the West End provided employment for physicians with interests in nervous conditions, and many of them made individually significant contributions to the study of nervous diseases. Yet neither ever developed the prominence that the Queen Square hospital eventually enjoyed.

The apparent driving force behind the creation of the National Hospital, the reclassification and subsequent differentiation of nervous patients from mental ones, did not find ready acceptance within wider medical London until the early twentieth century. The situation in the London teaching hospitals illustrates the point. Why it should be necessary to differentiate nerve patients from other groups was unclear to their consultants. As late as 1922, one author noted that the centralisation of nervous patients created the problem that 'more than one-half of the persons who seek relief at the neurological out-patient department of a general hospital are suffering from functional as opposed to organic disease.'[121] The intractability of that situation was further compounded by the fact that many patients manifested neurological symptoms as a part of their general disorder.

As the above makes abundantly clear, in Victorian Britain this movement towards specialist practice was contested and fraught with ambiguity. Even as physicians or concerned laity founded specialist hospitals with increasing frequency throughout the country in the nineteenth century, as Stevens in particular shows, the general perspective of medicine's elite and non-elite practitioners alike was one of qualified disdain for specialists.[122] Although many physicians engaged in scientific and clinical research, their interests often pulled them in diverse directions. William Broadbent, for example, a physician at St Mary's Hospital, was once alarmed to learn that some of his research had landed him the dubious title of 'cancer specialist', when, in fact, he had published several reports on various subjects, including many 'memorable contributions' on the nervous system.[123]

The British, of course, were aware of the process of specialisation as it was occurring abroad. At the close of the nineteenth century, the specialist in nervous and mental diseases had become a more common member of the crowded corridors of British medicine.[124] Across the Atlantic Ocean, perhaps somewhat earlier, the American Civil War had been filling hospitals and dispensaries with soldiers afflicted by injuries of the central and peripheral nervous systems.[125] Scholars have viewed the environment of American medicine as uniquely favourable to medical specialisation. By 1875, as Bonnie Blustein has so ably shown, physicians had founded the American Neurological Association.[126] One member was the American pioneer of the treatment of nervous diseases, Silas Weir Mitchell. Mitchell made his medical name in studying gunshot injuries to the nervous system during the Civil War and also by his infamous rest cure. But he probably also came to the public's attention through his publication of popular novels that included descriptions of his neurotic patients.[127] Meanwhile, medical students from across the globe had been flocking to Paris to spend time in the clinic of Jean-Martin Charcot (1825–93).

Edwin Bramwell, for example, would follow that pattern, albeit a generation later.[128] Charcot had been appointed to La Salpêtrière in 1862, a hospital remembered as a veritable 'museum of neurological material'; by 1892, he was appointed to the world's first Clinical Chair of Diseases of the Nervous System in the Paris Faculty of Medicine and just as similar trends in neurology were unfolding in Germany.[129] Renowned as a lecturer on nervous diseases, Charcot would present neurological cases to his students, highlight their interesting symptoms and distinguish those characteristics required for making proper diagnosis. By far his most famous cases were patients suffering from hysteria.[130]

By the 1880s, the international communication of physiological and pathological research on the nervous system was common in Britain. So too were translated textbooks focused on the diseases of the nervous system. The Sydenham Society, for example, had translated Charcot's lectures on the diseases of the nervous system into English by 1881.[131] In spite of these international and local developments, great ambiguity surrounded the practices of the physician with interests in nervous diseases in Britain in the late nineteenth century, including the work of John Hughlings Jackson, now often regarded by neurologists as the father of contemporary British neurology.[132]

Overview of the volume

Initially, then, neurological knowledge began as the apogee of general medical and scientific understanding. That is, physicians and scientists in the nineteenth century did not regard neurology as a medical specialty or scientific discipline. Instead, they emphasised the broadness – the all-encompassing spirit – of inquiries into the nervous system. In some sense, they modelled themselves upon the great naturalists and philosophers of their age. Such professional ambiguity in self-identity ultimately proved untenable.[133] As lay people and physicians formed departments of nervous diseases (and then departments of neurology) in the general hospital system in the twentieth century, a professional identity more restricted to the somatic complaints and diseases of the nervous system became increasingly common. The doctors central in that story, however, continued to see patients with mental conditions and continued to research questions of broader significance.[134]

When they did deign to define their practices as neurological in the late nineteenth century, British physicians adopted the broadest terms possible. As Chapter 1 reveals, few physicians desired that their practices should have specialist status equivalent to, for example, ophthalmology or medical electricity.[135] Discussions about nervous conditions flourished everywhere; discussions in the Ophthalmological Society of the United Kingdom, for example, were integral to the foundation of the first British neurological society. There were numerous commonalities between the Ophthalmological Society and the Neurological Society of London, and the formation of the former in 1880 provided a stimulus for the foundation of the latter in 1886.[136] Whereas members of the Ophthalmological Society were unapologetic in their political aims, the members of the Neurological Society defined their membership and subject loosely and located its practices within those of general medicine. Medicine, these physicians argued, should remain whole. Thus, the general physicians frequenting the Neurological Society's meetings did not think of themselves as specialists per se, but fashioned themselves as general physicians of broad scientific – especially physiological – and medical interests. This self-presentation allowed these physicians to tout their neurological knowledge while simultaneously aligning themselves with the mores of a medical culture that remained firmly hostile to specialisation.

The uncertainty of determining who the generalists with specialist interests were, as opposed to the specialists possessing generalist aptitudes, created tensions between the traditional values of general bedside medicine and the emergent idioms of social rationalisation, which by that time promoted medical specialisation as a corollary to social progress. By 1906, the opposition to medical specialisation had become so intense that calls to unite medicine had resulted in the formation of the Royal Society of Medicine. This moment, the focus of Chapter 2, was an apogee for medical generalism, which thereby heralded its decline in medical culture as well. Historians have often cited the existence of this new society, described as an amalgamation of various specialist societies in London beneath one roof, as explicit endorsement of specialisation.[137] It was, however, nothing of the kind. The incorporation of those various societies effectively curtailed the former societies' political autonomy and financial independence and removed their right to copyright their proceedings. However, there was no controversy about the Neurological Society's dissolution into the Royal Society of Medicine (RSM), where it became known as the Section of Neurology.

If these institutional transformations were less significant than has been recognised, the changes exacted by the conditions of First World War were pivotal for medical specialisation.[138] Whereas, before the war, general physicians with interests in neurology were common, by the 1920s a younger generation of self-described neurologists were entering medical practice. Many saw opposition to medical specialties as rather calculated and no more than a cost-saving convenience benefiting the British government's coffers. Nevertheless the move towards specialisation arose out of a broader political need for rationalisation, efficiency, and economy in medical organisation under the conditions of total war. Practitioners of medicine later claimed this social and political transformation as a revolution in medical practice and therefore a change in science and understanding. This social alteration – a conversion that occurred in the interwar period – was integral to the formation of neurology.

In consequence, as Chapter 3 describes, British neurology in the interwar period achieved remarkable international status, and the clinical methods and research, especially those characteristic at the National Hospital in Queen Square, were romantically adulated abroad.[139] The British Medical Research Council established a Neurological Clinical Research Unit at the National Hospital for Nervous Diseases, Queen Square, and this Research Unit was further supplemented by grants from the Halley Stewart Trust for research fellowships in neurology. Despite these changes, neurology's institutional ambiguities endured. If the interwar environment promoted changes in neurology's structure, then internally those changes were constrained by establishment traditionalism – the desire to produce and reproduce the best generalist practices of the previous age.

That problem appeared for American and European neurologists as well. At various international meetings neurologists attempted to move their specialty towards greater political and economic autonomy – i.e. independent and separate status within hospitals, universities, and licensing boards.[140] Interwar British neurologists, perhaps feeling frustrated by the political inadequacies of the RSM, used the prestige of these international scenes as one pretext for criticising its organisational structure. Claiming to be dissatisfied by its London-centric nature, and threatened by its seemingly unchecked expansion (by 1933 the Section of Neurology had over three hundred members), a small group split from the Section and formed the Association of British Neurologists, an elite club consisting of merely fifty-one members.[141]

This new association began to take some steps towards formally addressing neurology's institutional ambiguities. Chapter 4 describes how the association advocated the formation of a Committee on Neurology at the Royal College of Physicians and lobbied the Ministry of Health to appoint an Advisor in Neurology, which occurred finally in 1958.[142] When not engaged in political matters, the members of the Association of British Neurologists held scientific meetings yearly. Theirs initially remained an eclectic membership: pathologists, physiologists, psychiatrists, general physicians with an interest in neurology, and neurologists comprised its core, but few of its original members actually held official positions in hospitals or medical schools as neurologists.

Nevertheless, the formation of the Association of British Neurologists marked a point of transition for the neurologists. Whereas the earlier practices of British neurology had been broad and all-encompassing, this Association selected new members with greater care and restricted them to a specific type of clinical practice. Likewise, where political engagement in neurology had not been considered proper conduct, the new Association protected the specialty and took steps to defend its interests in negotiations with the government, medical profession, or licensing bodies.

Some neurologists perceived a crisis in the field in the years between 1950 and 1960. Leaders voiced concerns that the numbers of neurologists were shrinking, and that few new graduates were entering the field. They claimed that funding for research was drying up, and in many fields the most talented and renowned practitioners were retiring.[143] The peculiar and idiomatic logics of neurology's practice increasingly located the field in an imagined past. This nostalgic frame of reference was predicated upon a past that had never existed. In hindsight, the irony of British neurology's crisis in the 1950s was that it entered a period where its practitioners had defined their identity. The definitions, however, were institutional, political, and practical. Most neurologists felt nothing but disdain for simplistic, overly rational definitions. Now that they had defined their sphere of practice, a previous individualism that had been available to them diminished.

In relinquishing the privilege of ambiguity for professional stability, neurology had entered into a new relationship with the British state, a relationship that would define British neurology and thus represent neurologists' acquiescence to limitations in practice.

Did the rise of the specialised clinical neurologist mean that the Renaissance man or woman of science and medicine vanished from the landscape of clinical neurology? As the concluding chapter discusses, the integrative practice that neurologists cultivated permitted such an identity to remain in place. Over two centuries, they had fashioned an identity for themselves that allowed them to be concerned with the philosophical status of man.[144] Neurologists had come to require languages to express the historical, psychological, and sociological status of their patients, with the consequence that for the neurologists the normal products of the nervous system – those elements that constructed their patients' professional and private lives – became as much an object of their analyses as disease states. Patients who showed uncharacteristic habits could be diagnosed in a wide variety of ways. Such discrimination required a neurologist's discerning eye, cultivated imagination, and broad outlook – a habitus that was as capable of distinguishing individual genius from madness as it was from separating civilisation from its decadent discontents.

These characteristics never vanished from the practices of clinical neurologists. Indeed, as the neurosciences became a recognised field of interdisciplinary inquiry in the 1950s, they brought biological science, social science, and medicine closer together. Pharmacology, physiology, and genetics were perhaps the most actively involved areas of science involved in broadening the disciplinary meaning of neuroscience, a development that spawned fields as wide-ranging as operations research, computer science, and cybernetics. Thus, while in this period clinical neurologists regarded their field as being in decline, it is apparent that the 1950s and 1960s marked a reconvergence between the scientific and clinical realms that facilitated new conceptions of selfhood.

As the numbers of neurologists and neuroscientists increased in the 1970s onwards in Britain and beyond, their research programmes diversified in extraordinary ways. The cultural impact of those decades of the brain was far-reaching. It was in the era of postmodernity that people became their brains. Selfhood and brainhood collapsed together. The promise of downloadable brains seemed to offer the holy grail of immortality. But it was the Renaissance-style self-fashioning underlying the transition from physician to neurologist that made such ambitions plausible. If humans had become their brains, then the new philosophers of postmodernity were bound to be those whose business it was to study the brain. Putting it differently, a long history of a carefully cultivated set of professional dispositions had come to define neurology and by extension neuroscience.[145]

• 1 •

Physicians in neurological societies; neurologists in general medical societies

Introduction

Among the many intellectual discoveries of late nineteenth-century physiology, one that has frequently drawn attention is David Ferrier's research on the cerebral localisation of function in animals, inaugurated in the 1870s and generally accepted by the early 1880s.[1] Celebrated for its demonstration of the scientific basis of phrenology, embedded in a long and powerful intellectual history of the mind, no doubt instrumental in ushering in the anti-vivisectionist movement, and encapsulated in a human story of priority disputes, Ferrier's research possesses the ingredients of a gripping tale.

Shortly after Gustav Fritsch (1838–1927) and Eduard Hitzig (1838–1907) demonstrated that muscle movements in the body of a dog could be stimulated by the direct application of electricity to its brain, Ferrier began analysing whether stimulation of specific areas of the brain might lead to repeatable motor behaviours *in vivo*. A Scotsman by birth and medical student at Edinburgh, Ferrier had taken a *wanderjahr* in Heidelberg on the advice of philosopher Alexander Bain before taking up a residence in London. His friend James Crichton-Browne shortly later invited Ferrier to join a group of young clinicians conducting research at the West Riding Lunatic Asylum in Yorkshire.[2]

This cohort shaped Ferrier's scientific perspective. He eventually dedicated his monograph *The Functions of the Brain* to one of them, John Hughlings Jackson, whom Ferrier acknowledged, 'from a clinical standpoint anticipated many of the more important results of recent experimental investigation into the functions of the cerebral hemispheres'.[3]

Ferrier cited Jackson's research many times throughout his work and always in complement to his own conclusion that motor centres existed in the brain, a hypothesis that while paralleled by Paul Broca's studies of aphasia as well as Fritsch and Hitzig's original work, did not sit well with many of Ferrier's peers in Britain and elsewhere. As historian David Millet recounts, 1874 – the year in which John Burdon Sanderson read Ferrier's lecture before the Royal Society – was filled with numerous critical appraisals, yet Ferrier appears not to have thought his evisceration significant.[4] Furthermore, his unwillingness to treat his critics seriously left uncertain the status of his manuscript, then under review at the *Transactions of the Royal Society* by Michael Foster, George Rolleston, and Thomas Huxley. It did not ultimately appear in print – although the society did allow publication of a short abstract of it, which Ferrier followed with many significant works in their journals.[5]

There can be little doubt that Ferrier's physiological research had a permanent influence on the science and medicine of the nervous system. The interest of this story rests not simply there, but also in the spirited resistance that members of the Royal Society and the scientific establishment initially mounted against him. Fellowship in the Royal Society was one of the highest honours accorded to scientists. Its original charter had been for the dissemination of scientific knowledge, but Fellowship in the society so enhanced personal prestige that by the close of the nineteenth century the organisation's members had largely become incapable of avoiding nepotism, politics, and conservativism. The Royal Society was, however, the model that other learned societies drew upon. In that sense, Ferrier's story directs attention, not simply to his discovery, but also to practices common to medical and scientific societies that might well have prevented his conclusions from ever reaching a wider medical public. Such disciplinary practices could work for or against the dissemination of specialist knowledge. They could also promote cultural values widely shared by elite physicians and scientists and were a means by which proponents of generalism could resist rampant specialism. Such observations thus provide a starting place for framing the context and origins of Britain's first society of neurology, the Neurological Society of London, and for examining how its members contended and overcame the widespread resistance to specialisation.

This chapter begins, however, not with the Neurological Society, but rather by setting up a contrast between it and its important specialist counterpart, the Ophthalmological Society of the United

Kingdom. The strategies that members of both societies adopted so that they would appear within the mainstream of medical culture were various and easily illustrated by contrasting the two. The members of the Ophthalmological Society, discussed in the first section below, advocated a wholly specialist profile; the members of the Neurological Society, described in the subsequent sections, never aligned themselves with a specialist identity and instead embraced an inclusive attitude and scrupulously cultivated a generalist appearance in order to mitigate any pejorative charge that neurology was a narrow field of enquiry. The records of both societies make it possible to view the values, knowledge, and practices past practitioners sought to transmit in both societies. They reveal as well the culturally dialectical experience of the early specialist societies, which emerged in a culture hostile to specialisation. Such societies typically sought to maintain the values and practices of their generalist peers while simultaneously instigating a quiet but radical change into the unified structure of medicine.

Practical origins: neurology in the Ophthalmological Society of the United Kingdom

Historian William F. Bynum traced the origins of neurology to psychiatric discourses that originated in the eighteenth and early nineteenth centuries.[6] Those origins, as suggested in the previous chapter, were important. Equally significant and much less recognised were influences from ophthalmology, especially the formation of the Ophthalmological Society of the United Kingdom in 1880.[7] The formation of this society was a significant moment for medical specialisation in Britain, and the published sources from it are rich and various.[8] The society published its proceedings in quarterly instalments as the *Transactions of the Ophthalmological Society of the United Kingdom*. Each completed volume of the *Transactions* contained lists of officers and the council, as well as lists of rules for membership and participation in the meetings. Each volume published a complete membership list and included mailing addresses.[9] Members received the *Transactions* of the society, and, disseminated in this way, the proceedings of meetings reached audiences throughout Britain. Members could offer communications to the society as presentations at the meetings or through submission for peer-reviewed publication.[10]

From its foundation, the society's leadership appears to have sought legitimacy for specialist ophthalmologic practice. For instance, the council began asserting a political role for ophthalmology by publishing policy reports and offering recommendations to improve the public's health.[11]

The publication of its *Transactions* indicated to sceptics of specialisation that by the common consent of its members, ophthalmologists intended to buck prejudices against specialisation. There were no pretensions to a wide medical outlook, although, as William Bowman (1816–92), the society's founder, patron, and first president, noted at the inaugural meeting, the society's membership was diverse: 'I am truly glad to see here to-night several physicians and surgeons who are very competent oculists, though not called by that name, some who have greatly advanced the knowledge of ophthalmology in its more recondite regions.'[12] Far from making an anti-specialist claim, Bowman's comments were actually those of a skilful medical surveyor, staking claim to an organ but recognising that visual fields in the eye eventually became cortical space in the brain. Bowman was thus not relinquishing disciplinary space for the sake of conformity; he was defining ophthalmology's plot of land.

If neurology was one of those disciplines that Bowman relegated to 'recondite regions', ophthalmologists would not deny the field's importance in the periphery. A 'large part of the total communications received', Bowman remarked in the society's second year, had come from physicians with an interest in ophthalmology but not engaged in its practice, especially 'physicians largely concerned with diseases of the nervous system'.[13] Indeed, some like the by then deceased Robert Bentley Todd had been close associates of Bowman. Physicians with interests in nervous disease were welcome in Bowman's circle and participated frequently in the proceedings of his society throughout its first decade. John Hughlings Jackson presented numerous papers in those early years. In 1881 he presented a paper titled 'On Eye Symptoms in Locomotor Ataxia' and another he had translated from Professor Franciscus Donders (1818–89) in Utrecht, 'On the Relation between the Movements of Objects and the Rotation of the Eyes'.[14] In 1883, Jackson presented yet another paper, 'On Ocular Movements with Vertigo, Produced by Pressure on a Diseased Ear'.[15] That same year popular interest within the society for neurological topics led to a special session on 'Eye Symptoms in Diseases of the Spinal Cord' at which the Professor of Clinical Medicine at University College London, William Gowers, and the physiologist Seymour Sharkey (1847–1929) presented papers.[16] By 1884, the normal schedule of the society's annual proceedings included one session on 'Affections of Muscular and Nervous Systems'.[17]

Physicians with interests in nervous conditions showed their greatest involvement in the Ophthalmological Society between the years 1885 and 1889. Indeed, in 1885 Hughlings Jackson was invited to deliver the Bowman Lecture on 'Ophthalmology and Diseases of the Nervous System', where he offered a spirited defence of medical specialisation.[18] Regarded by his first biographer, James Taylor (1859–1946), as one of his classic works, the address was made by Jackson to the society in early November.[19] He explicated his ideas about the evolution of the nervous system and remarked on how pathological conditions demonstrated states of devolution.[20] Most fascinating, however, was the way Jackson linked his comments on the evolution of the nervous system to a broader argument about the natural social evolution of society. There was in his argument a proliferation of analogies between the necessary complexity of the social organisation of medicine and the ultimate evolutionary organisation of the nervous system. Drawing through analogy on Herbert Spencer's (1820–1903) theories of cultural and social evolution, Jackson argued that the division of labour was a 'universal law'.[21] He was therefore able to join differentiation, complexity, progressing evolution, definiteness, and integration in the nervous system of organisms – all Spencerian concepts – with views that naturalised medical specialisation to the social body of medicine. There were parallels, Jackson argued, between the evolution of the nervous system, society, and society's highest social order, the 'body medical'. 'Differentiation', Jackson proposed, 'is well seen in the development of animal organisms, and is seen, too, in the social organism.' He then added, 'It would be very remarkable if there were an exception in the case of one part of the social organism, the body medical, – if in so great a field of work as the medical there did not arise more and more different parts of that field.'[22]

Indeed the 'body medical' for Jackson was a complex subject; its anatomy included 'alienist physicians, neurologists, obstetric physicians, ophthalmic surgeons, aural surgeons, dentists, physiologists, chemists, &c.; the specialty of each comes out of, and is a differentiated part of, a wide general knowledge.'[23] Each specialist made a distinctly different contribution to social evolution and progress. He noted, 'Specialists have to justify themselves – to justify their differentiation.' Increases in differentiation, definiteness, integration, and cooperation among these medical species would determine progress in medicine. Douglas Argyll-Robertson (1837–1909), for instance, had justified the specialisation of ophthalmology by integrating observations about the eye into a paradigm that physicians with interests in nervous diseases could use as a 'means of investigation of several important diseases'.[24] Jackson remarked:

> Each different worker, knowing one subject best, and having great integration of different, definite medical knowledge, of necessity cannot have the precise knowledge of other subjects which other different workers have. Division of labour necessitates the co-operation of labourers. The whole of one disease is better understood by bringing to bear on its direct investigation and treatment different workers in different fields.[25]

Jackson then turned his attention to the epilepsies and argued that the body's symptoms before, during, and after episodes showed the various stages of human evolution. As excessive nervous discharges temporarily terminated higher evolutionary functions, lower levels rose to the surface for observation. Jackson's theory of devolution was similar to contemporary embryological arguments, shortly to become popular. Just as the foetus was supposed to have passed through all of its pre-existing evolutionary morphologies, nervous diseases brought out older evolutionary manifestations. Symptoms were not signs of diseased states only. Inferring normal physiological connections from these symptoms was possible, and they were clues to the human evolutionary past. The result, which was contingent upon the disease, was that lower levels of evolution appeared uninhibited.[26] For Jackson, nervous diseases not only presented clues about the evolution of the body and the physiology of the nervous system, they also revealed that the medical body could – actually should – undergo a similar evolution.

Neurologists, Jackson argued, were supreme integrationists. They took the knowledge of the ophthalmic and aural surgeon, practitioners working at the lowest level of evolution, and then integrated that knowledge with the observations of alienists on mind, the highest evolutionary structure. Neurologists, as integrators, concentrated on the middle layers, the higher human qualities and the lower animal reflexes. 'Thus the neurologist, by availing himself' of the knowledge of these different workers, 'may hope to justify his differentiation'.[27] Neurologists could be specialists; indeed *ought to be*, to promote progress in medicine.

More polemic than informative, Jackson's Bowman Lecture employed metaphors of growth commonly used in the late nineteenth and twentieth centuries to describe and justify the growing and allegedly organic complexity of society. Jackson may in fact have originated much of this language in so far as it was used to rationalise medical specialisation.[28] His remarks, if somewhat reifying, articulated a broader defence both of specialisation and of the social agenda of the Ophthalmological Society. Not only was specialisation rational and necessary for progress, Jackson had also argued that it was natural. His reliance on Herbert Spencer was more than the happenchance application of a theory to the nervous system.[29] Spencer's theories constructed a universalistic cosmic bridge between the nervous body and the social body, and specifically the 'body medical'. The individual's brain and behaviour were inextricably linked to society and culture, and in turn, society and culture were a part of nature and the universe. Jackson, moreover, was adding a further bridge to the social body of medicine. He was arguing that the heterogeneity of the nervous system justified and necessitated a heterogeneous pool of medical practitioners – each group would have a special interest in an evolutionary layer and consequently would coordinate and correlate their knowledge and practices together. This coordination and correlation would advance medicine.

Jackson had provided a fundamental, theoretical justification for all specialists in medicine, especially for specialists in nervous diseases. But whether anyone made note of his ideas is unclear. Nevertheless, if they wished, ophthalmologists, aural surgeons, neurologists, and alienists, hitherto perceived as outside the fold of general medicine, could find in Jackson's cosmology an argument not only locating them within the vast spectrum of medicine but also making them proponents of heterogeneity. Social heterogeneity was a sign, according to the philosophy of Spencer, of social and cultural progress – so too were medical specialists.

Unsurprisingly, Jackson's urge for medical specialisation through the creation of divisions of labour mirrored already emergent medical expertises, neurology among them. Scarcely three months later, in January 1886, the Neurological Society of London was formed at Jackson's house. He became its first president.[30] After holding that office for two years, Jackson became president of the Ophthalmological Society, with Thomas Buzzard (1831–1919), his friend and fellow physician with interests in nervous diseases, as one of his vice-presidents.[31]

It would be simplistic to attribute the formation of the Neurological Society of London solely to Jackson's arguments in his Bowman Lecture. But it was important, and other noteworthy connections between ophthalmology and neurology existed. Both specialist societies had important similarities. Firstly, theirs was a shared intellectual interest. Neurology and ophthalmology were somatic subjects, or what historical sociologist George Rosen later described as specialties derived from organ localism, i.e. the idea that a bodily organ justified a specialty for that organ.[32] The former was interested in nerves, while the latter was interested in ocular innervations, function, and diseases. For physicians interested in the nerves, the eyes were diagnostic windows into the central nervous system and the only outcroppings of the central nervous system they could study in the living subject. There was secondly a shared technology. The ophthalmoscope was a device used to diagnose conditions both of the eyes and of the nerves. Physicians noted its diagnostic utility for diagnosing nervous diseases early, especially syphilitic disorders, ophthalmic or cerebral cancers, and cortical blindness. An early example was Clifford Allbutt's (1836–1925) monograph *The Use of the Ophthalmoscope in Diseases of the Nervous System and of the Kidneys and also in Certain General Disorders*, which appeared in 1871.[33] William Gowers, the later author of a textbook on nervous diseases, published in 1879 *A Manual and Atlas of Medical Ophthalmoscopy*.[34] Hughlings Jackson made his own contributions as well, publishing, for instance, a note in the *Lancet* titled, 'Value of the Ophthalmoscope in the Investigation and Treatment of Diseases of the Brain'.[35]

One final point of comparison can be made by examining the membership lists from both societies in 1905. This analysis reveals that fifty-one physicians held joint membership in both societies, or 21 per cent of the Neurological Society's membership and 11 per cent of the membership of the Ophthalmological Society. Judging by the archival records of the Neurological Society, members holding joint membership in both societies formed the active core of the Neurological Society.[36]

There were, however, significant differences. When the Neurological Society of London formed, its members and council made little effort to create distinctions between neurology and medicine. It seemingly lacked the proselytising zeal for specialisation that characterised the Ophthalmological Society. There was no attempt to homogenise neurology's community. Indeed, the diversity of its professional membership was the society's central strength and the challenge of its subject.

Medical practices within the Neurological Society of the United Kingdom

With these origins in mind, a fuller exploration of the practices of the Neurological Society of London is possible. It was founded in 1886 and renamed the Neurological Society of the United Kingdom in 1905 (hereafter it shall be referred to as the Neurological Society).[37] From the society's archival sources – manuscripts, letters, membership lists, minutes, and financial records – it is possible to reconstruct some of the ways these physicians understood their work and the role of their new society. These sources also allow some general inferences about, for example, the way a medical culture opposed to specialisation moulded the cultural and social practices as well as outlook of the clinicians and scientists who made up the society's membership.

The first meeting held by the Neurological Society was in January 1886. In retrospect, this first meeting appears an eclectic gathering: the founders of the society were not only clinicians but were also scientists and political theorists. The president of the society, as has been already mentioned, was John Hughlings Jackson; its vice-presidents were Samuel Wilks (1824–1911) and James Crichton-Browne (1840–1938). The council, a veritable *Who's Who* of the London medical elite, included Henry Charlton Bastian (1837–1915), Sir William Broadbent, John Bucknill (1817–97), Thomas Buzzard, David Ferrier (1843–1928), Jonathan Hutchinson (1828–1913), George John Romanes (1848–94), and Edward Albert Sharpey-Shäfer (1850–1935). Francis Galton (1822–1911) was also an original member of the council. The secretaries were Alexander Hughes Bennett (1848–1901) and Armond de Wattevilles (1846–1925).[38] In addition, one of the council's first acts was to elect Herbert Spencer an honorary member of the society.

Records of the first council reveal that the founders adopted an expansive view of the definition of a neurological society: they did not wish their interests to seem restricted to narrow clinical problems and studies. As Thomas Buzzard recollected in 1908: 'It was decided to establish the Society on no narrow basis, and arranged that the President should represent one year special neurology, another general medicine, another surgery, another psychology, another physiology. Each with special leanings upon the subject of the nervous system.'[39] Nor did the society desire to appear overtly missionary. Thomas Buzzard recalled in the same letter that the scrupulous aim to avoid publication of the society's proceedings in a journal was 'a protest against a tendency to advertise which some thought was inclined to show itself in Society work.'[40]

The council might have had the unapologetic aims of the Ophthalmological Society in mind when they constructed their policy, but there were other candidates as well. Specialists had relied on membership in societies, publications in journals, entries in the Medical Directory, and even notices in newspapers, to alert the public to their practices.[41] With its elite membership, the Neurological Society could easily have had its transactions placed in either the *Lancet* or the *British Medical Journal*, undoubtedly drawing interest to any specialists desiring public attention.[42] However, at the second organising meeting, held in February 1886, the council members expressed the opinion 'that this was inadvisable except with special sanction of the council.'[43] It is easy to imagine why. For many of the Neurological Society's members, such a posture would have smacked of advertising and therefore a lack of social respectability. Circumstances, though, did change in the following years.

It is important to understand the distinction between this society and the Ophthalmological Society. The Neurological Society, although now easily cast as a specialist organisation, was not imagined by most of its members, save perhaps Hughlings Jackson, to have any aim of demarcating a sphere of clinical practice or monopoly. To use the terminology of late twentieth-century sociology, specialisation or community formation was not its purposes per se. Instead, the society created a venue for the integration of multiple fields of knowledge. Though some of its members, like Hughlings Jackson, had called the specialisation of medicine natural, an enormously important nuance is lost if his views are taken as a clarion call for a narrowing of focus. The specialisation of neurology was the formation of a human science with all of the ambitions thus implied.

In any case, a less self-promotional and therefore more culturally appropriate place for publication of the proceedings of the society was the journal *Brain*. John Hughlings Jackson, James Crichton-Browne, David Ferrier and John Charles Bucknill – all members of the aforementioned West Riding Asylum cohort – had founded it in 1878 (two years after the journal *Mind* appeared). In 1887, the organ's publishers, Macmillan and Company, submitted proposals to the society suggesting a business affiliation. It is possible to infer from records that with its limited circulation, members felt publishing in *Brain* hardly qualified as advertisement. There were also some financial advantages to the new partnership.[44] Macmillan and Company suggested profits from the publication be split, allowing the society to subsidise the journal.[45] Hitherto the expense of publishing illustrations had commonly fallen on the authors' shoulders. Plates were expensive, and subsidies from the journal's profits meant a decrease in costs to the authors.[46] By 1888 *Brain* had become the official organ of the Neurological Society.[47] Nevertheless, it should be noted that the proceedings of the society in *Brain* began appearing only after 1894. Its members thus continued their studious avoidance of the appearance of advertising.[48]

Membership in the society was originally by invitation only.[49] By 1887, the society had created an application process whereby the applicant had to find 'at least three members of the society' willing to 'append their names' as sponsors on the membership form – a form that appears uncommonly reminiscent of that used for application to the Royal Society.[50] Once accomplished, a completed form practically ensured membership. Between 1887 and 1907, the society received over 353 applications. In 1907, the council scrutinised two applications submitted by women – Helen Stewart and Mary Sturge – and accepted them, but only grudgingly.[51] It was a short-lived openness. Shortly thereafter, the Neurological Society dissolved, to be replaced by the Section of Neurology of the Royal Society of Medicine. The women saw their membership revoked, the councilmen of the Neurological Society demurring that their status would be resolved once the Royal Society of Medicine considered the 'question of election of women members' until the time 'when the Neurological Section of the Royal Society of Medicine has had an opportunity of voting upon the matter'.[52]

Although concentrated in London, membership was not restricted simply to the metropolitan elite. In 1902, 123 members lived in London, while another seventy-three lived elsewhere in England. Ten were from Scotland, five from Wales, and an additional sixteen from other nations.[53] The council elected, for example, Adolf Meyer (1866–1950), a psychiatrist in America, to the membership in 1897.[54] Meyer found membership personally advantageous because he received *Brain* for the small cost of the membership, one pound.[55] The society's membership continually increased. In 1889, there were 133 members. By 1907, the year the society dissolved, there were 256.[56] Despite representation from the provinces, members attending ordinary meetings were mainly from London.[57]

The Attendance Book of the society offers access to many details, such as locations, minutes, the broad range of topics, and how the choice of topic determined the location of meetings. The most popular venues were the National Hospital, Queen Square, and the Physiological Laboratory, University College London.[58] Clinical demonstrations were typically held at the National, whereas physiological meetings occurred at the Laboratory. In the spring of 1886, for example, the minutes of the society recorded that the council decided to hold an ordinary meeting at the Physiological Laboratories 'devoted to the physiological relations of neurology' with E. A. Sharpey-Shäfer and Victor Horsley demonstrating 'their most recent researches on the subject of cerebral localisation'.[59]

Other meetings on functional nervous diseases occurred at the Paddington Infirmary. Physicians at St Mary's Hospital demonstrated electrical therapy for nervous diseases. Meanwhile, general meetings were commonly held at the rooms of the Medical Society of London. George Savage, a member of the council in 1886 and its president in 1897, was asked to arrange one meeting at Bethlem Royal Hospital in the autumn of that year, provided subjects were available for 'demonstrations and discussions' of the mental aspects of nervous diseases.[60] In 1899, the anthropologist William Halshe Rivers Rivers (1864–1922) invited the society to Cambridge for a special lecture on the results of his 'recent investigation at the Torres Straits'.[61] Such a various and expansive programme of topics was typical.

Less frequent were meetings intended to improve communication with members in the provinces. In 1903, to celebrate the change of the society's name to the Neurological Society of the United Kingdom, the

University of Edinburgh sponsored an extra-metropolitan meeting.[62] Professor E. A. Sharpey-Schäfer, formerly of University College London but by then in Edinburgh, invited the society to Scotland with the promise:

> We can arrange those who come a very hearty welcome and I have not doubt that most of those who do us the honour of visiting our ancient city will be asked to accept private hospitality. The President of the Royal College of Physicians has promised his active cooperation and I am sure I can speak for the medical side of the University that every facility will be afforded the members to see whatever is most interesting in the neurological way.[63]

Nonetheless, travel to Edinburgh was neither a trivial matter nor desirous, for only thirty-four members attended the meeting. Most were from London.[64] Thus, the first provincial meeting of the Neurological Society of the United Kingdom resembled more a meeting of a travelling medical club than it did a gathering of provincial members who found it difficult to access the capital.

Perhaps recognising its lack of success in the first attempt, the society's council planned a second meeting for provincial members in 1905. Extra-metropolitan members received special letters of invitation from metropolitan members. They were offered an elegant supper, paid for by a guarantor's fund, as a further incentive to come.[65] Members from London, by contrast, were required to pay twenty-five shillings for their food and drink.[66] The meeting was on clinical and pathological subjects. The supper was extravagant.[67] As they supped through eleven courses, including *terrine de volaille à l'Ancienne* and *filets de bœuf Richelieu*, members offered numerous toasts to the society and the guests washed these down with a steady stream of fine wines and liqueurs.[68] The minutes of this meeting recorded it as an outstanding success, with eighty-four members in attendance, forty-seven from the provinces.[69]

Such ostentation was not typical of ordinary meetings. Although the society's members were the academic and medical elite, meetings were not really venues for advertising personal attainments, distinction, or wealth. Instead, what was on display at these meetings was an eclectic array of medical and scientific knowledge(s), technologies, hypotheses, and experiments – all designed to inquire into the structures and functions of the nervous system in all manifestations.

Not only was new knowledge being disseminated, methods of presentation were also being invented. As D'Arcy Power recalled of earlier medical societies in 1939, in the past written papers had often been 'illustrated by diagrams and by chalk drawings upon a blackboard, but as science advanced, by lantern slides, by epidiascope and by moving pictures'.[70] In 1893, the society, following this general pattern, held photographic exhibits of current experiments. A comparative series of photographs showing 'degeneration of the medullar and spinal cord following ablation of the cerebral hemispheres in mammals' was available for inspection, and Charles Sherrington presented photographs demonstrating the dermatomes of upper sensory roots.[71] At a meeting in 1897, Fred Batten offered a study on 'The Muscle Spindle under Pathological Conditions' and illustrated his presentations with lantern slides and by specimens under the microscope. Two further demonstrations that year also utilised 'lantern slides' to finesse lectures. E. A. Sharpey-Schäfer's lecture 'Is there a Direct Relationship between the Motor Paralysis Produced by Lesions of the Cortex and Loss of Sensibility, Muscular or Other,' was 'illustrated by Lantern Slides, three living monkeys and the brain of a fourth, which had been killed'. Professors Boyce and Warrington employed slides to illustrate their comparative anatomical discussion, 'Contributions to the Anatomy of Some of the Ascending and Descending Nerve Tracts in the Fowl'.[72] Such 'cutting-edge' presentations were only for physiological and anatomical discussions. The clinical presentations fell back on an older method, that of parading actual patients before an audience.

The clinical meetings of the society were reminiscent of medical school and post-graduate teaching in ward rounds. These were a typical highlight of meetings of medical societies in this period. Usually young physicians presented patients (called specimens in this context) with rare or interesting nervous diseases to the audience, members of which then discussed the neurological elements of the conditions. Typically, a junior physician began by presenting the patient's case history to the audience. He then proceeded with a physical examination intended to demonstrate the interesting signs. When possible, the audience saw multiple examples of the same conditions so that they understood the variability of the symptoms. Sometimes the cases presented were of uncertain diagnosis, and on these the entire audience deliberated in an attempt to identify the condition.

The 113th ordinary meeting of the Neurological Society, which took place in the late evening of 30 March 1905, may serve as a typical example. Gordon Holmes presented a ten-year-old boy with a 'midbrain lesion' and possessing, so he described, an unimportant family history. 'Four years ago he became unsteady on his feet, and began to stagger like a drunken man.' The child's gait had become steadily worse, the usage of the left-arm was gone, the right arm was beginning to shake, and his head and eyes generally deviated to the left. While sight and hearing were normal, he had developed a squint and paralysis of the left eye. Holmes then ended with the simple statement, 'there is considerable mental defect.'[73] Unrecorded was any diagnosis, prognosis, or treatment.

At the same meeting, Wilfred Harris presented 'a case of chronic chorea':

> An engine driver, aged 63, while at work ten years ago strained his back, causing such pain in the left side of his back that he had to walk home doubled up. He has never walked properly since, and soon afterwards became unsteady in his gait. At the same time his articulation became altered and slow, and he was often accused of being drunk, though a teetotaller. He had not been able to do any work for the last nine years.[74]

Harris then outlined other symptoms, including: incontinence, poor memory, changes in spatial reasoning, and he added that the patient 'denies venereal diseases'. As he finished, Harris suggested that the case appeared similar to a combination of 'spastic paralysis and chronic chorea, and might be labelled *spastic chorea*'. Once again, there was no treatment, diagnosis, or prognosis recorded.[75] The discussions of family history and constitution hinted at a broader Galtonian outlook.

Hidden behind these mildly written minutes were many deeper social practices. Part of these presentations was deliberate showmanship.[76] The skills of the physicians presenting the case were often a fusion of rhetorical imagery and medical knowledge. Metaphors, analogies, and similes were utilised to accentuate messages but were deployed less frequently to describe actual symptoms and signs. Precise language was a measure of precise clinical skills. The manners, maturity, and acumen of the physician's bedside practices – the art (and bread and butter) of medicine – were part of the display. A strong or weak performance would leave a lasting impression with the audience. The disciplinary power of British professional societies lay as much in their ability to acculturate as in their ability to exclude.

Although there is no evidence, it may be inferred that there were discussions at these clinical meetings following the presentations. These might have been similar to the conversations later recorded and extant in the *Proceeding of the Royal Society of Medicine*. In those records, physicians ask questions about patient histories, sometimes challenge diagnoses, and at other times enter into broader dialogues about the underlying pathologies. Some contemporary records suggest that the focus of these clinical demonstrations in the Neurological Society gravitated towards scientific inquiries: the physiology and anatomy of the nervous system contrasted with broader theoretical, even philosophical, musing. Alternatively, the clues that diseases provided to the normal functioning of the nervous system might have been a topic. With its diverse audiences, the society's clinical meetings provided multiple points of view and questions about allied diseases and disorders. The exchanges would have been frank, the dialogue accordingly sometimes heated, for physicians and scientists often aligned themselves with specific positions and medical perspectives.[77]

Meetings could also be strictly educational.[78] Physicians would introduce new theories, techniques, and occasionally therapies. Typically, the inaugural lectures of the presidents of the society described or took positions on the latest changes in scientific and medical knowledge about the nervous system, techniques, and therapy (almost exclusively surgical). In 1893, Professor E. A. Sharpey-Shäfer gave his presidential lecture on 'The Nerve Cell as the Basis of Neurology' and defended the neuron theory against reticular schools of thought.[79] Alexander Hill (1856–1929), Master of Downing College Cambridge, addressed the society on the topic of 'The Chrome Silver Method: A Study of the Conditions under which the Reaction Occurs and a Criticism of its Results'.[80] In 1896, Victor Horsley presented a surgical analysis of a 'case of removal of a cerebellar tumour, two years and five months after operation'.[81]

Although we could frame the formation of a neurological society purely in terms of specialisation and professionalisation, there is a striking absence of records of any public agenda for the society. The officers and council of the society did not concern themselves with legislation, political organisation, or neurology education. Nor was any code of conduct for neurological practice ever drafted. Neither are efforts to homogenise the occupations of the membership of the society evident: physicians, surgeons, alienists, philosophers, and scientists were all welcome. These facts contrast with the proceedings of the Ophthalmological Society. That society published public reports and attempted to implement changes in government policy that directly benefited ophthalmological practice. During the Neurological Society's twenty-one-year history, only one action seemed fundamentally intent upon creating a lasting tradition – the creation of the Hughlings Jackson Lectureship in 1897.[82]

The creation of an honorary lectureship while Jackson was still alive was a rather peculiar decision on the part of the council, although, as Walter Coleman (1864–1934) pointed out at the time, it was not without 'precedent', because the Ophthalmological Society had done this for William Bowman – yet further evidence of the close relationship between these two societies.[83] The council announced in early 1897 the establishment of a lectureship celebrating the discoverer of 'Cortical Epilepsy and its relation to cerebral localisation' and noted that Hughlings Jackson had consented to deliver the first lecture.[84] In December 1897, Jackson spoke on the 'Relations of Different Divisions of the Central Nervous System to One Another and to Parts of the Body'.[85] Lectures followed subsequently every three years: Eduard Hitzig (1838–1907) gave the 1900 lecture; William Broadbent (1835–1907) the 1903; and Victor Horsley (1857–1916) delivered the 1906 lecture – the first to honour Jackson's contributions specifically in the title: 'On the Illustration by Recent Research of Dr Hughlings Jackson's Views on the Functions of the Cerebellum'.[86] The tradition of the lecture continued, even after the Neurological Society disbanded.

The Neurological Society restructured with the 1907 formation of the Royal Society of Medicine and became the Section of Neurology. How this happened will be briefly recounted in the next section. In any case, the council of the society actively participated in planning the Royal Society of Medicine from the moment it was proposed. This is an indication of the ways that the Neurological Society always stood at crossroads between clinical and scientific generalism and specialism. It was a practical equilibrium, one likely predicated on the demography of the society.[87]

Further crossroads: the membership of the Neurological Society

The social composition of the sciences and medicine of the nervous system in nineteenth-century Britain is difficult to grasp with any certainty and the membership lists of the Neurological Society constitute one important source. While it falls outside the remit of this study to discuss the limitations of membership lists as sources, it should be obvious that only minimal inferences from them may be drawn and through comparisons only. The lists are, however, a useful index for understanding the richness and enormous overlap in the spheres of late Victorian science and medicine, which had implications for the science and medicine of the nervous system.

No visible college existed for neurology prior to the creation of the Neurological Society.[88] Some common past relationships between the individuals belonging to the society can be identified from a study of the biographies of its members. Many founding members of the Neurological Society could identify one of two figures as being especially important in their training. One was Thomas Laycock (1812–76).[89] Laycock had been a student of both Charles Bell (1774–1842), a figure who had inaugurated the modern secular approach to the scientific study of the nervous system, and Marshall Hall (1790–1857), the early pioneer for the physiological approach to medicine. Over the course of his clinical and scientific career, Laycock had published several original studies and theories on the organisation and function of the nervous system that accommodated and expanded upon the perspectives of Bell and Hall.[90] Although his relationship with many members of the Neurological Society was partially a consequence of his appointment as Professor in the Practice of Physic at the University of Edinburgh, his work piqued the interests of many, including John Hughlings Jackson. Jackson was not alone. Laycock, his biographer alleges, may also have exerted some influence on the clinical and scientific perspectives of David Ferrier, James Crichton-Browne, Thomas Clouston (1840–1915), Jonathan Hutchinson (1828–1913), Byrom Bramwell (1847–1931), and Thomas Lauder Brunton (1844–1916).[91] All were founder members of the Neurological Society.[92] Brunton, Ferrier, Hutchinson, Jackson, and Crichton-Browne were also elected into the Royal Society, a point explored shortly. (Note that all references to the Royal Society below refer to the elite scientific body, and *not* the Royal Society of Medicine, which was a medical body.)

The second figure, equally prominent in the background of many of the founder members, was Michael Foster (1836–1907), the first University Professor of Physiology at Cambridge. Foster had studied medicine at University College London. After succeeding Thomas Henry Huxley as Fullerian Professor of Physiology at the Royal Institution in London in 1869, Foster had been appointed to Cambridge, where he remained active from 1870 until 1900. Early publications by Marshall Hall, Robert Bentley Todd, William Bowman, and John Hughlings Jackson, among others, had begun linking the physiology and pathology of the nerves by the time Foster came to Cambridge.[93] Foster's school of physiology, however, represented tacit acceptance of the connections between physiology and medicine, and that physiological approach characterised many of the scientific and medical approaches to the nervous system and its diseases. Several of Foster's students focused their attention almost solely on the science and medicine of the nervous system. Among Foster's most prominent pupils were: Walter Gaskell, John Newport Langley, and Charles Sherrington. Others worthy of mention included Henry Head, Hugh Kerr Anderson, Henry Dale, William Hunter, William Ransom, Edward Reid, William Rivers, and Howard H. Tooth. All were graduates of Cambridge; all published articles in the *Journal of Physiology* between 1878 and 1900; all were founder members or became members of the Neurological Society.[94] In addition, all but Tooth were Fellows of the Royal Society.

From this cursory prosopography, it is apparent that a connection existed between the Neurological Society and the Royal Society. Eight of the Neurological Society's original council were Fellows. Yet the overlap in membership between the two societies was significantly larger. Comparison of their membership rolls reveals that forty-four members of the Neurological Society were elected Fellows of the Royal Society, or would become so after the Neurological Society's dissolution. A perusal of the many biographical sources on these Fellows, furthermore, makes self-evident the claim that this group had academic interests that were extremely wide ranging, encompassing chemistry, botany, histology, physiology, pathology, zoology, biology, and medicine and surgery.

From the Royal Society's Certificates of Election and Candidature, it is further possible to infer the existence of socially engaged networks – although to what extent they had any effectiveness we cannot judge.

From these documents, it is clear that while 194 Fellows of the Royal Society cast 622 votes for the forty-four candidates, the average number of votes cast was only three, and the median merely one. It is noteworthy that thirty Fellows consequently cast 293 of the total votes for the Fellows who were also members of the Neurological Society. This group of electors was not simply powerful within the Royal Society but also extraordinarily powerful in British science and medicine (see Table 1).

Although it is not within the remit of this chapter to discuss each elector's biography fully, it is possible to discern some general features within the cohort. Fifteen held some illustrious medical or surgical appointment; twelve held a position in academic science. Almost all were medical and scientific educators. John Burdon Sanderson, one example, had been the Professor of Practical Physiology and Histology at University College London and then Waynflete Chair of Physiology at Oxford in 1882.[95] It was Burdon Sanderson who read Ferrier's paper to the Royal Society. Several others had connections to Thomas Laycock or Michael Foster. A much less representative circle within the Royal Society can also be seen. Members of the X Club, a Victorian dining club that advocated for evolutionary thought, scientific research, and naturalistic frames of reference cast votes.[96] George Busk, anthropologist and vice-president of the Royal Society, was the only member of the X Club to appear in the group of thirty electors, yet it is noteworthy that his fellow X Club members John Tyndall and Thomas Henry Huxley (who do not appear in Table 1) voted for five others and that William Carpenter was a noted Darwinian.[97] Finally, one other group appears prominent: four – Jackson, Bastian, Gowers, and Ferrier – held appointments at the National Hospital for Epilepsy and Paralysis.[98]

It is easy to imagine that the circle represented by the physicians from Queen Square was the most important in fashioning the clinical side of the Neurological Society.[99] Charles Édouard Brown-Séquard (1817–94), also a Fellow of the Royal Society, had been the first physician appointed at the National Hospital and had apparently recruited Hughlings Jackson there in 1862. By 1863, Brown-Séquard, an incessant traveller, had departed for America and eventually a Professorship in Physiology at Harvard.[100] Subsequent appointments at the National Hospital included Thomas Buzzard, Henry Charlton Bastian, David Ferrier, Joseph Omerod, Charles Beevor, James Taylor,

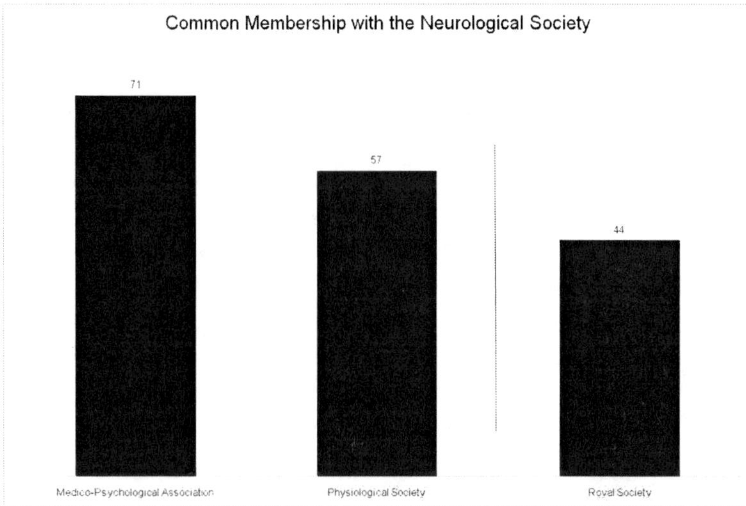

Figure 1: Numbers of members held in common with the Neurological Society

There were 242 members of the Neurological Society. Twenty-nine per cent of them held membership in the Medico-Psychological Association, which in 1905 had 597 members. Twenty-four per cent of members of the Neurological Society also held membership in the Physiological Society, which in 1905 had 275 members. Eighteen per cent of the Neurological Society were members of the Royal Society. Some individuals – for example John Hughlings Jackson and Frederick Mott – were members of all three. *Sources*: Membership Roll of the Medical-Psychological Association (*Journal of Mental Science*) and the Physiological Society of the United Kingdom (Wellcome Library for the History and Understanding of Medicine.)

mental illness. His obituarist recalled that, 'Between the physiogenic and psychogenic schools of thought he endeavoured to keep a due balance, and foreign visitors to his hospital...had occasion to comment on the "polypragmatic" spirit of [Horton].'[102] The obituaries of these members suggest that polypragmaticism was the spirit of the group. From a twenty-first-century perspective, it might be tempting to see the potential for occupational antagonism, or – to use sociological language – dynamic interactionism.[103] Actually, the situation appears exactly reversed. The Neurological Society cultivated all perspectives; neurology was a highly inclusive form of knowledge.

In this way, members of the Neurological Society accommodated the traditional structures of medicine. In their view and practice, medicine was whole. And they were, moreover, deeply invested in that perspective. Several members of the Neurological Society were (or became after the society disbanded) presidents of the Royal College of Physicians or Surgeons in London and Edinburgh. Others were presidents of the Medical Society of London (see Table 2). As we shall examine in Chapter 3, sixty-two members of the Neurological Society were members of the Association of Physicians of Great Britain and Ireland.

Beyond these demographic indices, it is very difficult to infer much from membership lists about lived experience, self-fashioning, occupational identity, or even specialisation. Whereas biography can describe the complexity of a life lived, a sweeping account of an entire scientific and clinical field might beg for simplicity and parsimony. This section has sought to ground an alternative reading, one that turns the story of specialisation upside down and asks not how it happened but rather whether that narrative describes much of anything. The fascinating aspect of these collective features is that they reveal that many people lived, worked, and practised in a world not bounded by late modern logics but rather by their own. The more important story is how the more contemporary logic came into being and constructed such a rigid view of the workers in the past.

The temporary equilibriums of practice

That it was embracing complexity does not fully explain what happened in the Neurological Society. There is scant evidence in the archives of this society or in the reports of its proceedings offering many clues. Hughlings Jackson's Bowman Lecture to the Ophthalmological Society had fashioned neurologists as arising out of a wider social cosmology. They became a part of the anatomy of the medical social body and thus linked the division of medical labour with a story about the progress of medicine. If the Neurological Society's origins were underpinned by such rhetoric, why had the rhetoric of differentiation not continued? A clue is the society's second rule for membership. It stated that, 'The objects of the Society shall be to promote the advance of Neurology and to facilitate intercourse amongst those who cultivate it, whether from a Psychological, Physiological, Anatomical, or Pathological

Table 2: Positions of prestige in British medicine occupied by members of the Neurological Society

Royal College of Physicians	*Date*
Samuel Wilks	1896–98
Thomas Barlow	1910–14
Moore Normal	1918–23
John Rose Bradford	1926–30
William R. Dawson	1931–37
Royal College of Surgeons	
Jonathan Hutchinson	1889
John Tweedy	1903
Rickman John Godlee	1911
Royal College of Physicians (Edinburgh)	
Byrom Bramwell	1910
Edwin Bramwell	1933
Medical Society of London	
William Broadbent	1881
John Hughlings Jackson	1887
Jonathan Hutchinson	1892
T. Lauder Brunton	1905
Charles A. Balance	1906
J. Mitchell Bruce	1911
David Ferrier	1913
William Hale-White	1920
William R. Dawson	1922
Donald Armour	1929
Robert Arthur Young	1930

Sources: Obituaries of the members of the Neurological Society in the *British Medical Journal*, the *Lancet*, and *The Times*.

point of view.'[104] The society adhered to this expansive principle. Its presidents represented a diverse range of professional experiences, and included surgeons, physicians, anatomists, alienists, and physiologists. This diverse representation in turn had significant ramifications, not the least of which was that there was never any discussion about what delineated a 'neurologist'. In the absence of a professional definition, the society defaulted to another position best articulated by two of its rules: 'Anyone engaged in researches on Neurology, or manifesting interest in such researches, shall be eligible for the Ordinary Membership.' And, 'Men of distinction in science, who have contributed to the advancement of Neurology, shall be eligible for the Honorary, or for the Corresponding Membership.'[105] Such open-ended rules embraced a broad spectrum and handed no particular authority to medical practitioners. Physiologists and anatomists could occupy authoritative positions in this society, just as surgeons and physicians could. The neurologist was anyone researching 'nerves', a fact that made precise delineation impractical. In any case, delineation was never an issue.

However, without recourse to some professional definition, the professional designation of 'neurologist' was accorded to very few members of the Neurological Society. If used at all, it seems that 'neurologist' implied status and distinction of merit. The early character of the society was fluid. Its presidents, like its members, brought their own fleeting view of what constituted neurology to the society's meetings. This fluidity, though, was a sign of generalist acumen and members' prowess in medicine and science.

Such judiciousness and mutability undoubtedly left a rich treasury for any heir-apparent to neurology (such as internal medicine, psychology, neurosurgery, and psychiatry) to plunder. Certainly by the turn of the century there was already within this medical system the potential for what sociologist Andrew Abbott termed jurisdictional conflicts.[106] At the same time, applying too much focus to the volatility within the medical system neglects its other feature: the foundations underlying neurology's scientific and clinical pluralism. Neurology was a special subject. It demanded a special occupational relativism. Neurology described a series of practices, paradigms, and focuses in a variety of disciplinary arenas. Each had historical roots. As historian George Rousseau has pointed out, each derived much from a past rich with cultural traditions.[107] Equilibrium in these values, even at the turn of the twentieth century, was always temporary. If anatomical structures bounded neurology – the nerves – then it remained true that an unbounded mind governed the nervous subject. Dividing the nervous system's various portions into any disciplinary stew simply encouraged a narrowness of medical and scientific perspective. An equilibrium between general and specialist values protected neurology from devolving into a reductive conversation.

To be sure, there were certain ideological motivations for this definitional ambiguity. The temptation to make mind and body one and the same threatened whole centuries of idealist thought, an issue germane to many Oxford and Cambridge classically trained physicians and physiologists, who made up the base of the membership of the Neurological Society. As historian David Millett has pointed out, the rise of a physiology of brain without a physiology of mind in Britain – in other words, the special secularism of British physiology – was markedly in contrast to that in Germany.[108] Still the concomitancy of behaviour, psychic states, and simple reflexes suggested a state of efficiency optimised through evolution, upon which one might lay the foundations for a monist philosophy, one in fact eventually embraced by James Crichton-Browne. Few neurologists or physiologists adopted such a seemingly extreme philosophical position, yet because such intellectual opportunities were available and because there were so few concrete facts, physicians in Britain conceived neurology broadly. This practice prevented neurology from being usurped by political theorists.[109]

This equilibrium between specialist and generalist practice, between physiology and neurology, and mental and nervous conditions, appeared for other reasons. The lack of uniformity allowed neurology to flourish in the social light of respectability. Active members, for instance, who were or would become presidents of the Royal College of Physicians – men like Thomas Barlow (1845–1945) or John Rose Bradford (1863–1935) – could be members without signalling to constituents, admirers, or adversaries, any divisive inclinations. Historian George Weisz has argued that the ascendance of the specialist in British medical culture can be seen in the appointment of specialists like them to the Royal Colleges of Physicians or Surgeons. He offers, for example, that, 'in 1903, the ophthalmologist John Tweedy was elected president of the College' of Surgeons.'[110] Such a claim requires this important caveat: Tweedy was also an active member of the Neurological Society.[111] As the then Johns Hopkins Professor but later Regius Professor at Oxford, William Osler argued in 1892, 'the student of internal medicine cannot be a specialist. The manifestations of almost any one of the important diseases in the course of a few years will "box the compass" of the specialties.'[112] Osler might have been speaking of neurology. The parallels between the total natures of both subjects were apparent to any of neurology's heterogeneous enthusiasts.[113] The subjects balanced generalist intuitions against specialist perspectives – a fact obviously true of the proceedings of the Neurological Society.

In retrospect, the location of the Neurological Society appears comfortably and conveniently situated between the mores of a culture opposed to medical specialisation and the generalist reality of medical practice. As sociologist Marc Berg has remarked on medical practices, their 'rationality speaks a plural tongue'.[114] To be otherwise, the Neurological Society would have had to buck the medical mainstream, emulate its ophthalmological twin, and thus 'dirty the hands' with commerce. There was no such agenda. There was no need for such an agenda. Such political action would have been difficult in any case; the control of the medical establishment rested firmly in the hands of professors of medicine and hospital and university authorities incapable of or unwilling to concede the need for specialists. The society's conservatism was not a wise course of action – no one really saw another option.

By 1906 concerns to prevent specialisation reached their high point. A coalition of physicians, including neurologist Henry Head (there by the request of the council of the Neurological Society), proposed the formation of an umbrella medical society, which, although divided into specialist sections, granted access to a vast non-specialist audience.[115] Each section originated from a former specialist society that had appeared in the nineteenth century. The amalgamation of these societies was absolute: libraries (remnants of now long-past circulating scientific book societies), money accumulated in their coffers through membership dues and bequests, and the members of these societies all passed under the aegis of the new Royal Society of Medicine. In exchange, this new society's members possessed a new building, a larger medical library, and, most importantly, access to knowledge that had previously been scattered at all places and scheduled in all times.

The pressure on specialist societies to amalgamate with the Royal Society of Medicine must have been enormous.[116] What the consequences of not joining would have been is difficult to know, but declining to join was tantamount to exclusion from medicine. In any case, the Neurological Society's members relished the opportunity. Without even a hint of concern about their professional standing, the society's members voted unanimously to join. In 1906, the Neurological Society of the United Kingdom dissolved, and the Section of Neurology of the Royal Society of Medicine was formed.[117]

Interestingly, the Ophthalmological Society of the United Kingdom followed an alternative road – one that the Neurological Society might also have adopted.[118] Claiming that total dissolution would unfairly exclude their overseas members, the council of that society opted for a comfortable middle ground. The Section of Ophthalmology of the Royal Society of Medicine became its London-based chapter. Yet, the Ophthalmological Society would still hold an annual general meeting, which all members might attend. This meeting would take place in various cities across the United Kingdom, and consequently members unable to benefit from the London-based meetings would still have access to the society. Members of the Section of Neurology would eventually cite the model of the Ophthalmological Society when they parted company with the Royal Society of Medicine to form the Association of British Neurologists, twenty-five years later.[119]

Conclusion

Fellows of the Royal Society greeted with scepticism David Ferrier's conclusions on the cortical localisation of function. It is tempting to attribute the dual existence of the Neurological Society and its journal *Brain* to such social resistances. It is tempting also to look for higher intellectual currents. Herbert Spencer's largely transcendent view that society was organic and that the measure of progress was society's growth, evolution, and differentiation, could be an example that had as much import for physicians and scientists as Ferrier's physiological research. Metaphors and analogies are some of the simplest and yet most complex ways to define human existence – indeed some philosophers have pondered whether we think with language or whether language thinks through us. It may be parsimonious to claim that specialists and the specialisation of medicine and science arise from natural processes, or to attribute their existence to certain factors like the growth of knowledge or the formation of the organised society. Yet there are multiple reasons to be sceptical of such language, not the least of which is that one must deny enormous social and cultural complexity in order to concur with it. The power of history in all of this is that only the future provides the key to the past. It is obvious only to posterity that the Neurological Society was a specialist organisation. That, of course, is the important story, but it is one that becomes vastly richer with recognition that for most of its members that was an unrealised fact and unintended consequence.

• 2 •

The First World War and the transformation of neurology

Introduction

Could there be two more promising names than Henry Head (1861–1940) and Walter Russell Brain (1895–1966) for a history of the science and medicine of the nervous system? By happy coincidence, both figures were neatly emblematic of their generations. Head's period of influence was approximately greatest between 1895 and 1925; Brain's came a generation later, approximately 1930 to 1960.

The men bore striking similarities to each other. They both practised at the London Hospital, a medical teaching facility located in the capital's East End. Both figures left striking documents from their early lives: Head's correspondence with Ruth Mayhew, later his wife, must be one of the more remarkable collections of letters from the late Victorian and Edwardian eras. The scraps from Brain's life, if less extensive, are equally remarkable. His unpublished diary is one of the few sources on the experiences and thoughts of a conscientious objector in First World War Britain.

Each, as suggested by his personal papers, had humanistic aspirations. Head, as his biographer L. Stephen Jacyna has recounted, fashioned himself privately as a poet, literary critic, essayist, and a great admirer of literature and music. Brain, like Head, wrote lines of verse, reflective essays, and competent treatises on philosophy. It is clear also that the wives of both men played a significant role in the shaping of their careers and personality. Ruth Head (née Mayhew) is perhaps more famous, but Stella Brain (née Langdon Down) appears to have been enormously influential in the shaping of her husband's career, opinions, and sensibilities.

Professionally, too, Head and Brain had similar dispositions. They saw patients with mental and nervous diseases and were both interested in mental phenomena. Both treated famous patients; Head,

Virginia Woolf; Brain, Winston Churchill. Each had research interests in aphasia as well as diseases of the peripheral nerves. Likewise, they both possessed interests in medical politics, as evidenced by their editorship of *Brain*. Head's inclinations admittedly took him more towards research into the function of the nervous system, while Brain's inclinations were more towards political organisation – he would become president of the Royal College of Physicians London.

Nevertheless, in both men, clinical acumen, scientific ability, political perceptiveness, and cultural taste combined, fashioning their prominence. More important for the purposes of this study, however, is that the biography of each man frames one side of an extraordinary period of change for clinical neurology in Britain, the first half of the twentieth century. Head's was a medical world avowedly generalist; Brain's medical world eventually embraced specialisation. It was the conditions of the First World War that stimulated these changes, and for neurology, as their contemporary Edwin Bramwell observed, 'the Great War constitute[d] a convenient if arbitrary dividing-line between the present and the past.'[1] Head spoke to both worlds. He had advocated for medical generalism before the war; he advocated for specialism after the war. His younger counterpart advocated for and practised a general approach to medicine and science, even as he endorsed and aided efforts remake Britain's medical culture.

The work and attitudes of both men thus serve to frame the wider chronological scope of this chapter, which begins before the war and with the foundation of the great general medical societies of the Edwardian era and ends in the interwar period and with the rise of state medicine. Many people understood that their world was different after 1918. The following sections thus trace a world moving from generalism to specialism. The sources from this period – archival documents, official reports, correspondence, published papers, proceedings of society meetings, and retrospective memoirs – capture the dialectical interplay that unfolds between contexts and individuals, war and peace, age and youth, and most especially tradition and change.

Simplifying professional life: the Royal Society of Medicine

Henry Head was involved in the negotiations that ultimately led to the Neurological Society of the United Kingdom's dissolution in 1907.

At that same time, a new society appeared in the London medical scene, the Royal Society of Medicine, which had a section devoted to neurology. How is this change to be regarded? What was the nature of Head's involvement?

Typically, historians and sociologists of British medicine have described the event as an amalgamation of sixteen specialist societies into a more rationally defined umbrella organisation. In this sense, scholars construed the formation of the Royal Society of Medicine as an explicit recognition of specialties.[2] Historian Rosemary Stevens, while conceding that the Royal Society of Medicine did not grant specialist sections 'exclusive rights over admittance to each specialty', argued that the society's creation of sixteen separate sections in medicine and surgery implicitly recognised the legitimacy of specialist practice.[3] Historian George Weisz largely concurred. Like Stevens, Weisz acknowledged, however, 'that [the Royal Society of Medicine] was also meant to combat excessive specialisation'.[4] The caveats of both arguments underscore a very real puzzle. It strains credulity to describe the dissolution of sixteen independent specialist societies and the subsequent amalgamation of their assets into one body as advancing (belatedly or otherwise) the cause of clinical specialisation.

Certain facts about the Royal Society of Medicine's proceedings and structure are important to consider. Firstly, the sections had independent meetings, and in this they did promote specialist practice. Yet the *Proceedings of the Royal Society of Medicine* carried transcripts of the meetings of each section so completely that any physician unable to attend the meeting of one section could – if so inclined – be aware of all that had transpired elsewhere. In other words, transparency through wide dissemination of information to all physicians was the central motivation and official policy of the society.

Secondly, while the sections had independent meetings, the society also sponsored joint meetings of multiple sections, as well as large events like the annual address of the president of the society.[5] In addition, members could attend meetings of any of the sections, and the more elite of its membership became presidents of multiple sections, a position of less prominence than the presidency of the entire society but prestigious nonetheless. As has already been mentioned, Edward Farquhar Buzzard was president of the Medical, Psychiatry, and Neurology Sections. Macdonald Critchley and Charles Symonds, two more examples, were presidents of the Neurology and Psychiatry Sections. Francis Walshe was one-time president of the entire society.

Thirdly, while each section had its own organisational committee, elected representatives from these committees sat on the society's council. That council determined solutions to larger management questions. Costs of membership and publishing decisions, for example, were in the hands of this higher-level administrative body. All of these potential issues of independence would have represented lasting conflicts in specialised practices had the tacit recognition of specialties been an aim.[6] It is not apparent that such an aim existed.

Analysis of Henry Head's activities on the committee of the Union of Medical Societies (the committee that established the Royal Society of Medicine) might provide hints of that committee's ultimate motivations. As the Neurological Society of the United Kingdom's representative on that committee, Head would certainly have made formal report to the Neurological Society that might appear in the archival record. However, the only record is of his appointment is from a 1906 report:

> The question of amalgamation of the Society with the Union of Medical Societies came again before the Society in an amended form, and at a Special Meeting held on December 6, 1906 the following resolution was passed: 'That the Neurological Society of the United Kingdom agrees to take part in the Amalgamation of Medical Societies and appoints Dr Head as its delegate to the New Committee.'[7]

No records of the work of the committee of the Union of Medical Societies have been located. Nor do any clues appear in Henry Head's correspondence with Ruth Head from those years, but there are other elements in Head's letters that suggest a strong material motivation for creating such a union: the number of hours available in the average day of a London consultant were too few.

Looked at differently, the formation of a union of medical societies can be considered in economic and cultural terms. Head's circumstances were likely typical. Economically, like most London physicians, Head's income came mainly from his private consulting practice rather than his hospital work. There were multiple ways for Head to grow that practice, and all of these paths had to be taken. As a young practitioner, Head had needed to move up the medical ladder within a hospital of good repute. A position as assistant physician and then full physician within a hospital could constitute public evidence of his growing expertise.

Yet clinical expertise in Edwardian England was routinely established through scientific achievements that were lauded by medical peers, most of whom were older and had little inclination for clinical specialisation and much sympathy with tradition. The acclaim of one's peers had thus to be earned in the multiple sites of club culture and bourgeois society, and hither and thither were Head's days and evenings consumed. In what were after all intended as love letters or as the letters of a devoted husband, certain hints of these activities appear, as well as their stresses, advantages, and the passions they sometimes engendered in Head. A 1904 letter is particularly illustrative:

> I expected a dull evening...but spent a delightful time in the most ancient social medical club in the world. How you would have enjoyed their Silver. They have an officer called...a keeper of the cups. Such a collection. Every time a member is elected his name is engraved on a small medal and attached to the rim of a cup. As room on one cup is fully occupied another is begun. A tortoise shell walking-stick set with gold but properly of a defunct eighteenth century member is one club relic handed round after dinner: another is a portion of the temple of Aesculapius set on a pedestal. I sat between Byrom Bramwell and Clouston – the former representative of clinical neurology, the latter the famous professor of mental diseases in the university. Bramwell said 'How well you are looking' and I answered 'I have got the secret of Cortical Sensibility and that acts as a tonic'. But I did not tell him that there was another more secret elixir of youth working in my body. For it is more good fortune than any man has a right to be in love, madly in love and at the same time to have made a discovery that men have been wanting for 50 years.[8]

In between these private and professional musings, Head gives us some slight insight into his world. Bramwell and Clouston were powerful medical statesmen, and to be a guest at the Aesculapius Club was no small invitation for a rising member of the medical establishment. Head's later letters to his wife contain additional allusions to such activities, scientific or traditional. Head makes passing reference to meetings of a 'neurological club', the Physiological Society, and the Association of Physicians, as well as more than a few occasional international meetings. Given the personal nature of his letters, there are few reasons to believe that much from his professional life found its way into them.[9] But based upon these documents, as well as the archival records from the London Hospital, the Neurological Society, and the Section of Neurology of the Royal Society of Medicine, it is clear that Head made his presence felt within the medical community and that his schedule was crammed full of social obligations.

A union of medical societies would have possessed enormous advantages to one with his schedule. For one, most of the clinical meetings of the various societies would, like those of the Neurological Society, have formerly been held in different hospitals, laboratories, or universities throughout London. Now they occurred at one location. In addition, rather than spending the money to be a member of the many societies (to say nothing of finding the time to renew annual subscriptions), Head needed only to pay for and renew one subscription. Membership in the Royal Society (i.e. the scientific society) as well as the Physiological Society would still have entailed payment of dues, but a union of medical societies meant that it was no longer necessary for a consultant to keep up with the proceedings of all of the many medical societies.

Can Head really be considered representative of the London consultants? Yes and no. His scientific attainments and interests, clinical ability, and editorial responsibilities (to say nothing of his cultural and literary interests) appear greater than those possessed by the average Harley Street or Wimpole Street consultant with a private practice, but for those of his peers firmly established in the medical teaching hospitals, such busy days and evenings were commonplace. And even those consultants with specialist interests located on Harley or Wimpole Street or beyond, and without hospital appointments, would have needed general medical knowledge. How else could they have known which conditions to treat and which to refer on to others?

It is within this organic milieu that an understanding of the dissolution of the Neurological Society and the formation of the Royal Society of Medicine can be reached. It was not a tacit recognition of specialties, but rather an attempt to organise rationally the values of a culture that still embraced, no matter how haphazardly, an ideal of generalism. This ideal became even more concrete in those years following the formation of the Royal Society of Medicine. It would take more than the existence of actual clinical specialists to transform that culture. Indeed, it would take a war like none ever seen before.

Generalist practice in Edwardian Britain

Judging from its archival records and published proceedings, the Royal Society of Medicine in the pre-war years was an uneventful venue. The proceedings of the Section of Neurology, for instance, maintained a schedule not varying greatly from that of the previous Neurological Society of the United Kingdom. There were the usual president's addresses, research communications, notices of new methods, as well as routine clinical meetings at which young physicians presented interesting patients to an audience. Unlike the earlier society's meetings, however, there were also joint sessions between two or more sections of the Royal Society of Medicine. The Neurological Section met jointly with the Ophthalmological Section, the Section of Medicine, and the Section of Psychiatry in the years between 1907 and 1914.[10] In addition, other sections commonly solicited contributions from council members of the Section of Neurology (although it is worth noting that those individuals rarely extended the reciprocal privilege to other sections' council members). The first notable event took place at a 1916 council meeting, where 'The question of enemy aliens, who are Corresponding Members of the Section, being allowed to retain their position, was considered, and the Council was unanimously of the opinion that their names should be expunged from the list at the conclusion of the War.'[11] By 1916, emotions everywhere ran extremely high but the proceedings of the Section of Neurology before 1914 were routine.

The former Neurological Society had set itself the mission of providing a venue for its provincial members, a mission that culminated in the aforementioned grand meeting of 1905. One unforeseen consequence of the 'amalgamation' of the specialist societies was that provincial members had little choice but to attend meetings in the capital. The sections of the Royal Society of Medicine were unlikely to hold meetings in the provinces.

This London-centric nature of the Royal Society of Medicine would have worn thin with consultants practising and conducting research elsewhere. Had it not been for the foundation of a national association of physicians in the same year as the Royal Society of Medicine's formation, it is possible that new provincial organisations would have sprung-up in medical centres beyond the capital. The idea for this new body was the brainchild of an illustrious figure in medicine: the Oxford Regius Professor of Medicine, William Osler, had first suggested the new association to some friends, known as 'the gang', in 1906.[12] Osler, Archibald Garrod (1857–1936), Humphrey Rolleston, William Hale-White (1857–1949), John Rose Bradford, and Jonathan Hutchinson (note that the last three had been active in the Neurological Society) envisioned it as a 'pleasant gathering' and 'nucleus' for the medical men 'actively engaged in research'.[13] According to a history kept in the association's archives, they circulated their idea to professors of medicine scattered throughout the country, who all agreed to sign a letter of invitation to ordinary members. Late that year they sent letters to a limited number of physicians engaged in medical research. In perhaps yet a further indication of the apathy members of the former Neurological Society felt about their specialist status, sixty-two of its past members became original members of the Association of Physicians.

The Association of Physicians of Great Britain and Ireland thus formed in 1907. It had 232 members.[14] The *Quarterly Journal of Medicine*, the official organ of the society, appeared in the same year, and its objective was 'the advancement of Internal Medicine, and the promotion of friendship among physicians'.[15] Both the association and the journal intended to be representative of every 'division of the Kingdom'.[16] The association's first president was Richard Douglas Powell (1842–1925), then president of the Royal College of Physicians, and the former chair of the committee on the Union of Medical Societies, the body that had established the Royal Society of Medicine.

Considered together the Association of Physicians and the Royal Society of Medicine thus appear as two faces of a Janus-like medical generalist. The Royal Society of Medicine created an implicit outlet for specialist research while watchfully governing the structure of unified medicine. At the same time, the Association of Physicians provided a high-level national forum for consultants engaged in medical research to share their knowledge of internal medicine. Henry Head, for example, present at the first meeting, demonstrated how the spinal cord recombined sensory impulses from the surface of the body.[17] Since he presented this information to a general audience, few in the room could have deemed his presentation information for nerve specialists only.

Even though membership was open for all physicians conducting research, membership clearly connoted privilege and power.[18] Most members in 1907 had entries in *Who's Who*. Furthermore, a perusal of their obituaries suggests they shared, to borrow historian Christopher Lawrence's choice language, patrician tastes in food, wine, music, and other cultivations appropriately tailored to middle-class values.[19] The association's members were influential in medicine and the politics of local communities, and ambitious young practitioners sought to emulate them.

Initially the meetings of the Association of Physicians were cordial affairs, and very much like those that had occurred in the Neurological Society years before. The association's rules mandated attendance, and thus the social elements of the annual meeting had great import before the First World War.[20] At meetings, members presented their research; the audience discussed the contribution. Following morning sessions, there would be a lunch, and then some demonstration or lecture, usually on pathology, but sometimes technological or historical.[21] For example: 'Dr Mellard shewed microscopic slides of the blood from his case of leukanaemia,'[22] or 'The University Librarian shewed certain rare Medical Books from the Hunterian Collection.'[23] 'Professor J. H. Teacher [1869–1930] demonstrated William Hunter's Anatomical and Pathological Specimens.'[24] On one occasion there was an 'extensive historical exhibition given by the Wellcome Historical and Medical Museum'.[25] In the evening, the throng would gather for a dinner and smoker.

While ideally members of the Royal Society of Medicine could attend meetings of any section at whim, participation in meetings of the Association of Physicians implied much more. It denoted distinctions in medicine and medical research, thus indicating acumen and aptitude, as well as 'respectability and social standing' within medicine.[26] Whereas the Royal Society of Medicine allowed its membership to attend what they wished, the Association of Physicians, by mandating attendance, presumed its members were interested regardless of the subject discussed. In retrospect, the existence and aims of both societies manifested a contradiction: the explicit anti-specialist origins of both organisations could not push back the reality that both were becoming venues for narrower conversations.

The Royal Society of Medicine was too London-centric. The Association of Physicians too exclusive. There were far too many provincial physicians not benefiting from the proceedings of either. These limitations may have stimulated interest in forming more inclusive, even specialist societies. Any such suggestion, out of line with the original agendas governing both societies, required the right stimulus, and doubtless one stimulus was that the Association of Physicians did not hold meetings during the war. Its meetings resumed in 1919 at the urging of William Osler, who jokingly warned that otherwise 'we shall forget what we all look like'.[27]

No part of tradition: pacifism and specialisation

Everyone had forgotten. Or, putting it differently, the losses during the First World War were so great that the remaining members could do little else but look forward. While the older members of the Association of Physicians might have believed in its original founding ideals and principles, as well as Victorian codes of honour and duty, they could not comprehend the bitterness of the few survivors of the younger generation of men. Nor could they imagine the experiences the younger generation had internalised in the theatres of war.[28] The implications for medicine and neurology mirrored the social and cultural circumstances between the generations.

The loss of life took a toll on everyone. Yet to ignore the social divisions between the generation that fought and the generation that had pushed the younger into the trenches would be a mistake.[29] The leaders of British society (and British medicine) were men, and sometimes women, whose professional, political, and social lives had been well advanced before the war began. For them the rallying-cry 'back to 1914' sounded ennobling. Their attitudes, prejudices, appreciations and perceptions reflected a normality that to the younger generation appeared little better than nostalgia and indeed hypocritical given the horrors to which their actions had led. Their apathy could not be forgiven either: Enid Bagnold, later author of *National Velvet*, heaped scorn in her extraordinary 1918 *A Diary without Dates* on the concerned ladies who had charitably found the time to pass through hospitals filled with wounded men but could muster little more than surprise that some of the soldiers could walk.[30] Like Bagnold, the new artists and philosophers of modernity – such figures as Henri Bergson, Ernst Kirchner, and James Joyce– gave the brave new world its vulgar casting, a relativism that shocked the conservatives in Britain and that was later deplored by the Fascists in Germany, Italy, and Spain. The post-war moderns had lost their faith, as Joyce wrote in *Ulysses*, in everything including, 'orthodox religious, national, social, and ethical doctrines'.[31] Here Walter Russell Brain, aged twenty in 1915, may illustrate the discontents to which the period gave rise.

Walter Russell Brain was unique among British neurologists, indeed rare among British civilians from this period, for having been a conscientious objector during the war. Historian Arthur Marwick noted that there were approximately 16,000 absolutists imprisoned during the conflict in Britain. Brain was not among their radical number, but as a member of the Friends' Ambulance Unit in York he joined around 6,000 others in the non-combatant corps.[32]

Because Brain was with the Friends' Unit between 1915 and 1916, it might be tempting to think of him as being a Quaker for all of his life. In fact, Brain converted to Quakerism only in 1931, a fact that George Pickering, his biographer, makes little mention of in Brain's Royal Society obituary.[33] There is in consequence no extant clue to the convictions that led Brain to pacifism – no evidence of familial connections or of radical academic mentors. Autobiographical documents in his personal papers also provide few clues. The one source from this period of Brain's life, a diary that he kept while in York, offers no hints. As a biographical source, consequently, it is of little value; but as a record of the divide between Britain's generations, it is highly illustrative.

In July 1915, Brain found himself in a hospital opposite the Rowntree's Cocoa Factory in York. The hospital was then 'fairly comfortable' but 'at present entirely unfurnished except for the orderlies quarters, and these are somewhat bleak'.[34] The building consisted of a large hall, with cement floor and tiled walls. 'Placed round the walls and head to head down the middle are some forty beds, each furnished with a mattress, a pillow (no pillow case) and three blankets, very large and very rough. This is all except some trestle tables and some benches.'[35] Such were Brain's surroundings for the next year.

Brain had joined the Friends' Ambulance Unit that month, having been turned down for a position in Oxford at a medical unit (he had been studying history at Oxford). At the time he possessed an amateur's knowledge of x-rays and photography: 'I had bought a book on x-rays and visited the x-ray department of the Royal Berkshire Hospital.' To his surprise, this knowledge provided him with more radiological knowledge than anyone else at the hospital possessed and thus he became 'orderly to the X-Ray department'.[36] But his initial activities were not spent there. Initially many of his days were spent being taught by physicians on hospital techniques like asepsis. When not learning, he and others were cleaning and preparing the hospital to receive the wounded.

It is clear from his diary that Brain felt happiest when preparing the x-ray facilities and was looking forward to a time when his energies might be devoted to more intellectually stimulating tasks.[37] By the time Brain received his first x-ray duties, he could not conceal some elation: 'Today is memorable for our first patient is in the X-ray department. The man had a Turkish Shrapnel bullet enter his knee. We took one photograph.... The bullet is about the size of a marble and quite round.'[38] He added, 'Having taken the photo we...retired to the basement where I developed the plate. It is very satisfactory. I propose to buy some printing paper and take a print of every photo we take. I think it would be very interesting.'[39] By September, Brain was routinely in the x-ray facility. The number of patients he was seeing was steadily increasing: 'we X-rayed four men this morning and I developed the photos this afternoon.'[40] Brain's responsibilities further increased as the physicians in the hospital recognised his talents. November 1915 found him not only working away busily in the radiological facilities but also as clinical clerk to the physicians, a position Brain described as 'exceedingly interesting work – in fact the best the Hospital has to offer'.[41]

By January 1916, Brain had become confident enough in his work to experiment with the x-ray protocols. He recorded, for example, perfecting the bismuth meal technique.[42] The results of such experimentation were 'a great success'.[43] This routine continued for another six months, at which point he was transferred to the x-ray department of King George's Hospital in London, where he stayed for the remainder of the war.[44]

While Brain felt enthusiastic about his growing medical expertise, in his diary he remained stoutly pacifistic. His pacifism emerges in his diary in three ways: he frequently obsessed over the horrors of war he was seeing in the hospital and provided lucid accounts of the wounded that, while not gratuitous, were obviously intended to justify his dissenting position. Less frequent, but no less heartfelt, were direct indictments of the madness he saw around him. Finally, there was occasional reference to others who agreed with his position, and he gained confidence from their solidarity.

The first wounded soldiers arrived in early August 1915. Cases of shrapnel wounds, gas injuries, and broken bones were serious, but Brain chose instead to note one case in particular: 'In the case of one of the others this is the eleventh hospital he has been in. He tells me he has had seven operations for his arm, which is shattered. The bone refuses to knit and he does not expect, or indeed hope, that his arm will be saved. It is his right arm too. He says he wishes they would take it off and have done with it so that he could get well and go home.'[45] That his focus should be on a man who preferred to lose his dominant arm rather than to go back to the front can be construed as indicative of Brain's willingness to bear witness to the lengths men would go to in order to avoid the conditions of war.

In mid-September further observations of the strange violence of the world appeared in the diary:

> The most remarkable [case] is that of a boy with, literally, a broken neck. He is quite young, not more than 17, I should say, and has been hit by shrapnel in the neck, the third cervical vertebra being fractured – the spinal processes into several pieces. He walked to the X-Ray room but wept at the prospect of entering and refused to lie on the table. We had rather a job with him. It is, to me, a strange psychological problem that a boy like that, little more than a child, should go through a Campaign at the Dardanelles, and yet weep with sheer nervousness in Hospital.[46]

It is noteworthy that among this budding interest in the organic features of neurological disease, Brain's curiosity coalesced around the enormity of the 'boy's' past experiences and the psychological simplicity of the boy's fear. The coldness of his analysis, empathetic as it appears now, suggests also that Brain little understood the realities of the war. Convictions were not experience. Another case was no less daunting.

> I had this evening a very interesting talk with a man who had been wounded at the Dardanelles by a Turkish bullet.... He told me that

> for some time one side of his face was perfectly black, from the explosion, in the same way, he explained, as men can be detected, who shoot off the fingers of their own right hand, by the blackening caused by the cordite. I asked him if he had seen many do that, and he said a good number – when they saw what they had to face. He said he did not blame them, for to send young men into it was simply murder.[47]

By 1 October 1915, his respect for the soldiers' experience and their turmoil was deepening into gravity; he seems to have become aware of the naivety with which he had originally viewed the war. A convoy had arrived around midnight. 'It consisted of 80 men, all sitting cases, and all of them were in the trenches when the advance began. We had never had a convoy so directly from the trenches before. They came with all the grease of trench soil on their uniforms, and all the weariness of war in their eyes. One, I noticed, had wire-cutters hanging from his belt. Most of them limped, some could hardly walk.'[48]

Such reflections undoubtedly reinforced his pacifist convictions, but it is interesting to note that over time his empathy for the wounded became increasingly objective. Whether this was because the wounded had become mundane and commonplace, or whether it was because his scientific interests and medical responsibilities had grown, is difficult to say. In any case, the figure that emerges in his diary becomes ever more clinical and less inclined to polemics.

When Brain was not describing the wounded in his diary, he still found ways of denouncing the war. In August two 'delightful letters' arrived, and one was from a woman who described herself 'of the Peace Party'. Brain noted that she was 'interested to hear that I am a pacifist. She believes that the war has achieved nothing and can achieve nothing.'[49] Perhaps this voice from outside the confines of the hospital confirmed, however minutely, that he was not alone in his views of the crisis. Later that August he would write polemically, emphasising the passage with an underline, 'War in all its aspects, can be expressed in one word – waste.'[50] The statement, a seemingly frustrated remark, was not belied by anything he witnessed around him. And similar unrestrained resentment was echoed a few days later, but this time it was wrapped in Christian disbelief at the illusions, hubris, and nonchalance of the older non-combatant generation:

> Today I got the morning off, and went to Salem Chapel again where I found for York, quite a large Congregation gathered to hear a former pastor, Rev. F. A. Russell of South Port, preach. The sermon, nominally on 'Family Prayers' developed into an assertion that 'we in this war are fighting for all that is Christian against all that is devilish' whereat there was quite a murmur of applause and I feared a man on my left was going to clap. I think that war fever must be really an infectious mental disease, a sort of epidemic hysteria. Does the man really believe that there are no Christians in Germany, or no devils in England? War seems to convert ordinarily sane people into raving lunatics.[51]

But for the few letters of encouragement he received from others, the world seemed to have gone mad. The only sensible people were the wounded soldiers. 'All the patients are doing well, but I have not met one so far who wanted to get back to the front. The vast majority are anxious to be just sufficiently disabled to prevent their being sent out again, and ask me very pathetically "my left won't [sic] get well enough for them to send me out again, will it?" There is often little enough fear of that, poor fellows!'[52] By September, Brain was convinced that he had seen enough to understand the true nature of war. 'I can only say again what I have said before, that no one outside a hospital who has not been to the front can have the faintest possible conception of the meaning of war. How words would fail one to express the horrors that one sees even here.'[53]

By December, as already noted, clinical objectivity had begun mitigating Brain's empathy. Indeed, he had even become moderately sceptical of some soldiers' complaints: 'Another busy day in the X-Ray room. I have had more cases these last two days than for a long time. Particularly interesting was a case of suspected renal calculus. At least the man declared that his condition had been diagnosed as such, but Dr Eastling suspects him of malingering. The X-Ray were able to show that no calculus existed.'[54]

That Brain suspected the soldier too and did not sympathetically and simultaneously attribute his mental condition to external forces is perhaps indicative of the ways in which he was being transformed by his medical experiences. The lack of recognition of the irony that he, an objector, should readily accept the clinical classification of malingerer for another is utterly absent from his diary. Its absence, however, allows us to shift our focus away from Brain's experiences in York to ones more generally common for his contemporaries in combat. It is only necessary here to mention briefly that Brain left York for St George's Hospital in London in 1916, and from there at the close of the war he completed a medical training at Oxford and the London Hospital. His ascent professionally thereafter followed rapidly, as evidenced by the fact that he was a president of the Section of Neurology of the Royal Society of Medicine, the Association of Physicians, and – perhaps most importantly – of the Royal College of Physicians London from 1950 until 1957. He became a hereditary peer in 1962 – a seemingly unpredictable outcome for someone with his youthful ideological convictions.

Specialist or not? Head wounds; nerve injuries; both?

It is important to remember Brain's ironic acceptance of malingering, for that topic was one of great import in his day. His diary, however, captured the sensibilities of many of his generation. Attitudes like those most famously held by the war poet Siegfried Sassoon were perhaps less commonly spoken among the enlisted men, but a letter between Charles Symonds – Brain's friend and medical officer in France – to his fiancée, suggests that the attitudes were nevertheless widespread among the young. Symonds observed that the quality of commentary in London newspapers was proportional to the number of 'stupid and pompous old buffers' back home.[55]

Little can be gained here from a full account of the tragedies that caused such resentments and political engagement – they are well known. It is worth mentioning only that the scale of casualties, especially in France, was so enormous as to call for a new system of logistics in the field.[56] These new management technologies, as many historians have elaborated, infused specialist practice with a new legitimacy.[57] The conditions of war created divisions of medical labour in Britain: the economy of wounded bodies became a mass-production economy of specialised bodies.[58] The soldier with peripheral nerve injuries, head wounds, or organic and functional nervous diseases was but one instance among many.[59] Yet the legitimacy of these specialised bodies had not translated even by the close of the war into an immediate acceptance of the necessity of neurology, a fact that Brain and Symonds' contemporary, Francis Walshe, discovered much to his apparent consternation.

Walshe had returned home from Egypt in 1919 and was rendered speechless when he learned that the War Office, despite having commissioned him as a 'specialist in nervous diseases', was refusing his request for a demobilisation bonus as a medical specialist in neurology.[60] Responding perhaps to what became the famous sharpness of Walshe's pen, the War Office eventually recanted its position, 'in view of the fact that your original offer of employment was as "specialist in treatment of nervous diseases" it has been decided to sanction the extra 2/6d per day.' But the letter also noted, 'Neurology is not one of the subjects in which specialist appointments are usually made.'[61]

To a returning veteran like Walshe, the reticence of the War Office to accept neurology as a specialty probably smacked of a rather convenient financial-mindedness. But the number of physicians commissioned even as specialists in nervous diseases is rather difficult to uncover – I have found no official statistics. Most physicians served as general medical officers.[62] James Purves Stewart, author of a popular textbook entitled *Diagnoses of Nervous Diseases*, completed changes for the fourth edition of this book while stationed in Malta and practising as a consulting physician with the rank of captain. His autobiography, however, records no incidences of his treating nervous conditions in the field, and he seems to have served in a general capacity.[63]

Ignoring for the moment the perspective of the practitioners, even the question of the number of wounded suffering from nervous injuries is a difficult one to address. Military statistics offering clues to the number of wounded with neurological injuries are vague in their estimates.[64] Surveying a total of 1,043,653 wounded soldiers, the official statistics record that between 1916 and 1920 the number treated for epilepsy (mainly caused by shrapnel and bullet wounds) was 2,652; for organic nervous diseases, 1,020; for diseases of the spine, 304; and finally for head wounds 34,313.[65] All of these injuries occurred mainly in France and Egypt.[66] Statistics on functional nervous diseases are equally murky. Many soldiers suffered from neurasthenia; the estimate from these statistics is 21,549.[67] Yet, according to the authors of the statistics, there was 'unfortunately little information regarding the wastage due to disorders in France other than that for the period of August to December 1914 and for 1915'. Data from 1916 through 1918 are simply incomplete.[68]

These retrospective statistics do not communicate the immediacy of the problems caused by the war. To reiterate: it was not the numbers of wounded soldiers only that made rationalisation of field medical services necessary; it was also the speed with which casualties were created. During the Somme advance there were a million Allied casualties with 420,000 British, and perhaps, as historian Eric Hobsbawm noted, as many as '60,000 on the first day [1 July 1916]' alone.[69] For a crisis of this scale, divisions of medical labour were the most expeditious means of organising treatment.[70] Rational organisation moved the wounded from the field to special centres where physicians increasingly cared for specific types of injuries. By creating these specialised centres, physicians developed practical experience of specific wound types.[71] From their mistakes they developed a deeper empirical intuition about which patients could be saved, which were likely to return to service, and which needed to be sent home to a hospital like the one where Russell Brain volunteered. Though unemotional and pragmatic – and no doubt the resentments and cynicism of the soldiers was partially a response to these machine-like conditions – such a system saved lives that might otherwise have succumbed to the arbitrary logics of field triage. Whether the state recognised neurology or any other specialty or not was of little import, for these conditions nevertheless prepared a young generation of practitioners for specialist practice.

Such was the case for William John Adie. Adie began his service as a medical officer to the 1st Northamptonshire Regiment.[72] When the Germans destroyed his regiment in the retreat from Mons, he was transferred to the Leicestershire Regiment as a medical officer.[73] They too were decimated, and he was 'later given medical charge of the 7th General Hospital, also acting as consultant to the 2nd Army centre for head wounds'.[74] In the head wounds clinic he collected 'valuable neurological material' that he never published.[75] Adie's path to the head injuries clinic was therefore circuitous, but once there he established himself as a specialist in nervous diseases, although it is doubtful that he ever achieved a recognised military status in the specialty.[76] These were circumstances true for Gordon Holmes as well. Indeed, if biographical details from Walter Russell Brain's experiences illustrate in the extreme the way in which the younger generation was steadily alienated from the values and dispositions of the older one, then Holmes' experiences in France illustrate some practical outcomes of that shift for the science and medicine of the nervous system. More disconcerting, those outcomes permit us also to see how the science and medicine of the nervous system became useful to the British state and was thus co-opted by the forces of tradition even as it remade the status quo for specialists.

A nerve specialist in France: Gordon Holmes' research, patients, and legacy

It is interesting to contemplate why so many sources exist of Gordon Morgan Holmes' career in France, as well as to ponder why he has been so routinely the subject of hagiography. In many ways, Holmes was no more representative of British neurology than Henry Head or Russell Brain. He was approximately fifteen years younger than Head, but older than Russell Brain by nineteen years. However, while most of his later contemporaries in neurology worked as general physicians in field hospitals in the many theatres of war, Holmes' practice and his wartime research chiefly concerned soldiers with head, spinal and peripheral nerve injuries. His research on these patients was later renowned as a major contribution to clinical neurophysiology. Perhaps, precisely because Holmes was not representative, his wartime service and research seemingly created continuity between the older medical culture – he possessed its cultural values and embraced its medical generalism – and the new emergent culture of specialised medical practice of which he was one venerable product.

Holmes came to France circuitously. Because he suffered from myopia, the British services had initially rejected him and the British Red Cross commissioned him instead as a surgeon. He worked with the Red Cross from 30 September 1914 to 5 November 1914.[77] That month was spent near Paris, where there were four Red Cross hospitals served by only '10 Motor Lorries and 10 Motor Bicycles' but required nearly ten times that number to handle the casualties.[78] By 7 October 1914, Holmes was in a unit with perhaps fifteen other surgeons and fifty nurses.[79] He later remembered:

> I went to France in October 1914 and stayed there until America came into the War in April 1917. I had to deal with the nervous troubles of the men at the front. There were quite a lot of such cases. The strain of being in the trenches for long spells under heavy bombardment by

the German guns, and seeing so many of their friends die, took a toll on their nervous system.[80]

In November 1914, Holmes received a military commission to No. 13 General Hospital, a makeshift hospital in a former casino just south of Boulogne with approximately one thousand beds.[81] There he remained until his marriage in 1917.

At No. 13, Holmes and Percy Sargent (1878–1933), a surgeon, saw countless cases of head wounds and spinal injuries. Holmes' sphere of political influence, however, went far beyond treating these injuries, and he became increasingly influential in dictating policy on soldiers suffering from psychiatric breakdown.[82] He appointed Charles Myers (1873–1946) as a 'specialist in nerve shock', and together they began organising special treatment centres for functional neuroses.[83] By October 1917, Myers had returned to Britain, disgraced for his belief that special psychoanalytical centres should be created near the field for cases of shell shock and, as historian Ben Shepherd recounts, 'from then onwards the direction of all the army centres was in the hands of Lieut.-Colonel Gordon Holmes' until he requested transfer home.[84]

Very few of Holmes' notes survived the war. Those that did include fifty-seven handwritten entries describing soldiers with spinal injuries.[85] Although they are some indication of the survival rate for paraplegic and quadriplegic soldiers, they are only modestly illuminating about Holmes' practice in France. Notes like these undoubtedly formed the basis of his papers and lectures from this period, many now considered classics of neurology.[86] His Goulstonian Lecture in 1915 was on spinal cord injuries, his Montgomery Lectures in 1919 were on disturbances of visions caused by bullet and shrapnel wounds, and his Croonian Lecture in 1923 on war injuries to the cerebellum. For Holmes, as he would later explain, these injuries always indicated ways 'the normal functions of the nervous system' could be understood. This information could be used to 'arm ourselves and our successors with knowledge, which is always the most potent instrument at our service in our lifelong contest with illness and suffering'.[87]

Holmes' tenure in France exerted a lasting, profound impact on his professional outlook. He became dogmatically opposed to Freudian psychoanalysis in the treatment of shell shock, suggesting to the young British-born, American-based neurologist Foster Kennedy (1884–1952) that he 'go back...to America...and see to it that the care of functional and organic cases there be put on the right basis – which basis is almost anything, rather than Freudian'.[88] Holmes and his younger associate, William Johnson, preferred moral management and disciplinary methods for treating psychological conditions, and both tended to consider the causes of the disease to be defective morale rather than an acute psychic injury.[89]

The American neurosurgeon Harvey Cushing published a diary of his experiences during the war that provides further glimpses into Holmes' practice in France. In May 1915, Cushing observed a number of 'amazing' cases of head wounds and spinal injuries on a visit to Gordon Holmes at No. 13, and he estimated that: 'with the proper backing these two men [Gordon Holmes and Percy Sargent] have an unparalleled opportunity, not only to be of service to the individual wounded, but, when this is all over, to make a contribution to physiology, neurology, and surgery which will be epochal.'[90] For Cushing and many other Americans, the British neurological experience was profound, and many young aspiring nerve specialists like Foster Kennedy were driven by ambition to be involved in the project.[91] The war, it seems, would establish future medical careers even as it destroyed a generation.

This study of Holmes reveals experiences that specialists in nervous diseases might have had in the field. Nonetheless, putting that knowledge and skill to use back in Britain was difficult, since the lack of an organised neurological service created substantial problems in the organisation of medical care for nerve casualties at the home front.[92] Cushing observed in his diary that, 'the Neurological [British] Home Service is all at cross-purposes with patients scattered at Tooting, King George's, Queen Square, Maida Vale, the London, and 200 incurables at the Star and Garter, Richmond.'[93] There were also theoretical differences, and these mirrored circumstances in neurological, psychological, psychiatric, and general medical organisation for patients with injuries of the nervous system.[94] In his memoir Cushing described 'Dinner with several neurologists and neurosurgeons, among whom there was little agreement about heads, spines, and peripheral nerves – except that there is an immense lot of work to be done on the incompletely treated cases which gravitate over here from France.'[95]

Disagreements were not merely theoretical problems for nerve specialists. They reflected and paralleled an increasingly incoherent homeland service for nerve patients. The institutional provision for wounded soldiers was beginning to assume the shape of a political wedge. On one side were cases of visible injuries requiring long-term if not permanent management. Head wounds and spinal and peripheral nerve injuries were permanent visible scars of the atrocities of war. In contrast, despite the pleas of a compassionate public, neurologists like Holmes could muster only slight sympathy for victims of shell shock. That juxtaposition would frame future neurological views of functional and organic nervous diseases.[96] The fissure between psychiatric and neurological knowledge appearing in the interwar period could be reduced to debates about whether visible head wounds were equivalent to invisible injuries of the mind.[97] Holmes entertained no doubts at all: for him conditions of the mind were failures of character, signs of hereditary degeneracy, or simply evidence of malingering – a medical condition that, it should be remembered, the young, pacifistically inclined Russell Brain had even begun recognising.[98]

Shell shock and malingering: the political legitimacy of neurology, 1918–23

The spectre of the malingerer haunted wartime and post-war discourses. The returning wounded, many incapacitated for life, saw for themselves only the prospect of economic dependency upon the state.[99] It was perhaps predictable that questions would arise about notions of deservedness. An increasingly important determining role for government became commonplace: individuals, and families, required assistance that only the Ministry of Pensions and the newly created Ministry of Health could provide.[100] No one wanted the undeserving to receive aid, and thus one of the effects was a further demand for medical specialists. Everyone needed expertise. The public, largely filled with empathy for the returning soldiers, commonly held that patients suffering from psychological problems deserved special treatment and aid.[101] Meanwhile, the state required competent physicians for assessing the worthiness of claims for full or partial disability – physicians able to spot malingerers exploiting public goodwill were in especially high demand.[102]

These circumstances created a new economy for medical specialists, among them neurologists.[103] While an American author could bemoan in 1921 the fact that 'war neuroses were essentially problems of neurology, and neurologists as a whole had very little to do with the attempt at the solution,' neurologists in Britain spearheaded efforts to diagnose and treat a range of conditions, including psychological ones.[104] Treatment and the provision of care for soldiers with spinal cord injuries were but one instance.[105] Importantly, neurologists routinely found that somatic injuries had not damaged the nervous system; what had appeared at first to be somatic paralysis turned out to be neurasthenic or hysterical symptoms. Foster Kennedy remarked in 1917, 'The neurosis of war is intrinsically Hysteria.'[106] Such a differential diagnosis was possible through rigorous neurological examination only.

Scholars often overlook the growing political significance of neurological knowledge following the war, and even the secondary literature on shell shock usually casts the condition as mainly germane to the history of psychiatry.[107] Yet there were broader theoretical stakes in this issue for neurology than is typically realised. On the one hand, if psychological trauma manifesting as shell shock had organic components, then the implication was that mind and brain were one and the same. On the other hand, since no physical features were ever observed in cases of shell shock – that is, since pathological, biochemical, or physiological research never revealed lesions correlating with aberrant behaviour – then it was felt that this disease of the mind could only nominally be connected to the condition of the body. Unlike the shocking head wounds Holmes and others encountered in the field, psychological injuries struggled to achieve similar legitimate corporeality in medicine. Pathologies of the mind were simply not holes in the head.

The realist logic of neurology mandated if unseen then unproved. It was easy therefore for others besides Holmes to explain psychological trauma as an inherited degeneracy, a failure of moral character, or malingering.[108] A letter from Francis Walshe to his commanding officer testifies to the archetype: 'I am strongly of opinion that although a neurotic individual of poor morale and most unwilling to work, he is fit for his duties as clerk….' He added grudgingly, 'It becomes very difficult to deal with men of defective morale when Medical Officers are in such a hurry to pronounce them unfit for service.'[109] To interpret neuroticism, poor morale, and an unwillingness to work under the umbrella of simple defective was the conservative counterpoint to the sweeping and radically individualist claims of the psychoanalytic movement.[110] Burgeoning psychological knowledge, epitomised by the work of Sigmund Freud, had been expanding into unknown territories, challenging the mores of Victorian and Edwardian medical thought.[111] Like neurology, psychoanalysis and psychopathology began to emerge in this period, and their success with the Freudian model meant that interwar neurologists (although mainly beyond the shores of Britain) toyed with psychoanalytic therapies.[112]

Unsurprisingly, somatic and psychological perspectives found favour in different political quarters.[113] Political conservatives saw the stoic British character as the normative standard and appropriate bearing of every man, especially a former soldier. For them, neurological knowledge contested the legitimacy of psychological diseases such as shell shock. They depicted pensions for such cases as evil tools binding free individuals to dependency upon the state in perpetuity. Political leftists, though not necessarily receptive to Freudian ideas, were unprepared to disavow the psychological trauma that industrial warfare had visited upon the minds of soldiers.[114]

Both positions appeared in the 1922 *Report of the War Office Committee on Shell Shock*. The report's committee interviewed a number of specialists in nervous diseases, many of whom had worked in the head injury centres of France and were by then regarded as leading authorities. The report referred to them as consultant neurologists, despite the fact that the title had not been recognised in the field.[115] Most interviewees asserted that shell shock, though it might exist, was reified. William Johnson stated, for example, that: 'so-called "Shell Shock" consisted of a motley of conditions.'[116] Although a few specialists, like William John Adie, were prepared to claim physical concussion caused it, clinical research had not found physical lesions or somatic features of the disease, despite extensive investigations.[117] Many thought that the dominant feature of the disease was an underlying desire to flee the continual hazards of the trenches, and that as the disease came to be adopted in the popular vernacular, it also came to seem inevitable.[118]

The self-fulfilling prophecy shell shock represented, they argued, stimulated normal emotional desires for removal from the stress, strain, and boredom of the trenches. Gordon Holmes insisted: 'the "will and wish" factor had considerable influence. [The troops] recognised they would escape further service in the line for the time being...the great increase in these cases coincided with the knowledge that such a condition as shell shock existed.'[119] It was, nevertheless, difficult to determine whether the patient was malingering or traumatised. As

Arthur Hurst noted, the 'signs of genuine neurosis and simulation are identical and that simulation can only be diagnosed with certainty in very few cases.'[120] All specialists agreed that the stress of the trenches could break down military discipline and duty, and they thought that most patients so affected simply required a hot meal and quiet bed for a few days. Asked whether the breakdown in morale was unavoidable in conditions like those of the past war, most specialists demurred and hedged that too 'little was known.'[121]

The report's conclusions benefited from neurology's relativism – all the interviewees agreed that traumatic experiences were real but exaggerated by public sympathy.[122] Public concerns had been raised initially by the alleged shooting of men who had disobeyed orders in the field. Such military actions the committee deemed repugnant because, rather than punishing deserters, it might have meant executing mentally distressed soldiers broken under the stress of war.[123] The refusal of a soldier in the field to follow orders the committee considered an ambiguous action requiring serious deliberation, including evaluation of his mental condition. Executing deserters, the committee estimated, was a morale-breaking, possibly mutiny-causing activity, dangerous for recruitment. If the public believed that shell shock was inevitable when conditions were like those in the trenches, and if it was widely recognised by soldiers that exhibiting symptoms of shell shock might lead to their execution, then a large disincentive was being introduced to civilians to join the armed forces.[124] Likewise, the committee noted, another symptom appearing in officers suffering with the condition was risk-taking behaviour. Bravery was one thing, but an officer seeking his own death might lead his men to theirs, with dire consequences for a campaign. If officers believed symptoms of mental breakdown would lead to their execution anyway, they might attempt a desperate and suicidal act of bravery to free themselves from the conditions of war. That would be an untenable and chaotic behaviour in the discipline-requiring armed forces.

Nonetheless the War Committee argued that it was difficult to distinguish soldiers actually suffering from shell shock from those who were malingering.[125] The triumph of neurological knowledge was that it had produced – or at least could claim to have produced – a scientific justification for not caving in to the demands made by the psychological and psychiatric profession, some of whom were determined to see the condition as inevitable and thus everywhere.[126] As historian Ted

Bogadaz contended, the committee members constructed a halfway house in which Freudian ideas were refuted but simultaneously used to solve this problem. 'In a sense the committee which had dismissed Freud may have unwittingly demonstrated how impossible it had become by the early 1920s to speak of mental illness without some recourse to his theories.'[127]

Neurological knowledge, however, justified political pragmatism – and vice versa. The question was not whether shell shock existed, but to what extent it did so and could be proved the patient's malady.[128] The neurological answer, in contrast to the Freudian one, offered a seemingly commonsense political expediency which, while not ignoring or delegitimising the status of psychologically traumatised soldiers, also avoided giving them the benefit of the doubt as well.

In this way, British neurologists demonstrated the political utility of their knowledge of the nervous system. Of the report's fifty-nine interviewees, fourteen were presented as possessing a neurological status – though their actual professional status during the war had been more ambiguous than the report implied.[129] Even if British neurology had politically demonstrated the legitimacy of the organic aspect of its occupational knowledge, still to be tackled were broader barriers preventing the emergence of clinical neurology in hospitals and universities as a legitimate professional distinction.[130] Only a continual political campaign for neurology would achieve that aim. In their own ways, both Henry Head and Walter Russell Brain took on that burden, but their efforts did not solely establish neurology as an independent and necessary clinical specialty. Rather, the war had shifted social and political priorities in favour of a rational – Taylorist might be a more appropriate word – organisation of medicine and society, and thus that new sense of relations provided the first real foundations for the social transformation of neurology from a general to a specialist practice.

'Doing my bit': Henry Head inaugurates the interwar specialty of neurology

If the period between 1918 and 1923 was politically important for neurology, then 1918 to 1920 was a period of personal and professional import for Henry Head. While the old don of medicine William Osler was urging the Association of Physicians to return professional relations to how they were before the war, Head appears in the record to have been looking forward to a new progressive age for medicine and neurology. He may moreover have been accustoming himself to the view that his contributions to the science of neurology were approaching an end. In 1918, Head was president of the Neurological Section of the Royal Society of Medicine. By May of 1919, a note among many later compiled by physician Donald Hunter on Henry Head revealed sadder circumstances:

> A tragedy beyond description today overtakes The London. Henry Head with early but definite signs of Parkinsonism has retired from the staff. This shatters the plan whereby it was hoped to make him the first Professor of Medicine to implement the Flexner Plan. Poor Henry, poor us! What a distinguished professor he would have been.... A Medical Unit under Henry Head would have been renowned the world over.[131]

Head's letter of resignation had actually been sent to the hospital governor in January. In it there was no mention of impending illness, only expressions about shortages of time, a desire to resume private practice, and a hope of putting 'together during the few years of activity that remain to me' some of the observations he had made during the war.[132]

Throughout the next five months, administrators at the London Hospital made significant efforts to keep Head as director of a new medical unit within the hospital that would have created a stronger synergy between academic clinical research and clinical medicine. This medical unit, had it been formed, would have ranked as one of the first of its kind in Britain. Doubtless it would have advanced the process of reorganising medicine throughout the country, a process already proposed by the Haldane Commission and continued with the 1913 formation of the Medical Research Committee (this government body became the Medical Research Council in 1920), which continued these developments throughout the interwar period with the establishment of clinical research units. Head, however, was not tempted by the offer and set conditions for acceptance too large for the hospital to meet. While it is likely that his illness determined his decision to turn down the offer, there are reasons to believe that Head was not persuaded that the culture of the London Hospital was prepared to accept the full implications of modernisation, a subject upon which he would dwell in an important 1918 presidential address before his peers in the Neurological Section of the Royal Society of Medicine.[133]

There is no way of knowing how many heard Head's address. Nor is it possible to determine whether it had any immediate or long-term effects. It is perhaps noteworthy that Head appears (I have found no other example) to have been the only British neurologist to have made such a speech since John Hughlings Jackson delivered his Bowman Oration on the appropriateness of specialisation in 1885 at the Ophthalmological Society of the United Kingdom. Head's speech, moreover, was one of the most impassioned the section would hear in its entire history. It consequently seems appropriate to understand it as both provocative and inaugural.

Head chose to speak on the place of neurology in the new world, and his opening declaration that 'to-night we hold the first meeting of this Section after the close of the greatest war in the history of the world' signified his intended solemnity.[134] He embraced the notion of a conflict between the generations, portraying the war as the causes and follies of old men and the devastation of youth. 'This victorious peace has been won by sacrifice of innumerable young lives; and for us older men the future must be dedicated to making the world a better place for those who are to take up our burden.'[135] The gauntlet, then, was not thrown at the feet of the younger generation. Head instead aimed his comments at the older generation. Younger men, he insisted, already rued the inadequacies of their elders.

> The cataclysmic events of the last four years have shaken men's belief in the old order, and medicine has not escaped the universal demand for a restatement of current values. The young are looking to us to enunciate the principles on which our teaching is founded. They are not disposed to accept without criticism conventional explanations.[136]

Head claimed, moreover, that little had happened in neurology during the last twenty-five years of his career. He prophesied, however, a future period of intense questioning, research, and speculation. Neurology in the younger generation would pass beyond the vanity of eponyms. Neurologists of the interwar period would frame disease in terms of function, perhaps Hughlings Jackson's theories on the evolution of nervous function would combine with Charles Sherrington's physiology. Because Sherrington had articulated principles of neurology more clearly than Jackson, he had shown convincingly that Jackson's evolutionary principles of neurology merited collective attention.[137] Head continued by arguing for a refinement of scientific neurology. Jackson and Sherrington's principles of neurology, he suggested, were not merely theoretical fancies, but the essences of clinical practice. 'Clinical diagnosis is a by-product of scientific investigation.'[138] For a pinprick, touch of cotton wool, or olfactory test to acquire clinical meaning, a whole canon of underlying anatomical and physiological knowledge had to be written and disseminated to students and practitioners.

> The charm of neurology, above all other branches of practical medicine, lies in the way it forces us into daily contact with principles. A knowledge of the structure and functions of the nervous system is necessary to explain the simplest phenomena of disease, and this can be only attained by thinking scientifically.[139]

Head then articulated the underlying principles of clinical and scientific neurology. The most evolutionarily complex functions were the first to disappear. Wherever a lesion appeared, a correlative defective function would arise; a lesion could produce 'positive' effects by releasing otherwise restrained functions; the central nervous system had been slowly evolving; and finally, integration of nervous functions was always based upon a struggle of expression 'between competing physiological activities'.[140] He ended provocatively:

> We neurologists are brought into daily contact with these diverse functional reactions. We work in the passage-way between the physical universe and the dwelling-place of the mind. We can watch the processes of evolution, visible in the actual behaviour of the central nervous system. We see the coming and the going, and we alone can record which of the many aspirants has conquered the right to enter or to leave that council chamber of human activities.[141]

Many features of Head's address, including his choice of title, 'Some Principles of Neurology' sounded programmatic, even prescriptive. The dichotomies in Head's lecture were many: age versus youth;

general medicine versus neurology; form versus function; clinical practice versus scientific knowledge. In all cases, he sided with the second element. Youth, neurology, function, and scientific knowledge trumped the actual conditions of neurology, which, as Head saw them, were: old, medical, anatomical, and clinical. All were superficial in relation to the future Head foresaw. His prescriptive was not for the younger generation of neurologists – medical officers just beginning their training as housemen or medical registrars. Instead, it was a less than stark warning to the older generation not to be obstructionist.

Head was acknowledging that the younger generation would challenge the rules of the older. He implied, moreover, that they were right to do so. Twenty-five years of his professional life, he argued, had seen few changes either scientific or political; the next twenty-five years would see many. The generation of physicians trained in the theatres of war would introduce radical social, political, and scientific reforms to medicine. It would be better, Head was urging, to welcome these changes rather than fortify the forces of tradition aligned against them.

There is no record indicating why Head decided to adopt such an expansive tone. The portrait provided by his biographer L. Stephen Jacyna is of a man rarely inclined towards such public remonstrations. Yet from his retirement speech, delivered in January 1919, it is clear that the war had made a substantial impression upon Head. As he thanked the London Hospital for allowing him to establish a Department for War Injuries of the Nervous System, Head claimed to have seen it as a means of 'doing my bit' and added:

> These injuries were in some cases so definite and circumscribed that they resembled some horrible human vivisection. Such injuries were never seen before – will never be seen again – but out of it all, one after the other, new facts emerged with startling clearness. Indeed, I may say that instead of 'doing my bit' for the War, I have been in reality heavily paid. During the last four years I have been given opportunities such as nobody ever had before, and will never have again.[142]

It is not conjecture to imagine that Head was cognisant that his experiences were typical of his younger colleagues. Thus perhaps his intention in his 1918 address was to give a new articulation and (in consequence) a new legitimacy to the younger generation's perceptions of their work and practice.

Specialist neurology in interwar Britain

The proceedings of both the Neurological Section of the Royal Society of Medicine and the Association of Physicians changed perceptibly in the years following the end of hostilities. In 1919, Head, in one his last public appearances in the records of the Royal Society of Medicine, urged that the Section of Neurology join an 'International Association of Neurologists'.[143] That same year the Hughlings Jackson Lecture was revived, having not been delivered since William Gower's 1909 oration on 'Special Sense Discharges in Organic Disease'.[144] A year later, a national union of neurologists was apparently created, with a roll of names enclosed in a now-lost letter to the council of the Neurological Section.[145]

Intellectually, the proceedings of the Neurological Section following the war were also eventful. Papers presented in 1919 were almost all related to war injuries of the nervous system. William Aldren Turner's (1864–1945) presidential address, 'The Influence of Psychogenic Factors in Nervous Disease', was followed by many others that derived much of their content from investigations of wounded soldiers' minds and bodies.[146] Edward Farquhar Buzzard presented on cases of spinal cord injuries caused by the war.[147] Alfred Carver offered comments on 'Some Biological Effects due to High Explosives'.[148] E. G. Fearnsides described the 'Essentials of Treatment of Soldiers and Discharged Soldiers Suffering from Functional Diseases' while even Henry Head elaborated on the meanings of a case of 'Shell Wound of the Head'.[149] Arthur Hurst described 'The Hysterical Element in Organic Disease and Injury of the Nervous System'.[150] George Riddoch (1888–1947) outlined neurological complications arising from bullet wounds to the throat, while Percy Sargent mused upon 'Some Lessons of the War Applied to Spinal Surgery'.[151] T. A. Ross (1875–1941) presented on 'Certain Inter-Relations of Peace and War Neuroses', and his colleague, R. G. Rows, outlined his hypotheses on 'Anxiety States'.[152] Francis Walshe considered the epidemiological picture of 'Forms of Peripheral Neuritis among Troops Serving in the Egyptian Expeditionary Force, 1915–1919'.[153] The trend was largely the same throughout other British medical journals that year, and for a couple years following.[154] Such an out-pouring of research led some, like American Harvey Cushing, to marvel at the 'valuable contributions to neurology by Englishmen'.[155] Such energy fomented the sense, to which Edwin Bramwell later spoke, that the war had marked the end of an age for the medicine of the nervous system.[156]

If the war produced this rush of neurological papers in 1919, then it made other contributions for neurology possible as well. In an unprecedented move following a 1919 clinical meeting, members proposed and passed a resolution that the president of the section approach the Ministry of Pensions. The resolution, as recorded in the committee minutes, stated, 'That in view of the difficulties of estimating the severity of disability following injuries of the nervous system, the Director-General of Medical Services, Ministry of Pensions, be approached by the President with the offer of assistance in the shape of a report from a Committee of the Neurological Section.'[157] Although it is unclear if anything came of this resolution, the minute is startling: it is the first recorded instance of British neurologists formally seeking to advise government.

In terms of its representation in hospitals and universities, neurology changed substantially in the years following the war. No better evidence exists of these changes than a report, undated but likely from around 1945, composed by Walter Russell Brain.[158] Brain, by then a significant figure in London medical politics, adopted a negative view of neurology's organisation. But his description captures how substantially neurology had reorganised in the interwar period, and fittingly contrasts it with those observations Harvey Cushing had made on the neurological service in 1917 in his diary of the war.

As Brain described, the three specialist hospitals provided a growing but inadequate service for London. The National Hospital, with 150 continually occupied beds, had grown in size through the acquisition of a small convalescent home in East Finchley with an additional thirty in-patient beds. The hospital had twelve physicians, three surgeons, and one pathologist on staff, as well as numerous medical officers and nursing staff.[159] The Maida Vale Hospital for Nervous Diseases had eighty-five beds, nine physicians, two surgeons, six psychiatrists and medical officers and nursing staff.[160] The West End Hospital for Nervous Diseases had seventy-six beds, a staff of six physicians, three surgeons, and 'a large number of psychiatrists and psychotherapist, as well as medical officers of special departments'.[161]

Beyond the specialist hospitals, Brain noted, many of the London County Council hospitals had begun providing treatment for a vast number of 'acute and chronic neurological cases'.[162] These patients, other documents make clear, were sometimes seen by Francis Walshe, Charles Symonds, Samuel Alexander Kinnier Wilson, James Purdon Martin, Macdonald Critchley, Edward Mapother, [Thomas] Grainger Stewart, and Cecil Worster Drought.[163] Brain found their organisation wanting as well: 'The L.C.C. arrangements were wasteful of time.... The Medical Superintendent was left to decide which neurologist on the panel of consultants he would summon, Dr. A. might be called to St Charles Hospital, Notting Hill at the same time that Dr. B. was summoned to St Mary Abbots Hospital, Kensington, a mile away, while Dr. C. on the same day would receive calls to the Western Fever.'[164] This situation, in Brain's view, was deplorable. His larger point was that the number of beds allocated for neurological cases in the capital was ridiculously small, as were the numbers of physicians practising in neurology. But the number of beds he described in the specialist hospitals, as well as the London County Council arrangements, the general growth of departments of neurology, and indeed the very view that Brain adopted of the circumstances of neurology were without precedent. If Henry Head had inaugurated a new era for neurology, then the appearance of Russell Brain's rather gloomy report was one of those definitive moments that marked the ultimate formation of the specialty.

Certainly the general hospitals had changed, and indeed therapeutic innovations had likely begun the process in the years before the war. The first officially designated department of neurology founded in Britain was at St Mary's Hospital.[165] There Wilfred Harris (1869–1960) in 1907 had changed an electricity department, founded in 1881, into a neurological department.[166] Equally typical of these early changes in the structure of the general hospitals was the 1912 appointment of Herbert Campbell Thomson (1870–1940) to a special department for 'Diseases of the Nervous System' at the Middlesex Hospital. In the history of the hospital that he later authored, Campbell Thomson reflected that his appointment as physician and lecturer in nervous diseases occurred because of growing demand for neurological teaching among undergraduates. The new position, he noted (grumbled might be closer), did not bring many advantages. The hospital administrators did not create an in-patient service but only recognised services he was already providing in his outpatient clinics. Thus burdened by new teaching responsibilities but provided with no additional beds, it seems that all his new title provided him was occasional referrals of nervous patients.[167] But it was a start. Douglas

McAlpine (1890–1981), Campbell Thomson's 1926 replacement, used the position to convince his father, the wealthy industrialist Sir Robert McAlpine (1847–1934), to endow twenty-four beds, creating an in-patient neurology ward in 1930.[168]

What is clear is that wartime conditions both promoted these changes but also caused physicians and administrators to conceive these positions originally in the broadest of possible terms. Few efforts were made to follow the model fostered at the National Hospital that discriminated between nervous and mental diseases. The experience at Guy's Hospital is illustrative, and William Johnson, then a young recruit to Arthur Hurst's (1879–1944) outpatient nerve clinic there, was typical. Johnson, having worked in a head injuries clinic in France, was recruited to Guy's Hospital in 1917. Hurst had demanded a senior registrar with a talent for treating neurotic patients to care for Hurst's psychoneurotic cases at Seale Hayne Asylum in Devon. Johnson's knowledge of the psychoneuroses apparently made him qualified for working with cases of both mental and nervous disease. Like his mentor Hurst, Johnson thus never felt comfortable claiming specialist status. His obituarist remembered him as never being 'an exclusive specialist' and ruminated that he was 'one of the lessening band of general physicians, at home in all aspects of medicine and with wide practical interests'.[169]

Johnson's younger colleague, Charles Symonds, was appointed at Guy's Hospital as an Assistant Physician in Nervous Diseases in 1920. The history of his appointment, as recorded by documents in the Guy's archives, requires an even fuller exposition. H. C. Cameron, historian of the hospital, noted that between 1908 and 1913 a committee at the hospital had reviewed the entire question of specialist departments in order to recommend their future development.[170] Some physicians on that committee had then argued against the teaching of undergraduates by specialists, on the grounds that it would bog the elementary medical curriculum down in the swamp of details. Students, they felt, would leave insufficiently prepared for the rigors of general work. In contrast, others on the committee argued that for the hospital to continue its proud tradition of contributing to the progress of medicine, specialist research had become requisite. Divisions of medicine, they deemed, were necessary for the advancement of science. The traditionalists could only understand this as eroding the teaching hospital ethos – the tension between bedside practice and science is ever on display in these records.[171] Nevertheless, as a 1908 report reveals, the committee ultimately advised the creation of a department on diseases of the nervous system even as they averred that 'the Physicians on the Committee do not feel...convinced of the necessity of a pure Specialism in Dermatology, Neurology, and Paediatrics.'[172] It is interesting to note that Charles Symonds, the first physician appointed under these circumstances, always kept his title, Physician of Nervous Diseases. It was not, as perhaps it came to seem later to his students and trainees, an anachronism.[173] It reflected instead the history of his appointment.[174]

Many similar stories of debates, acrimony, disappointment, and compromise in hospitals abound in histories and in archival records for the whole of the interwar period. Despite these difficulties, many London hospitals successfully established new appointments in neurology following the end of the 1914–18 conflict. King's College Hospital appointed Samuel Alexander Kinnier Wilson as assistant neurologist in 1919.[175] University College Hospital appointed Francis Walshe head of a 'newly established neurological department' in 1920.[176] In 1923, Anthony Feiling (1885–1975) established an open neurological teaching clinic at St George's Hospital in London.[177]

Similar stories abound for English provincial medical centres as well. In 1927, the Royal Victoria Infirmary in Newcastle appointed George Hall (1879–1955) specifically for his interest in neurology.[178] The General Infirmary at Leeds appointed Hugh Garland (1903–67) in 1937 as assistant physician with an interest in nervous diseases.[179] The Burden Neurological Institute was founded in Bristol in 1938 (apart from London, it was the most significant clinical research centre, and, unlike the National Hospital, embraced patients with mental and nervous conditions).[180] At Birmingham, Philip Cloake (1890–1969), the Professor of Medicine, and Arthur Stanley Barnes (1875–1955), Dean of the Faculty of Medicine, strove throughout the interwar period to establish a department. Barnes retired in 1941, unsuccessful in his endeavours. Cloake, however, persevered and attempted to create a tripartite division in the medical school encompassing neurology, neurosurgery, and neuropsychiatry. His efforts failed too, although the medical school gave him an honorary position as professor of neurology when he retired from his medical professorship in 1946.[181] Leeds established a neurological department in 1947.[182]

Generally, patterns of events in Scotland mirrored those in the south. The Victorian Infirmary in Glasgow appointed a physician in nervous diseases in 1914.[183] The Western Infirmary in Glasgow, by contrast, appointed its first neurologist in 1941.[184] Aberdeen did not have a neurological department until after the Second World War.[185] Circumstances deviated little from these well into the 1950s. There were three neurologists in the western region, three in the south-eastern region, and none anywhere else as late as 1958, although 'neurology work is undertaken by general physicians who have a particular interest in this branch of medicine.'[186]

Edinburgh University and the Royal Infirmary further illustrate this point. In an enclosure sent to American surgeon Harvey Cushing, the surgeon Norman Dott (1892–1973) outlined his desires for a never-realised neurological and neurosurgical centre. He noted, 'neurology in the wide sense of the term does not occupy quite the definitely recognised status of the special subject that it does in most American and many Continental Schools.'[187] Edwin Bramwell, Dott's colleague and the Moncrieff-Arnott Professor of Medicine at the university, though identifying himself as a neurologist, also practised as a general physician.[188] As part of the celebrations of his retirement, the university established the first lectureship in neurology at the university, to which Bramwell's former registrar, William Ritchie Russell (1903–80), was appointed in 1938 (he eventually became the first Professor of Neurology at Oxford).[189]

As in Scotland, there was little exclusive neurological practice in Wales throughout the interwar period and into the late 1950s. A 1948 government survey of specialist services in Wales noted, for example, the existence of minimal neurological services at Cardiff Royal Infirmary, Swansea General Hospital, and Wrexham Emergency Hospital.[190] Even after the National Health Service was established, the number of house calls made by Welsh neurologists in 1953 (there were three neurologists for all of Wales) was found to be 173 for the year.[191] This was hardly a sign of special Welsh resilience to nervous diseases; it reflected the substantial role general physicians played in treating neurological patients. As in Scotland, even in the 1960s, it was almost exclusively general physicians in Wales who saw patients suffering from neurological illnesses. They referred only the rarest cases to consultant neurologists.[192]

As certain idealised habits of mind and dispositions began to be cultivated around the identity of these workers, their places of work began to acquire defining features – a tendency to think of oneself as aiding a select population, as a reader of a distinct scientific and clinical literature, and as clinician reliant upon a specific set of diagnostic practices. In most cases, the local medical culture determined the outer limits of their occupational identity, and that expression was typically modest. Certain practical differences materialised out of these local perspectives and circumstances. Initially, many of these physicians had seen themselves as members of a common profession – medicine. At some point, however, they began increasingly to view themselves as members of a common occupation – neurology. That shift in identity was local, generational, and mainly occurred in the interwar period.[193]

Conclusion

Thus largely passed away a culture of medical generalism and thus also arose the culture of specialist practice – a transformation that at the time had everything to do with political exigencies and social expediency. In the period before the First World War, the science and medicine of the nervous system was differently constructed. So too were the mentalities of practitioners with interests in the nervous system. If some focused their work purely on diseases of the nervous system, then this in no way stipulated that they necessarily conceived of themselves as specialists. Rather they saw themselves as consultants, better able – it may be true – to treat some conditions over others, but consultants nevertheless. To us their organisation – the Neurological Society of the United Kingdom – appears cast in specialist metal. But there is little evidence that members of that society ever understood its purpose in those terms. Indeed, evidence points to a contrary view, especially with that society's dissolution into the Royal Society of Medicine. That event marked the ascendance of generalist culture in Edwardian medicine, an event also reflected in the foundation of the Association of Physicians.

Perhaps the formation of those societies was a reactionary movement, a response to deeper forces pushing for divisions that crept ever forward within society and culture. Such events signify or symbolise a society in steady upheaval. Yet specialisation was a force derived of liberal economics. The medical generalists possessed a powerful monopoly, costly especially to consumers, but also costly to younger practitioners. The forces of tradition commanded enormous obligations and stood in the way of social, technological, and therapeutic change, or 'progress' – reform defined in liberal terms as opportunity for work and income. Nor need these facts be construed as economic reductionism; there were measurable benefits from specialisation. Harnessed scientifically, it increased the pace of scientific research and the speed with which patients could be treated and cured. In the case of shell shock, while it created controversy in diagnosis and treatment, it also permitted civil servants and bureaucrats some latitude in fulfilling government obligations.

In this sense, the First World War had revolutionary facets. It challenged every aspect of the status quo, and gave rise to a culture inclined away from traditions and the static qualities that defined the Victorian age. The consequences would be significant in many ways: for the people, universal suffrage for men and women in 1918; for medicine, specialisation, initially state funding for research and ultimately, by 1948, universal healthcare; and for neurology, the formal establishment and formulation of limits in practice and scope. Henry Head's 1918 presidential address unconsciously spoke to this wider context; Walter Russell Brain's report was one of its ultimate manifestations. The next chapter expands upon these insights through its focus on neurological research and neurological internationalism in the interwar period.

• 3 •

Neurology in interwar Britain

Introduction

There is a story that has unfortunately become more of a legend of neurology than it ever was a reality.[1] It is a sad story – one that involves egos, recrimination, and chauvinism. In 1928 a researcher at the Westminster Hospital came to the attention of the Medical Research Council (MRC), then a relatively new body supporting basic clinical research.[2] Kathleen Chevassut had studied science at Bedford College for Women and had completed graduate work at the Westminster Hospital Medical School.[3] But, like many women in this period, she had failed to qualify in medicine.[4]

At the Westminster Hospital she had been mentored by neurologist James Morgan Purves Stewart. He advised her to give up medicine and devote herself to clinical research, where she had already shown promise with her biochemical analysis of cerebrospinal fluid. Purves Stewart paid for her research and encouraged her to examine samples of spinal fluid from his patients with multiple sclerosis. Versed in the literature on filterable viruses and knowledgeable about the latest techniques in bacteriology, Chevassut began examining his samples.[5] In a few of these she claimed to have discovered an organism, which she and others suspected as being aetiologically significant in the disease.

Purves Stewart used Chevassut's research as the basis for pioneering human trials of a vaccine against the dreaded disease – a vaccine that Chevassut alone could produce. Both Chevassut and Purves Stewart, whose relationship deteriorated by 1930, published their findings in the *Lancet*.[6] Concerned both with the publicity that the preliminary tests had created and the appearance of Chevassut's lack of autonomy, the decade-old MRC took what was an unusual step for it, of funding a medically unqualified researcher. It simultaneously hired another researcher and clinician, Edward Arnold Carmichael, to confirm her preliminary findings.

Carmichael failed to reproduce Chevassut's results. He reported his negative findings at the Section of Neurology of the Royal Society of Medicine in December of 1931. Purves Stewart and Chevassut both denied Carmichael's findings but medical opinion turned against them. Chevassut ultimately determined not to continue her research under the patronage of the MRC.[7] Stewart then disclaimed his relationship with her. Yet it was commonly held that he had significantly enriched himself and that Chevassut had faked her results on his behalf.[8]

The common perception was simpler than the reality. Chevassut may well have made mistakes and have been dishonest but the record on these points is murky. She was certainly naive. And accordingly she comes across in the historical record as a rather sympathetic figure: a woman working in a world of male science and medicine, an easy target in comparison with her powerful and in any case far from naive mentor.

It is clear that Chevassut believed that she had discovered the organism that caused the disease. But others worked against that view. Carmichael, for instance, worked at the National Hospital, Queen Square, where clinicians at the time were pioneering a new and thus competing fever treatment for multiple sclerosis.[9] At the same time, the clinicians at the National Hospital were also searching for philanthropic sources for neurological research.

Chevassut's perhaps most fateful decision was to abandon the MRC for the Bernard Halley Stewart Trust. This private philanthropy offered her new research facilities and £10,000 as a research endowment. Armed with such facilities and funds, Chevassut might well have been able to continue her research indefinitely. But the clinicians at the National Hospital, especially Francis Walshe and Edward Carmichael, as well as the secretary of the MRC, saw in the Halley Stewart Trust a potential benefactor for neurological research. As this chapter will show, they subsequently worked behind the scenes to discredit Chevassut and her research.

The outcomes for British neurology were substantial and material in the 1930s. They coincided with significant professional changes to the field as well.[10] The scandal, as it came to be regarded, had revealed the damage possible from unregulated research and professional misconduct. The Section of Neurology had carried no code of professional behaviour that could be used to censure individuals such as Purves Stewart for misconduct. Consequently, even as financial support for neurological research became available to neurology, British neurologists created as their new political body the Association of British Neurologists. This new organisation, from which Purves Stewart was permanently excluded, acted to safeguard neurological research from the temptations of personal interest and easy fame.

This story of domestic discord in neurological research cannot be fully understood without reference to several overlapping realities. The culture of British medicine had changed. Medicine was slowly becoming more centralised both in its governance by the British state but also in the local organisation of hospital practice. Medicine had also become more technologically complex. Moreover, the specialist, especially to young aspiring doctors, appeared an ever-more reasonable figure. There were other geopolitical realities: Britain was more stable than other European powers. Its enormous losses in life in the war had not been matched by losses of infrastructure, and, as one of the triumphant powers, it held a status that while fragile, was unmatched in Europe. In this sense, the institutions, domestic and international politics, and the developments in science and industry of interwar Britain were always bound to inspire comment. For these reasons, much about interwar British culture emerges to us through an international perspective, and this is especially true of British neurology of the period. While Chevassut's story might well have conveyed one impression of the professional circumstances of neurology in Britain, observers from outside the nation saw them differently. In a significant sense, British neurology was made as a result of that dialectic between domestic self-perception and international acclaim. To convey this view more firmly, it is perhaps best to follow another small vignette from the same period, before turning towards domestic and international developments.

Neurology's local realities and global conjunctures

Behind the Chevassut affair was a far wider and important context. Since the end of the First World War, the spirit of reform in British neurology, which had coincided with neurophysiological investigations of wounded soldiers, had led to an increasing global recognition of British neurology's distinctive clinical method and simultaneously suppositions about British neurologists' superiority in the practice of neurology. If British medicine as a whole was poorly situated to provide material support to this nascent yet now also prestigious specialty, then this was a fact not entirely understood beyond Britain's borders.

As the work of historian Delia Gavrus suggests, from the 1920s there were constant claims of underdevelopment in neurology in medical schools and hospitals across Europe and North America.[11] In part, these claims were elements in a movement to modernise hospitals and medical education. The National Hospital in Queen Square made an enormous effort to transform in the interwar period and, as has already been remarked, most of the London teaching hospitals created departments of nervous diseases or neurology in this period as well. Hospitals and medical schools in North America followed the pattern, and so did centres in Europe. The unifying feature of these movements was that clinicians and hospital administrators at the centre of these changes described circumstances for neurology in their local environment in terms of the development of neurology elsewhere. While British neurologists pointed to institutions in Europe and North America as models, both European and North American figures pointed to the British. The consequence was that British neurology in the interwar period had achieved remarkable international recognition despite local realities at odds with this picture.

One story clearly illustrates this trend. In the 1920s Johns Hopkins Hospital and Medical School in Baltimore, then arguably the flagship medical university in the United States, made a substantial effort to garner funds for the development of a neurological service. It approached a variety of funding bodies, including the Rockefeller Foundation, and in its preliminary applications and discussions continually contrasted the weakness of neurology in Baltimore with the excellence of the British model.[12]

The centrepiece of its applications was an effort to attract a world leader in neurology to head-up its new programme, a point that officials at the Rockefeller Foundation and other philanthropies subtly stipulated as necessary for their support. The dean of the Hopkins Medical School, Lewis Weed, consequently approached several figures to head-up the new department and did so by extending invitations to figures for temporary visiting professorships in neurology. In late June of 1924, Francis Walshe was invited to Baltimore and tempted with the offer of a position. He turned it down and the Hopkins effort collapsed. Lewis Weed spent several years reviving the proposal. By 1930 he and Hopkins had invited Gordon Holmes, Walshe's senior and mentor, for a visiting professorship. Holmes too turned down the offered position. Clinicians at Hopkins would not see significant institutional develop for neurology there until after the Second World War. The same was not true, however, for British neurology, especially at the National Hospital, Queen Square. The lesson British neurologists had learned was that powerful philanthropic bodies viewed them as leaders in their field.

State medicine and the rise of biomedical researchers

Much had changed in Britain since the war's end: the bustle of the modern world, its noise and electric lights, as well as its methods of producing, were new. Demobilisation and universal suffrage movements had contributed to the production of mass culture. But wages were down, productivity decreasing, and global demand for British exports falling.[13] Reconstruction was a topic in the political and social foreground. Finance and banking, historian Arthur Marwick notes, had superseded industry, and indeed it had become 'customary in all countries, including America, for the very successful in business to hope to slip into the cultured world of the aristocracy', and high finance seemingly crossed that social divide with the greatest of ease.[14]

So too did medicine, if perhaps in more farcical fashion. Medical men in this period garnered royal pedigrees and wore them proudly. Knighted and ennobled social climbers, these were figures of satire, as in the case of Sir Roderick Glossop, the comical nerve specialist in the writings of P. G. Wodehouse.[15] Neurologists were no exception. Purves Stewart – Sir James – never tired, many noted, of listing his military and medical accomplishments.

In retrospect, it seems that the badges of ancient world orders invented traditions of continuity to stabilise a rapidly changing world. For many physicians before the war, the difficulty of their work had been between publicly demonstrating scientific attainments in a specialty while maintaining proficiency in general clinical practice.[16] The environments of voluntary and teaching hospital wards, as well as their private practices, demanded general competence. Yet, important symbolic capital came through the cultivation of scientific expertise. Research publications and membership in scientific bodies brought not only admiration from peers but also a broader range of clients.

Each generated greater status for individuals within the medical establishment. Status included presidencies of medical societies, administrative positions in teaching hospitals or the Royal College of Physicians, and advisory roles in government.[17] It was an inefficient and impractical model for both research and medicine. In this context, specialisation made increasing sense but created explicit tensions between traditionalists and modernisers.

Archibald Garrod, Consulting Physician to St Bartholomew's Hospital, noted in 1919 the ambivalence of Victorian and Edwardian physicians about specialisation:

> No more beautiful examples of scientific methods and reasoning can be quoted than those employed by the neurologist in localisation of lesions of the brain and spinal cord, and in gaining insight into their nature. It is true that his conclusions are based upon anatomical and physiological observation, which enable him to carry in his mind a stereoscopic picture of the brain as transparent as the stereoscopic images of the radiographer, *but* the men who made those observations were, until recently, engaged in the practice of medicine or surgery, and some of them might even have been classed as 'popular physicians'.[18]

What was Garrod's point? It might be worth observing that James Parkinson's classic *The Shaking Palsy*, although a stunning example of anatomic-physiological reasoning and clinical inference, had been the work of a nineteenth-century general practitioner. In other words, Parkinson's genius had been wasted yet his neurology as a clinical method was exemplary of how bedside medicine could become 'as strictly scientific as the methods of the laboratory'.[19] Garrod's point was not simply that medicine ought to be scientific. It was also to make a claim that, while past 'popular physicians' might confirm the excellence of the British medical tradition, they also affirmed its underlying weaknesses. Past researchers had been forced to focus their energies on income. Garrod's modern vision of clinical research, by contrast, sought to bridge the gap between medicine and the laboratory by creating a new class of clinical researchers: men and women who would devote their lives to biomedical research.[20]

Garrod was advocating a transformation that was already ongoing within British medicine.[21] Following the rather toothless recommendations of the 1914 Haldane Commission, hospitals began forming departments and teaching divisions for various specialties, including neurology.[22] Soon after, the MRC (formed in 1920 from its wartime predecessor the Medical Research Committee) began funding research, marking the advent of state patronage of clinical research.[23]

Among the powerful figures in British medicine in this period was Thomas Lewis.[24] Lewis was a successful propagandist for Garrod's professional clinical researchers, and it was for this reason that he became a supporter of Edward Arnold Carmichael, a clinically trained neurologist who appeared to desire a career in research, but who in the absence of a patron would certainly be lost to private practice. During the Great War, Lewis had researched heart conditions. In the interwar period he received substantial support from the MRC and the Rockefeller Foundation and had cast their support as evidence for the value of clinical researchers.[25] His campaign for such a division of labour became somewhat bombastic. In a 1930 essay published in the *British Medical Journal* and entitled 'Research in Medicine: Its Positions and its Need', he had argued:

> [Research] in medicine is most compatible with specialism.... It is not possible in research to maintain full familiarity with general medicine, with its ever-changing devices and palliatives, when so much of both time and energy are concerned in studying matters that have no immediate relevancy to practice, and in laboriously and accurately collecting data and critically forming conclusions.... Ability to undertake research...is not a criterion of practical capacity; and experience in research, especially on the laboratory side, has little or no value in practice; consequently, when preliminary years are spent in large part in this way, they displace years of more valuable practical experience. The proper sequel to such research is not practice but further research – in short, a career largely concerned with investigation.[26]

In the same article, he claimed that 'young and competent men' could not 'be expected to hazard the best years of their lives in long and special training without reasonable prospect of corresponding careers before them'.[27] He might well have been writing about Carmichael (or, for that matter, the woman Carmichael would shortly discredit, Kathleen Chevassut).

Lewis' views, if held only by a minority, matched those of his more politically powerful friends, especially Walter Morley Fletcher, then secretary of the MRC. A scientific idealist but political realist, Fletcher's tenure at the MRC was markedly mandarin, despite his oft-stated position that science should be autonomous and not under state control. He viewed the progress of scientific knowledge and thus its patronage as a calling that would eventually 'destroy... death', provided that the state nurtured research.[28] Such utopian rhetoric when combined with *realpolitik* made him an extraordinary advocate for scientific and clinical researchers. It was that desire to support researchers that led Fletcher to back such investigators as Carmichael and Chevassut; it was his shrewd attitude that gave him no compunction in destroying Chevassut's career when it became apparent that there were material gains to be made for British science and biomedical research by doing so.

Modernisers like Fletcher, Garrod, and Lewis were working against their prevailing culture. But they appear now as great exemplars of the interwar transformation of British medicine and science. If they were not mainstream, they were nevertheless at the forefront of commonsense changes. And, for all of that, the changes they represented were part of a radical reordering of political, industrial, and ultimately public values for medicine.

Internationalism remakes British neurology

Those changes in neurology were already visible in medical society life by 1918. Following Henry Head's presidential address to the Section of Neurology at the Royal Society of Medicine, certain noteworthy changes appeared in the section's administration. The section's council, for example, moved to create a directory for a never-realised 'National Union of Neurologists' and this effort corresponded with other moves that markedly shifted the Section towards internationalism.[29]

Why did this movement towards internationalism occur? These efforts coincided with wider political developments, a fact perhaps best reflected in the formation of the League of Nations in this period. Yet internationalism for interwar neurologists offered advantages that cannot be ignored. The international sphere was an idealised space for creating disciplinary and epistemological unity. The appearance of international solidarity lent neurology – in Britain and elsewhere – the appearance of definitional stability. It concealed local uncertainties beneath the clothes of international styles.

International events functioned to create the appearance of commonalities between groups. Meetings were moreover useful opportunities for enacting changes in the dominant medical culture. For instance, the International Neurological Congress of 1935, held in London and sponsored by the Royal Society of Medicine, coincided also with British centenary celebrations of John Hughlings Jackson's birth. Jackson, as a figure of international stature, provided a national symbol that could be used in two worthy ways. He exemplified the greatness of the British medical tradition and thus the value of the old culture. He simultaneously served as a justification for turning away from that older world towards a new culture that saw value in medical specialism. In other words, older traditions of the British medical establishment were rewritten into the story of medicine's march towards modernisation.[30]

Organisationally, this was both a novel role for the Section of Neurology and an unlikely one. The Royal Society of Medicine's rules of practice were not aligned with new cultural modes. It was thus both an agent for and an obstacle to reform. While providing a venue for scientific meetings and celebratory events, as well as international congresses, the Section of Neurology lacked control over its membership. Like its elite counterpart, the Association of Physicians of Great Britain and Ireland, the section's council did not possess the inclination or wherewithal to lobby politically for its specialties. It lacked control over the publication of its proceedings. Thus, aside from slightly increased efforts to assert broader influence for neurology, especially in public and policy discussions surrounding shell shock, few changes actually occurred within the body between 1920 and 1925.

The two exceptions were in areas significant but adjacent to neurology practice: diagnostic technologies and surgery. Like most physicians, physicians with interests in the nervous system resisted technological changes in medicine. They regarded technology as being of dubious utility compared to the art of clinical examination. Neurosurgery, one of the areas responsible for changes in neurological practice in this period, proved more receptive to technology.[31] These differences of opinion were indicative of an obvious conflict growing between neurology and neurosurgery, the latter being an almost thoroughly

American phenomenon. Jefferson, as well as Hugh Cairns, Norman Dott, and others in this period, had trained under Harvey Cushing.[32] British neurologists, suspicious of Cushing's practices, disliked a surgical technique not reliant upon a neurologist's knowledge.[33] Such differences mapped onto the divisive idioms of the age: on one side stood surgeons with technology, modernity, and rationalisation; on the other, physicians with art and tradition.

The first change signalling modernisation and a new social order for neurology was thus the formation of the Society of British Neurological Surgeons in 1926. This event marked a distinct shift away from the generalist culture, and for neurologists, consequently represented an identity-making moment – one that heralded the decline of the Section of Neurology. Circumstances began changing in the summer of 1925.

In July 1925 American neurologist Theodore Weisenburg (1876–1934) invited the British neurologists to join the American Neurological Association in an Anglo-American Congress. Weisenburg, physician to the Philadelphia General Hospital, proposed the meeting take place in America in 1926. In October, Gordon Holmes, writing on behalf of the council, apologised: 'I am sure that many of the English Neurologists would like to meet you all in America, but I am afraid it would be quite impossible for many of us to get away during May and June as that is really the busiest time of the year, in the middle of the University term and just before the annual Examinations.'[34] In March 1926, the section's council returned the invitation, suggesting that the American Neurological Association meet with them in London in 1927.[35] James Purves Stewart, president-elect of the section for 1927 and 1928 (note that his disseminated sclerosis research with Kathleen Chevassut was just coming to public and professional attention),[36] wrote to Weisenburg expressing his regret that no members of the Neurological Section had attended the America meeting, adding, 'At our own Annual Meeting, however it was unanimously resolved to send a cordial invitation to the members of the America Neurological Association to attend a meeting in London in July 1927.'[37] The Americans accepted.

The joint congress was the first of its kind for British neurologists. Hence it represented an opportunity to demonstrate their national accomplishments. The organisation of the meeting's papers was consequently a delicate process. The balance between speakers from America and Britain, of course, needed to reflect both countries in equitable fashion. But drawing attention to Britain's neurological eminence was a central concern as well, because demonstrating the supremacy of British neurology in the best of the British clinical tradition also prepared the way for making claims countering the conservativism of the prevailing local medical culture. Such a balance could be achieved by showcasing the accomplishments of Americans who had studied in Britain.[38] Likewise, British practitioners who had received Rockefeller Fellowships for foreign study could bring positive philanthropic attention to the successes of British medicine.[39]

Certain privileges of playing host were of immediate benefit to the British – although no one saw it in such sharp terms. The schedule, so a letter from William Adie reports, was to be short talks on 25 July 1927, and a lengthy discussion on the cerebellum in the morning and then a clinical meeting at the National Hospital in the afternoon of the second day. And then a discussion on sensory disturbances in organic disease on the final day, which concluded also with a discussion of pathological papers and specimens, a topic bound to showcase Britain at its best.[40] Meanwhile, if the presentation of papers was stacked favourably for the British, the honour of a plenary address could be exchanged with the Americans. The British offered the Hughlings Jackson Lectureship, the ultimate gesture of British neurological diplomacy, to the president of the American Neurological Association, Charles Dana.[41]

If the strategy, which was less instrumental than the above suggests, was successful, then it was not due to the organisational advantages of the Royal Society of Medicine. Gordon Holmes, the chairman of the scientific committee of the joint meeting, was by now editor of *Brain*. He wrote to Weisenburg, 'I am doubly interested in the British-American Neurological Meeting next July, as in the first place I am Chairman of the Committee which has responsibility on this side for the scientific arrangements, and in the second place as Editor of "Brain".' To Weisenburg, Holmes subsequently complained of difficulties in publishing the proceedings: 'The Neurological Association is a Section of the Royal Society of Medicine, which claims a copyright for its Proceedings of all papers and discussions of the Section, so we must get permission to publish these elsewhere...I have intended to suggest that the Proceedings should be published in toto in "Brain".'[42] Holmes eventually succeeded in this activity and reported to Weisenburg: 'The Royal Society of Medicine will not require the Proceedings to be published,' and, he added – provided the American Neurological Association agreed – the proceedings would appear in *Brain*. 'I may say that this year we complete our fiftieth volume, and we are anxious to turn out something really good.'[43] It is difficult not to see Holmes' manoeuvres as coinciding with a rising dissatisfaction with the Royal Society of Medicine.

James Purves Stewart's behaviour was typical. No stranger to advertising, he was giving his fullest attention to orchestrating a celebration of Britain's neurological tradition. He wrote, for example, to Edwin Bramwell, soliciting Bramwell's aid in convincing his father, Byrom, to attend the meeting:

> I am especially anxious, if it is at all possible, to get Sir Byrom to be with us for one meeting, if he finds himself at all able. We should not ask him to tire himself by a speech of any sort; all we want is to have his presence as an inspiration, so that the members of the joint congress may go back and say to their pupils that they have had the honour of grasping Sir Byrom Bramwell by the hand. I will write myself to Sir Byrom in due course, but meanwhile I hope you will prepare the way. Sir David Ferrier is the other great pioneer whom we are trying to persuade on similar lines, and he has practically promised to come.[44]

Purves Stewart's effort to arrange for 'pioneers' to be present is particularly illustrative of the ways these occasions could subtly rewrite neurology's past. Byrom Bramwell's status as an eminent clinician placed him squarely in the older, generalist tradition of medicine. Purves Stewart's efforts to secure the presence of a living memory created continuity between conditions of the past and present that oddly denied the realities of both.[45] Nostalgia served to blur the lines between the two cultures of medicine, affirming the present by establishing a long tradition for neurology. A new world was necessitated by the progress of the old. Meanwhile, it was the old that was 'sold' to the Americans.

The Anglo-American meeting was a tremendous success.[46] The event was a veritable *Who's Who* of the science and medicine of Anglo-American neurology and psychiatry.[47] Adolf Meyer, an American neuropsychiatrist from the Phipps Clinic at Johns Hopkins Medical School, was, for example, among the crowd of the almost 250 neurologists and psychiatrists – 34 from America – enjoying a splendid repast of twelve courses and accompanying claret at the Café Royal at the official banquet.[48] *Science* reported later that 'Sir James Purves Stewart, president of the section, gave an address [that evening] on "Mount Athos, a Survival of the Middle Ages".'[49] Purves Stewart distributed copies of the lecture to the audience 'with the writer's compliments'.[50] For Meyer, and likely many others, the significance of the conference was emotional as well as professional.[51] For many of the figures from America, it was a sentimental sojourn to Old Europe. Many of the American figures in neurology had trained there. Many had returned again as medical officers during the terrible years of the Great War.

What is striking about this conference is how it connected the otherwise disparate and fragmented realities of neurological practice in both countries. Contact between these two nations seemingly allowed neurologists in both contexts to see themselves through the gaze of their colleagues. Neurology, epistemologically and institutionally, thus gained a new social reality and visibility to both parties. The result was an ideological consensus, one that derived much of its power from the flexibility of historical discourses – nostalgia, commemoration, and celebration – as well as tropes of progress. As one American neurologist later recalled, 'all of the Americans who attended the gathering returned to this country enthusiastic over the successes of this meeting and inspired to further such occasions on a larger scale.'[52] Inspiration was key: the formation of the International Congresses, which subsequently occurred, was an act of profound import, not just for neurology in Britain but also for the specialty throughout the world. It established an idealised global counterweight to the more distressing local circumstances neurologists often faced in their national contexts. By hosting the Americans, the British had raised the prominence of their own circumstances internationally. While local realities and institutions remained devotedly old fashioned, neurologists in Britain were nevertheless beginning to reform.

State support for clinical neurological research at Queen Square

It is likely that James Purves Stewart had not endeared himself to his colleagues during his presidency of the Section of Neurology. He was often described as exasperatingly megalomaniac. As word of his involvement in the ill-fated multiple sclerosis research spread – articles were published in the lay and scientific press heralding a cure for the dread disease – his prominence must have begun to appear a visible stain on the reputation of his contemporaries. In 1929 he became involved in the organisation of the First International Neurological Congress, which was to be held in Berne in 1931. By 1930 Purves Stewart and Kathleen Chevassut had published papers in the *Lancet* describing their research, and numerous London neurologists had quickly begun voicing concern about the legitimacy of his vaccine trials. Some thought their publications ought to be deplored, because they might give rise to false hope in their chronic patients. But Purves Stewart was too prominent for them to attack publicly, and the grumbling might have appeared petty professional envy. Behind the scenes, all that the council of the MRC heard from Chevassut were reports of failure and political intrigue. Carmichael, who had come to Walter Fletcher's attention in the mid-1920s, likewise reported a similar inability to find an organism causative in the disease. It was in December 1930 that Chevassut's research, and thus by extension Purves Stewart's, was discredited.[53]

Having received an ultimatum from the MRC and likely suspecting that there were few she could trust, Chevassut withdrew from both the MRC and Purves Stewart's patronage, in lieu of another, seemingly better and safer opportunity. The consequences of this decision would prove tragic for her. Purves Stewart immediately disclaimed his involvement with her and then spread rumours that she had misled him. His protestations, however, fell on deaf ears, and gossip and innuendo and accusations circled that he had enriched himself on a quack cure (it is easy to imagine that his presence at the 1931 First International Neurological Congress embarrassed his British colleagues). He would retire not long after, disgraced, and persona non grata in British neurology.

Chevassut's end would be worse; yet the influence of her failed research project exerted a longer positive impact on British neurology than many would ever acknowledge. Not long after Purves Stewart had abandoned her, a letter had appeared in the *British Medical Journal* by a young physician named Barnard Halley Stewart, recently appointed to take charge of his father's philanthropic foundation, the Halley Stewart Trust.[54] In his letter, Halley Stewart wondered whether Carmichael's failure to replicate Chevassut's work had done anything other than to raise further questions. No one, he argued, knew whether her work had been a waste of time and resources or actually fruitful. It was these circumstances that led him to declare the remarkable decision to support Chevassut's research by providing her facilities, salary, and funds for research. His letter announced a grant of £10,000 to secure laboratory facilities in a small house the trust had purchased for this purpose, 30 Chesterford Gardens.[55]

Not surprisingly, many received the news of this decision with great scepticism; the last thing that should happen, many felt, was the continuation of this research.[56] For his part, Francis Walshe could not sit by apathetically. Caustic, conservative, and Catholic, and a medical correspondent to the *Herald* and the *Tablet*, Walshe turned his pen towards writing condemnatory letters to Barnard Halley Stewart, Jr. To no avail: he eventually finished his correspondence with a flourish:

> as far as this research is concerned you are living in a world of fantasy in which I can make no contact with you. I fear that you may be inclined to take this view of mine somewhat amiss, but I would ask you to suspend judgment for a twelvemonth. Then re-read your letter of the 29th and my reply. I wager that by then we shall be marvellously in agreement in believing that feminine charm and inconsequence and a light-hearted disregard of accuracy are fatal endowments for one engaged in scientific research.[57]

The Halley Stewart Trust soon reached this conclusion.[58] It is easy to infer that numerous voices, not just Walshe's were calling Chevassut's ability into question. A letter in the MRC archives from late June of 1931 reveals that Walter Morley Fletcher had met with the elder Halley Stewart:

> The old man himself, who was completely unknown to me, gave a surprise visit last week and explained that he was thoroughly dissatisfied with the whole business by this time, and suggested we should take it over from him. He then learned for the first time all that we had previously done. I believe the Trustees are meeting to-day and will come to some decision...I am afraid it is become pretty plain that she was receiving money or promises of money from the Trustees while taking our research grant from public funds, of which an essential condition of course was that she should not receive money from other sources without our knowledge. In any case, she concealed altogether from the Trustees, when leading

> them into an expenditure of about £10,000, the previous help and opportunities we had given her. I think the various interpretations you give of her conduct can be easily extended without any undue charity to cover these lapses, but it looks bad from outside. Much the best thing she can do now is give-up this wild-goose chase, swallow the pride, which should never have been aroused, and go back to her medical work. I have nothing but commiseration for her. But I feel very strong resentment against Purves-Stewart and others at the Westminster Hospital.[59]

Not only does the record contradict many of Fletcher's observations, it is also unclear why Halley Stewart Sr would have claimed not to know that the MRC had supported Chevassut's research. Everything Chevassut had published stated that the MRC had supported her work previously. Her relationship with the MRC was public knowledge. Fletcher offered little evidence to substantiate his claim that Chevassut had been accepting money or promises of money while working for the MRC and the record does not support the claim. The record does, however, indicate that Fletcher met with Halley Stewart Sr throughout 1931.[60] Fletcher's accusations never took a more direct path than innuendo.

In January 1932, Chevassut resigned from the Halley Stewart Trust. Shortly after, Fletcher wrote to Francis Walshe, instructing him to prepare with Edward Carmichael a new proposal for 30 Chesterford Gardens, Chevassut's former laboratory. This activity, he wryly noted, would ensure that the Halley Stewart Trust would not have to 'scrap all the beautiful equipment' and 'throw away what has in all cost them about £12,000'. He added, 'You and Carmichael both spoke of investigating disseminated sclerosis or other diseases and of using that place, perhaps, as a kind of research annexe linked with Queen Square.'[61] Carmichael, according to Walshe, was the ideal leader for the job and required relief from 'hack work of the most demoralizing kind'.[62]

By February 1932, Fletcher had received Walshe and Carmichael's proposal. Noting that pathological research in neurology was becoming fairly common, they observed that biochemical and metabolic studies of the nervous system were not frequently conducted in the United Kingdom. Clinical material was always ready for investigation, but many problems still required deliberation, including: metabolic, biochemical, and physiological research on spinal cords showing signs of sub-acute combined degeneration. 'The organisation for such research', Walshe and Carmichael owned, 'is already available as it is being undertaken in the out-patient department at Queen Square on Saturdays. The facilities there are not good and it is impossible to control to the same extent as if the subjects were in-patients...the work is not perfect owing to lack of facilities.'[63] There were similar problems for research in myopathies, epilepsy, and myasthenia gravis. In order for the research to run efficiently, Carmichael and Walshe suggested that the facilities would require a minimum of ten beds, nursing staff, and kitchens. In addition, it would need a full-time neurologist, a dietician, a qualified medical officer with laboratory expertise, and possibly a trained biochemist, an expenditure that would be amply repaid, 'as investigation into the biochemistry of nervous diseases has not yet been undertaken'.[64]

This proposal for a research institute was genuinely remarkable. Not only was it unprecedented in Britain but, had it been realised, it would have been one of very few of its kind in the service of neurology the world over.[65] It was also strategic. Walshe, aware at the least of the Johns Hopkins approach to the Rockefeller Foundation, was preparing a competing bid to the foundation and for the benefit of the National Hospital.[66] In the best of possible worlds, the neurologists might get lucky and acquire both.

Before Fletcher could continue negotiations with the Halley Stewart Trust, he became seriously ill. Proposals for the Chesterford Gardens project lapsed while he recuperated (he never fully recovered).[67] By the time Fletcher returned to work, Walshe was glum about the prospects of major funding at the National Hospital: 'I should like to ask', he wrote to Fletcher despondently in May 1932:

> that if at any time you see the way clear for the establishment at Queen Square of a research unit, you will let me know so that our chances there may not be lost for lack of our knowing when to take them. Flexner was so disapproving of English medical educational methods last night that my hopes of some aid from the Rockefeller Foundation dwindled sadly away.[68]

Walshe was proposing the creation of a MRC research unit at the National Hospital by 1933 and his suggestion was not without promising possibilities. Fletcher, however, was soon disappointed to learn that legalities prevented 30 Chesterford Gardens from housing the patients necessary for clinical research.[69] Halley Stewart Sr also proved adamant that the facility be used for research only and voiced concern that Walshe and Carmichael intended it as a convalescent home.[70] As a compromise, he suggested that the trust support one or two researchers with fellowships instead. Fletcher in turn recommended that Carmichael would be an appropriate candidate for funding. 'He is a highly trained neurologist and really cares for nothing but research. He is now at the parting of ways and must either get some stable research position or allow his consulting practice to grow.'[71]

Fletcher, it appears, had come to regard Carmichael's research career as important to the MRC. He was not alone. He had received a letter confirming that many neurologists at Queen Square were of the same view.[72] Likewise, the Rockefeller Foundation European authority on science, Daniel O'Brien, had additionally mentioned in a letter from the same period that he regarded Carmichael as being of 'unusual promise and exceptional ability' because he was a member of a 'younger group... anxious to develop the scientific side of neurology'.[73]

In July 1932, however, it remained unclear where Carmichael would end up. That month, physicians at the National Hospital, concerned that their hopes for major philanthropic funding for research were not going to materialise, drafted a proposal to the MRC suggesting that they found together a clinical neurological research unit at the hospital.[74] The hospital would immediately pay for twenty beds, the services of a medical assistant, laboratory technician, and one house physician, and: 'Dr Carmichael would of course be the Physician chosen as Director.'[75] The National Hospital's proposal for the medical research unit had been put together by Francis Walshe, who was aware that Thomas Lewis' post at University College Hospital, which had been formerly supported by the MRC, was about to be permanently endowed by a capital grant from the Rockefeller Foundation, thus freeing up MRC funds.[76]

Meanwhile Carmichael reported to the MRC that he had toured the Chesterford Gardens facility with Halley Stewart Jr and been awestruck by how 'superbly equipped with apparatus' it was and had suggested that the 'fittings and equipment could well be transferred to' Queen Square.[77] Suggesting that the MRC receive a supplementary grant from the Halley Stewart Trust for Carmichael because 'we naturally shrink from direct responsibility', Halley Stewart Sr observed shortly thereafter that Carmichael's suggestion had come to him 'like plank pushed to a drowning man' and proposed that the MRC care for Carmichael completely and support him through a liberal grant from the trust.[78]

The agreement ultimately reached benefited Carmichael enormously. Halley Stewart and his son discussed the plans for the new unit, and Fletcher offered some advice on disposing of Chesterford Gardens.[79] (The trust eventually gave the property to the University of London as a facility for physics research.[80]) The elder Halley Stewart suggested a permanent supplemental endowment of £200 per annum to Carmichael.[81] He hinted that other funds might be available for research fellowships.[82] By October 1932, the proposal to form the clinical research unit was before the MRC. Carmichael's position, initially probationary, included a whole-time grant for his salary and additional funds to support the laboratory for five years.[83] The MRC council then fully supported the National Hospital's proposal, and the Clinical Neurological Research Unit was established.[84]

In winter 1932 Fletcher wrote to Halley Stewart Sr telling him of Carmichael's recent appointment. Mentioning the financial limitations the MRC faced, Fletcher promised that any additional investment the trust might make in Carmichael would not limit what the Council was prepared to give. Halley Stewart Sr subsequently proposed 'a Student Research Scholarship supplemented by the Trust for three years at £200, £225, and £250 per annum'.[85] In a letter Fletcher replied: 'If this were found possible, it would not only bring aid to the right kind of man, but by doing so aid the progress of the whole scheme.'[86] Shortly thereafter, the MRC announced the Halley-Stewart Research Fellowship. By 1933, candidates were applying for funds.[87] With the foundation of this unit, neurological research in Britain became one of the best supported in the world. In short, by 1933, British neurology had passed through a metamorphosis. Through Fletcher's *realpolitik*, a formal structure was given to neurology's research tradition. It would be further enhanced by the Rockefeller Foundation.

Global philanthropy and London neurology

Edward Carmichael's career directorship of the unit was tenable for five years. If he did not meet expectations, then either the National Hospital or the MRC could appoint a new director. It became evident shortly after Carmichael's appointment that some of his colleagues felt his younger independent collaborator, Derek Denny Brown, was more talented.[88] But for the most part, Carmichael achieved positive recognition. He had impressed the Rockefeller Foundation officers with his modern attitudes from the beginning of his appointment: 'He strikes me as a very high type and exactly the man for the place.'[89] Others concurred with this view. William Lennox (1884–1960), an American expert on epilepsy who was in Britain in 1935,[90] observed in a letter to the Rockefeller Foundation that Carmichael's leadership had improved research at Queen Square but noted tensions between Carmichael's clinical researchers and the hospital's full-time clinicians: 'Underneath the polite exterior, I sense a strong current of jealousy of the position and future of bedside neurology. The influential men of the staff have gained their reputation and knowledge by the use of pin, cotton wool, and reflex hammer and are a bit scornful (and fearful) of the new paraphernalia of the laboratory.'[91]

During the 1930s observers from the Rockefeller Foundation were frequently in London, and they reported such impressions to foundation officers in the United States.[92] It was a clear sign that British neurology's international prominence had grown substantially in the years following the Anglo-American Congress of 1927.[93] The foundation was aware that the Johns Hopkins Medical School had attempted to recruit British neurologists.[94] It was an open secret that Francis Walshe and Gordon Holmes had been offered the job of creating a new department at the prestigious institute and that both had turned it down.[95] The Rockefeller Foundation's officers had been watching events at Hopkins closely, perhaps waiting to see if they could attract a British neurologist. When Holmes visited, they had been particularly interested to learn how many American postgraduates had studied at the National Hospital in the 1920s.[96] It was clear that the bulk of American students studying the subject in Europe were receiving their training at the National Hospital, a fact that Holmes' work in planning the Anglo-American Congress had made clear as well.[97] It was becoming evident to figures at the Rockefeller Foundation that neurology required support, and they were considering a capital endowment for neurological research at the National Hospital.[98] By 1932 Gordon Holmes and Francis Walshe had begun working on a request for Rockefeller support and had heard informally that the foundation would consider their proposal with great sympathy.[99]

Rockefeller interest in British neurology dated from the 1920s. The foundation had, for example, been watching and considering supporting Edward Carmichael even before he became director of the MRC Neurological Research Unit.[100] Although by 1930 there were institutes of neurology in Belgium, Germany, France, and the United States, figures at the Rockefeller Foundation saw British neurologists as particularly talented, competent, and charismatic.[101] From a policy point of view, the foundation was increasingly concerned by the real lack of progress in treating asylum patients.[102] Asylums everywhere were overflowing, and many saw neurological research as a possible avenue to address this problem.[103] Neuropsychiatry, in particular, offered possibilities, and the figures at the foundation hoped research at the National Hospital might proceed in that direction if it were supported.[104]

From the beginning of its involvement in British neurology, it had been widely acknowledged at the foundation that there was a lack of institutional recognition for British neurology. It attributed this fact to a by-product of old British traditionalism,[105] yet its officers were uneasy about neurology's absence from academia. The National Hospital was not affiliated with any university. Nor did it have an academic chair for clinical neurological research. For that matter, no such chair existed anywhere in Britain. If the MRC Neurological Unit could be taken as a sign of government recognition of neurology, then that did not automatically translate into academic standing.

As a rule, the Rockefeller Foundation officers preferred to develop university research programmes in the German or American style. They did not support independent hospitals with good intentions but tenuous operating budgets – the temptation to use research endowments for other purposes in strained economic years was sometimes too great.[106] However, academic neurology was not a subject commonly recognised anywhere in the world. Moreover as the foundation officials contemplated endowing research at the National Hospital, it became obvious to them that to penalise an institution for belonging to the disparate system of London teaching hospitals was simply to sacrifice talented resources not existing elsewhere.[107] The organisation for medicine and medical research in London was known to be impractical and for complex historical reasons that had little bearing on the merits of the National Hospital's faculty.[108] Was it sensible to deny workers with great potential the resources they required because of inflexible policies?[109] Their conclusion was 'no', and by 1935 the National Hospital had received a grant for £60,000 for construction of new laboratories and teaching facilities. Another £60,000 was given as a research endowment.[110]

National unions of neurologists in Britain

There can be little doubt that part of the reason British neurologists bolstered their international reputation in this period was the formation of the Association of British Neurologists in 1932. As a new venue for the science and medicine of the nervous system, it was modern in comparison to its rival at the Royal Society Medicine. It was a social achievement too. Its membership was selective. Communications at its general meetings provided benchmarks of progress in laboratories now receiving support. The MRC Neurological Research Unit came into being at almost the same time as the association, and Carmichael's unit benefited enormously from this new venue. It provided his neurological researchers with an independent forum for presenting the results of research. Indeed, presenting at such a forum highlighted the achievements of young Halley-Stewart scholars as well. Although the Halley-Stewart trustees may have been unable to assess the quality of the research, they could infer from communications at the association, as well as publications, that their support was being put to good use. Carmichael cited such presentations to justify his request that a young registrar-turned-neurological researcher, Samuel Nevin, be reappointed to the Halley-Stewart Fellowship: 'An outline of what has been obtained was given at a recent meeting of the Association of British Neurologists and is now being prepared for the press. There is no doubt that he is working hard and doing good work.'[111] Communications were equally important bulwarks to Carmichael's career: 'Just off to Oxford for the annual meeting of the British Neurologists. Four papers from the unit to be given' was easy self-promotion to the MRC.[112] Judged statistically by reports given at the association's meetings, Carmichael and his group were the most active British neurological researchers in the 1930s and 1940s. Of the 136 communications presented to the Association of British Neurologists, twenty-three came from Carmichael's unit.[113] This is a staggering percentage when it is considered that of the fifty-three individuals presenting research at the Association of British Neurologists in the first ten years, only five worked in Carmichael's unit.[114] William Lennox was unequivocal about Carmichael's performance to the

Rockefeller Foundation: 'At the Association of Neurologists meeting at Bath, which I attended, there was none like him.'[115]

While Carmichael's unit benefited in material ways from the newly founded association, it is also likely that its establishment had little to do with his career. On this point, however, inferences only are available. The foundation of this organisation coincided with Stewart's bad behaviour as well as the initiation of the International Neurological Congresses, an idea born from the Anglo-American Congress of 1927. One provocative essay entitled 'International Neurological Congress, Berne' appeared in 1931 in the *Journal of Neurology and Psychopathology* – a journal Carmichael edited after 1937. The International Congress, the author reasoned, could only be a good thing for the progress of neurology, because:

> Rightly or wrongly, we often pride ourselves on being able to sum up the value of a man's contributions better after we have seen him and heard him speak. We take to him, or we do not. If we are every now and then reminded that the artist and his work are separate, or separable, that consideration of the one should influence us neither favourably not unfavourably in respect of the other, it is nevertheless legitimate to believe that his work is but the expression of what the artist has within him and that the two are not in point of fact dissociable. And the remark applies also to the scientific as well as to the world of artistry – perhaps with greater force. The reliability of the data in a scientific study cannot altogether be dissociated from what is learned of the author himself by means such as have been already outlined.[116]

It is difficult not to see the spectre of Purves Stewart's multiple sclerosis research forming a backdrop. If the artist or scientist and his work were separable, the most discerning eye viewed his practice not through what it was, but through who he was. The new International Congress could thus serve two agendas: it allowed study of the habits and attitudes of neurologist, both locally and globally. Secondly, it further served the cause of reform in British neurology:

> Can we regard the situation in England favourable when its position in the neurological sphere is given a glance? We have no cause for congratulation, be it fully and promptly admitted. The old Neurological Society of Great Britain was in the habit of promoting an

> occasional provincial conference over one or two days, but for years none of a comparable kind has been held. Although the latter Society [the Royal Society of Medicine] covers the whole field of medicine in its numerous sections, this has not prevented the development of distinct associations the prime feature of whose healthy growth is the conducting of annual meetings in different parts of the country. Without more than an allusion to the annual yearly congress of the British Medical Association, we may enumerate as somewhat more applicable to the point as those of the Association of Physicians, of British Surgeons, of Neurological Surgeons, of the Ophthalmological Society – and several more might be mentioned.[117]

These were early hints in 1931 of a rebellion against the status quo, an attempt to describe neurology's position in Britain and a nostalgic appeal to a perceived past. Was the author saying something new as well? On one hand, the appeal to the proceedings of the Society of British Neurological Surgeons seemed a symptom of a complaint. On the other, mention of the Ophthalmological Society was something new. It suggested a past fork in neurology's road, a conscious decision that had made all the difference. The juxtaposition of the Association of Physicians against the Ophthalmological Society seems now no simple accident. It emerges as a contrived rebuke against medical generalism. The reference to the meetings of the Association of Physicians was two-fold. On the surface, it was a justification calling for a cure to neurology's ailments. Beneath that was a more profound condemnation of the ethos that had created institutions like the Royal Society of Medicine and the Association of Physicians in the first place. All of the promise and all the successes of British neurology had simply aided the prestige of those institutions. But what did British neurologists have to show for those accomplishments? Neurologists could not even hold a meeting in the provinces, whereas their colleagues in ophthalmology had been doing exactly that since the 1880s.

> Then why not an Association of British Neurologists? Surely there is room and room to spare for the formation of such a group. The alternative would be for an annual meeting of the Neurological Section of the Royal Society of Medicine to take place outside London, and for several reasons, which it is not necessary to specify, the former suggestion is clearly preferable.[118]

Accordingly, there were at least three important impetuses underlying the formation of an Association of British Neurologists: an international movement, a desire to determine its membership, and a wish to acquire occupational autonomy. It is easy to imagine that a further advantage was perceived by leaders in British neurology: the new association delineated a professional jurisdiction that could impress their would-be patrons. In July 1932, Gordon Holmes held a meeting at his house.[119] Among those present were: William Adie, Edwin Bramwell, Henry Cohen, James Collier, Donald Core, Anthony Feiling, Ronald Gordon, James Greenfield, George Hall, Wilfred Harris, William Johnson, Frederick Nattrass, Cecil Worster-Drought, and Samuel Alexander Kinnear Wilson. Together these men formed the Association of British Neurologists. This new association's membership was to be limited to 'those actively engaged in any branch of neurology'. The association would hold meetings once a year. Its proceedings would not be published in the medical press. Officers were elected: the president was Wilfred Harris, the treasurer was Samuel Kinnier Wilson, and Gordon Holmes was secretary. During the months between July and December of 1932, Holmes and others sent out invitations to join the new association. By the second meeting of the council in December of 1932, Holmes reported that fifty-one neurologists had agreed to join.[120]

Conclusion

The formation of the Association of British Neurologists should be understood only as a small move towards reform. When the Aberdeen physician Ashley Mackintosh responded to an invitation from Edwin Bramwell to join the new association, he wrote, 'Although my claim to be a "neurologist" is now very meagre and I am getting more and more lazy as regards attending Meetings, I shall be delighted to join the Association of British Neurologists.'[121] Mackintosh's letter captures the enduring ambiguity of the neurologist in Britain. A claim to be a neurologist still required in 1934 inverted commas. It would take another generation before that situation was fully reversed. But the development of the association, the founding of the MRC Neurological Unit, and the endowment of the National Hospital, Queen Square, were events in the interwar period pointing towards that different future.

• 4 •

Neurology and state medicine

Introduction

Neurological science and clinical practice changed enormously between 1900 and 2000. In 1910, clinical practice would have involved a physician listening to a patient's history and then examining his or her body. Neurological technique was semiological (concerned with identifying and linking the body's signs to disease).[1] Using the patient's history and applying clinical acumen, the physician would derive a diagnosis of the nervous condition. It was this special act of diagnosis that determined the neurologist's practice and marked his (sometimes her) ability.[2] Beyond that, the options were few. If the illness was acute, some options – usually surgical – were available.[3] But although there was a wide range of therapies for nervous conditions, most nerve patients were chronic and in a state of progressive degeneration.

Circumstances by the close of the twentieth century were largely reversed. Diagnostic medicine had been transformed by developments in electroencephalography and imaging science.[4] If semiological approaches still played a role in the examination, then it was imaging technologies that held a pre-eminent status. Although therapeutics for many neurological conditions remained far from perfect, any number of neurological disorders that would have been permanently crippling or deadly in 1910 had all but vanished from clinics and wards.[5] Patient advocacy organisations, too, had developed around many neurological disorders, creating numerous support networks for families and carers. These improved the experiences of patients.[6] Pharmaceutical discoveries meant that new drugs managed neurological and psychological conditions in ways that would have been unthinkable a century earlier.[7] While many of the worst chronic disorders remained, optimism about their prevention was high and warranted. Thus, in the same period that neurology became an autonomous specialty, physicians and scientists solved many of the field's greatest challenges.

It would seem obvious, then, that science and clinical work must have proceeded together and that developments in the science of the nervous system would have found their way rapidly into clinical practice. That trend, however, is not obvious for several reasons, including the two world wars, which both halted much of the basic scientific research and brought more pragmatic clinical concerns to the foreground. More to the point, many physicians, even when they desired, could see little connection between clinical practice developments in anatomy, physiology, histology, biochemistry, and genetics.[8]

As historian J. Wayne Lazar describes, even the neuron theory, seemingly of self-evident import to the study of the nervous system and its diseases, failed initially to aid clinical neurologists in their diagnostic work.[9] The biochemistry and physiology of neurotransmitters and hormones – acetylcholine, adrenaline, and serotonin – was little understood, and it was only in the late 1940s and 1950s that scientists and physicians in Western countries began to consider the action of those substances germane to the diagnosis and treatment of neurological conditions.[10] Research in the physiology of the nerves and muscles, which developed so substantially between 1920 and 1960, only began to possess clinical relevance to neurologists once Hans Berger introduced the electroencephalogram in 1929 (and then the tool was mainly limited to the study of epilepsy).[11] Of this research, perhaps the most important discoveries advancing clinical neurology were Tracy Putnam and H. Houston Merritt's demonstration that the anti-epileptic Dilatin had fewer noxious psychoactive effects than competing drugs (hence neurologists could begin the hunt for drugs with therapeutic potential but limited psychological side-effects) and Jonas Salk's vaccine for polio, which was developed in the early 1950s.[12]

In other words, despite the appearance now that there must have been direct links between the proto-neurosciences and clinical neurology, the links were limited and typically more of intellectual interest than diagnostic and therapeutic utility. In part, these facts reflected generational differences and realities. For neurologists, the period between 1918 and 1945 was one defined by institution building, administration, and clinical work. The creation of research units devoted to neurological research such as Edward Arnold Carmichael's was a novel event. Only F. L. Golla's directorship of the Bristol-based and newly founded Burden Neurological Clinic truly rivalled the MRC Unit at Queen Square.[13]

In both cases, the *raison d'être* for neurological research remained enigmatic to patrons and clinicians alike, a fact captured rather sharply in the research agenda of the MRC Clinical Neurological Unit during the Second World War.[14] But for the young medical students and registrars training within the new departments and centres devoted to nervous diseases, the work their teachers, mentors, and colleagues had poured into creating new organisational configurations might have gone unrecognised even as these neurologists-in-training identified new research projects and combined them with clinical interests. With the passage of the National Health Service Act of 1946, the organisational and political work needed to continue, and so many of the most senior figures became increasingly disconnected from the scientific developments even as they continued to be involved in their own clinical work, and sometimes also editorships, professional committees, and university, hospital, and professional administration.

As described in the previous chapter, the formation of the Association of British Neurologists (ABN) was one response to these generational challenges. As this chapter will show, the members of the new professional association initially adopted a scientific posture. Their meetings included the by then long tradition of clinical pathological presentations but also provided a venue for studies in physiology, biochemistry, pharmacy, genetics, and bacteriology, as well as psychiatry and psychology that had import for clinical practice. It was at the ABN's meetings where scientific and clinical work merged together. Yet the ABN's original posture quickly transcended the scientific and clinical realms to enter political ones. As this chapter describes, by the 1940s neurologists – mainly leading figures in the ABN – had successfully created a working committee for neurology at the Royal College of Physicians. This committee was capable of organising on behalf of neurologists nationally – an essential activity as the government became active in hospital and healthcare service.

These features of neurology – the scientific research and the clinical practice – never found an easy alliance. The clinical work, the research, and the bureaucratic features and administrative needs of both often appeared as fragmented topics for action. Gains in clinical practice and hospital administration could be offset by declines in research organisation. By the 1950s, neurologists experienced real struggles with both the organisation of medicine and the opportunities for research. To the generation of neurologists who had made their names in the interwar period and were reaching retirement age, younger generations appeared somewhat adrift and perhaps even resentful. To most neurologists in the 1950s, the field appeared to be in decline, a professional discourse that was perhaps exaggerated by similar complaints in North America.[15] The reality was more complicated. The new generation's experiences, however, warrant consideration, for they illustrate the tensions that existed in a specialty that had at last found its own way.

The Association of British Neurologists: science and clinical practice

Was there anything about the ABN that made it different from its predecessors? One feature was its exclusivity; another was self-governance. But further distinctions in the early history of the association are difficult to demonstrate. Few records of the association exist for the 1930s and 1940s. Clearly, the creation of a new professional society of neurologists suggested that there were growing concerns about the limits of the Royal Society of Medicine's Section of Neurology. Indeed, neurologist Macdonald Critchley recalled that the Section of Neurology had been losing popularity as a social and scientific venue for some time.[16] Yet the Hughlings Jackson centenary celebration had been held at the Royal Society of Medicine in 1935, and the 1935 International Neurological Congress in London was hosted there as well.[17] Thus the Section of Neurology remained in 1935 the international face of British neurology. But the majority of the communications to the section were derived from clinical work. There was little new scientific research. Moreover, the audience was mainly drawn from London. It was not a national organisation.

The ABN appears to have been founded as a national version of the London-based Section of Neurology. At the time when the association was founded, 'a list of 51 names was prepared to whom invitations to become Original Members of the Association should be sent.'[18] That list of original members is no longer extant, but it was probably printed in an ABN membership book similar to those extant from the 1970s. The secretary updated that list every year and sent revised editions to members.[19]

Like the Neurological Section of the Royal Society of Medicine, the original membership of the ABN cast a wide occupational net.[20] Though there was by then the occasional full-time neurologist in Britain, the association in its early years remained made up of physicians with wider interests than just neurology, neuropathology, and neurophysiology. Yet the association was more occupationally homogeneous than any British neurological society had ever been. As Macdonald Critchley recollected, it was felt at the time that it was appropriate for 'the founding of a select neurological club...restricted to full-blown consultants'.[21] Peter Robinson, the association's first historian, observed from interviews that the ABN was founded by 'a group of neurologists' who 'wished to have their own forum to discuss clinical and research problems' distinct from more general discussions held at the Section of Neurology.[22] And with only fifty-one members, the Association was certainly exclusive. By contrast, in 1937 the Section of Neurology had 316 members. Nevertheless early presidents and council members (such as Edward Buzzard, Edwin Bramwell, Donald Core, Henry Cohen (1900–77), and Stanley Barnes) had been professors of medicine in their regional medical schools and would not have identified themselves as exclusive neurologists. Nor was membership absolutely restricted to those in clinical practice. E. D. Adrian, for example, although medically qualified, was a Cambridge physiologist. An entry in an undated Rule Book makes the point that: 'The object of the Association is to promote the advancement of the neurological sciences in the British Isles.'[23] The ABN Minute Book was equally ambivalent about whether only clinicians would be admitted:

> On July 28th 1932 a meeting was held at 9 Wimpole Street, London [Gordon Holmes' residence], at which it was decided to form an Association of British Neurologists, the membership of which should be limited to those actively engaged in any branch of Neurology.[24]

Membership therefore indicated growing consensus that a specialty of neurology existed and deserved independent status, but what that status entailed was not self-evident. The careful appeal in the minutes to the branches of neurology left the matter open-ended.

Founding the association was undoubtedly a 'movement towards neurological autonomy', but it is easy to believe that its original members would have found vulgar any activity publicly agitating for reforms for neurology.[25] Thus the tenor of the association in early years was one of subdued exclusivity and a club-like atmosphere. Indeed non-members presented papers but could only attend their portion of the meeting. They were asked to leave at the next break.[26]

Neurologists who remembered the early meetings readily recalled the terror they experienced in presenting their first paper to the association. The paper's quality of delivery was generally held to be decisive for election.[27] Communications were presented informally. The audience was solemn and sometimes pernickety.[28] When John David Spillane (1909–85) was elected president of the association in 1974, it was recalled that his first paper had been greeted by Francis Walshe's barbed comment: 'clearly *someone* [i.e. other than Spillane] will have to look into all this.'[29] When the association hosted the Society of British Neurosurgeons in 1959, Charles Symonds remarked dryly at the formal dinner: 'there was some difficulty in finding a time when they [i.e. all of the neurologists] were all on speaking terms with one another.'[30]

One meeting was held per year throughout the 1930s and 1940s. In 1950 a second meeting was added to the programme.[31] The annual meetings of the 1930s were uneventful. The minutes record mainly scientific communications. Rare was anything resembling broader political communication.[32] Usually the new president-elect would close the annual meeting by inviting the association to his home city. Edwin Bramwell, for instance, presided over the fourth annual meeting and had invited the association to meet in Edinburgh at the third meeting in 1935.[33] The council would typically meet in London early in the year and plan an administrative agenda for the coming annual meeting's arrangements. In January 1936, Bramwell and the council met in London to plan the coming meeting. By then, Bramwell had arranged for the general meeting to be held at the Edinburgh Royal Medical Society and the reception and dinner at the Royal College of Physicians, Edinburgh, and interestingly: 'It was decided to hold [the meeting] in the same weekend as when the Physiological Society meets...if possible.'[34] Commonly a second meeting of the council was held later in the spring, where new members were nominated and last details finalised.[35] The fourth annual meeting occurred in June 1936. After a new member – Samuel Nevin (1905–79) – was elected, the scientific proceedings began and were only occasionally interrupted by breaks for tea. Thirteen papers were presented, and although mainly clinical, these were representative of a broader scientific activity. E. D. Adrian, for example, presented a paper entitled 'Cortical Activity due to Electrical Stimulation'.[36]

Attendance varied. Only thirty-one members attended the fourth annual meeting (although some physiologists attended). Regular attendance would not be much larger until the 1970s.[37] In general, the association alternated its meetings between London and the extra-capital medical centres. In the former, the meetings were held at various institutions. Extra-metropolitan meetings tended to be in cities with universities. In 1937 the association held its first joint meeting with a neurological society from abroad.[38] That same year the ABN began recognising overseas members, although these could only be former members taking up 'appointments abroad'.[39]

The year 1939 was the last year the association convened its annual meeting until 1945. An administrative meeting was held in 1944, and the pattern of annual general meetings resumed in 1945.[40] Thereafter, business continued as usual and followed the pattern established in the 1930s. Only two noteworthy changes occurred from the pre-war circumstance: one was that attendance (as well as the number of members permitted to join) began increasing slightly. The second was that the council of the association began collaborating with the Royal College of Physicians to reform neurology.[41]

As already noted, few records of the ABN's proceedings and administration have been located. The minutes, though detailed, are not especially illuminating as to the social experience of the 1930s. Nor have many records pertaining to the association been located in the personal papers collections of its members. Edwin Bramwell's diary provides one of the few extant descriptions from the 1930s. It is therefore worth recounting. Bramwell describes his night train journey from Edinburgh to London. At the meeting, which was at the National Hospital, Edward Buzzard 'vacated the Chair' for Stanley Barnes, then Dean of the Medical Faculty in Birmingham. Bramwell then recorded:

> A very successful meeting: There must have been fifty present. Last year at Leeds there were only twenty-three. It has been suggested that the Association meets [sic] every second year in London. After the Meeting, Greenfield showed us round the new Rockefeller extension and laboratories. In the evening the Association dined at the Langham – an excellent dinner, twelve and sixpence exclusive of wines. We sit where we choose at these dinners; I sat between Farquhar Buzzard and Symonds. The dinner was very enjoyable.[42]

He noted the following day: 'Yesterday's meeting was continued at 9.30 at the National Hospital. There were six communications again today. The most interesting, I think, were Adrian on Electrical Stimulation, Graham Brown on Reflex Gait in Decerebrate Cats, and Riddoch on Phantom Limbs. I left Kings Cross at 1.20 arriving home at 8.45.'[43]

Bramwell's account, while succinct, draws attention to certain details of the association that might otherwise be ignored. Because it was a society for neurologists across Britain, travel to the meetings became one of the investments of membership. His mention of a tour of the new Rockefeller Wards at the National Hospital, which were finally operational, is also interesting. It can be taken as an indicator of a growing recognition of the changes and modernisation taking place within neurology. His reference to E. D. Adrian and T. Graham Brown's papers is particularly noteworthy since it calls attention to the physiological contributions presented at the society. Such a nod towards basic science shows that the clinicians recognised the growing importance of nerve physiology, chemistry, and physics even as those sciences' clinical implications remained unclear.

In general, it is difficult to judge whether papers at all of the annual meetings were scientific or clinical in their focus. Of 141 papers recorded in the minutes as presented at these meetings in the first ten years (1933–39 and 1946–48), fifty-seven neurologists presented papers, while sixty commented at least at once during the same period (it is noteworthy that whoever asked questions was mentioned in the minutes). Thirty-four members of the ABN presented at least two papers in ten years. Forty-four members took part in the discussions at least twice in ten years. In this decade, three women participated in the meetings: Dorothy Russell, Helen Dimsdale, and a Miss G. Griffiths. Each was introduced to the members during this period. None, in other words, had been an original member. Dorothy Russell was a pathologist and an original member of the Society of British Neurosurgeons. She may also have been the ABN's first woman member.

Scrutiny of those who presented and commented in the first ten years (1933–39 and 1945–47) tells us a little more about the power structure of the association.[44] On average, Gordon Holmes, unquestionably central in the association's proceedings, was involved in discussions three times at each meeting but presented only one original paper. Charles Symonds spoke twenty-three times at ten different meetings but presented only three papers in those years. Samuel Alexander Kinnier Wilson contributed no papers but spoke seventeen times at four meetings of the ABN (he died in 1937). His was by far the highest average contribution per meeting at a minimum of five times per meeting. Ritchie Russell offered eight original papers and participated in fifteen discussions. He had been appointed Lecturer in Neurology at Edinburgh University in 1938 following Edwin Bramwell's retirement (in 1949 the faculty at Oxford appointed Ritchie Lecturer in Neurology and in 1966 he became their first Chair of Clinical Neurology). Philip Cloake presented two papers in this period but participated in discussions thirteen times (he became Honorary Professor of Neurology in Birmingham in 1946). Likewise George Riddoch discussed the presentations thirteen times. He, however, presented four original papers. It is not surprising that these clinicians largely reported on clinical work. Nor is it surprising that they offered talks with less frequency than individuals with full-time appointments outside clinical medicine.

By contrast, for example, Joseph Godwin Greenfield, pathologist at the National Hospital, presented the largest number of original research papers at the ABN. He participated on thirteen different occasions in the discussion. While neuropathology was self-evidently relevant to clinical and scientific neurology, his contributions could also be cast as somewhat traditional in terms of basic science. Greenfield eventually founded the Neuropathological Club. E. D. Adrian, the association's one Nobel Prize winner, offered four papers on physiological topics. Edward Arnold Carmichael presented eight times. Doubtless his position as Director to the MRC's Neurological Research Unit made it impossible for him not to participate. Similarly, Swithin Meadows, a Halley Stewart Research Fellow in Carmichael's unit, presented four papers at these meetings.

What to make of these patterns that defined the ABN in the interwar and early post-war periods? The established members of the association spoke often but produced less. The younger members, by contrast, produced more but spoke less. One pattern is obvious: the most productive junior members were also those who eventually came to occupy positions of influence and leadership within the association and in the specialty. None of these observations is necessarily surprising. They do, however, reveal both a hierarchical structure in the making and also a burgeoning sense that young practitioners could make their careers through achievements in research. Other than an increase in the number of meetings per year and the mounting of a lobbying campaign for British neurological services, these trends continued into the 1960s. Indeed, except for an expansion in members, the ABN has changed little from these past configurations. The exception was during the Second World War, a time when the ABN met but little.

Wartime clinical practice and science and the political reorganisation of medicine

Britain declared war on Germany on 3 September 1939. A few days earlier the Third International Neurological Congress had convened in Copenhagen (from 21 to 25 August), where German, French, American, and British neurologists (among others) had been together.[45] The meeting in Copenhagen must have been tense. Preparations for war had been in the making in Britain since 1938 and many neurologists had been involved from the beginning in the small committees that came to engage in political and wartime organisation, a mode of organisation, which had, as historian Alan Young observed, several drawbacks.[46] Such committees had little power. While members could identify problems and propose corrections, they often lacked the ability to effect policy changes. In an interesting contrast, committees concerned with neurological research and treatment in this period were often highly successful.

As there were no meetings of the ABN from 7 of May 1939 until 29 January 1944, the question arises of how members of the association were occupied during the war.[47] Many of the ABN's members in London and across the nation were in constant contact with each other.[48] In addition to providing a neurology service, many sought to coordinate Ministry of Health provisions for soldiers with nerve injuries with a MRC clinical research study on the treatment of those conditions – i.e. science and clinical work merged around a pragmatic question. The remarkably successful direction of these projects aided the emergence of neurology under the National Health Service (NHS) and indeed may have even created important precedents for the regionalised plan that defined the new health service.

In Britain, government preparations for war throughout 1938 and 1939 had focused on a number of elements. These included evacuation plans for civilians during air raids and more generally arranging emergency medical services for large numbers of civilian casualties.[49] A Ministry of Health committee (which included Gordon Holmes) had drawn up a plan for the organisation of hospital services in war.[50] Anticipating the greatest medical crisis Britain had ever faced, the officials at the Ministry of Health began contemplating administrative policies that divided national health services into regionalised systems that could cope with military and civilian casualties and support a national blood transfusion service.[51] The London medical service was divided into ten sectors, each led by one of the teaching hospitals. Casualties flooding into those main hospitals would be relocated to outlying (usually municipal) hospitals, aiming to move the wounded away from further harm.[52]

Away from London, committees of voluntary and municipal hospital authorities coordinated regional services which would both respond to local conditions and implement national recommendations from the Ministry of Health.[53] One future effect of this regional and nationalised planning and general incursion of government into the voluntary and municipal hospital systems was the formation of the National Health Service.[54] A more immediate effect, according to Rosemary Stevens, was the creation of centres providing a range of specialist services for patients with war injuries.[55] These centres proved important for neurology in many ways and partially justified calls neurologists would make after the war ended for broader recognition of their specialty.

During the war, officials at the Ministry of Health and the MRC formed another set of centres throughout Britain to provide medical services to soldiers with brain, spinal, and peripheral nerve injuries.[56] These centres were initially formed for a broad research study being carried out by the MRC into the treatment of nerve injuries.[57] In an unprecedented inter-ministry collaboration, the secretary of the MRC offered to coordinate the MRC research project with a regionalised plan to provide services to wounded soldiers with nervous injuries being initiated through the Ministry of Health.[58] Three MRC committees had been formed to deal with research questions on brain, spine, and nerve injuries. Each committee had included neurologists, physiologists, and orthopaedic surgeons.[59] Eventually these committees were combined into one committee for nerve injuries. By then the Ministry of Health and the MRC had begun collaborating on treatment and research.[60]

Initially, the major research and treatment centres were Wingfield-Morris in Oxford, Winwick in Lancashire, and Botleys Park in Surrey.[61]

Facilities in Newcastle, Liverpool, Bristol, Sheffield, Edinburgh, Glasgow, and Birmingham were soon developed as well. By 1944, there were twenty-five facilities in Britain for patients with nerve injuries. All provided neurological services. Most of these later centres were treatment facilities only, but at least four were involved in the MRC's research programme as well.[62]

One general purpose of these treatment centres was outlined in a 1941 Ministry of Health memo:

> The object is to secure as much continuity of treatment as possible and to ensure that the patient who needs it is able to return to examination and, if required, treatment after a suitable interval. Ideally, all further examination and treatment would take place at the Special Centre where original treatment is given, but the distance of the patient's home and practical difficulties of travel and loss of time may preclude this in many cases.[63]

Missing from this mission statement was the additional provision that gainful employment for all of the wounded was the ultimate goal.[64] Also missing was a statement about the research goals of many of these centres, a point often lost upon uninformed physicians working in them.[65] The logistics of treatment at these centres was also difficult to manage. Coordinating treatment at these centres fell into administrative disarray, chiefly because two ministries as well as the MRC were involved.

The Ministry of Pensions was expected to pay transport costs of wounded soldiers seeking treatment and being followed up. The Ministry of Health was expected to notify the Ministry of Pensions that services were being provided and the expected rate for compensation. They were also to make sure that patients came back for additional examinations and treatment.[66] Finally the MRC had to coordinate with the two ministries to ensure that patients involved in research studies understood that they were supposed to return to their original treatment centres for follow-up examinations and that they could afford to come back.[67] The work of these centres has been judged to be of tremendous importance in terms of original research and effective treatment.[68] Certainly fulfiling the requirements of their general mission statement was no small administrative feat, but how happy patients were with the care they received, and what was the long-term impact of the research conducted there, are questions beyond the scope of this study.[69]

From 1939 until 1941, the Ministry of Health did not recognise neurologists working in nerve injury facilities as specialists. They were classified as general physicians.[70] This situation was eventually corrected by George Riddoch. Riddoch (1889–1947), born in northern Scotland and educated in medicine at Aberdeen University, had become house physician at the West End Hospital for Nervous Diseases in London, and served at the Empire Hospital for Injuries of the Nervous System during the First World War.[71] It was from that period that his interest in nerve injuries dated, and it had been partially stimulated by his mentor, Henry Head. Riddoch was one of the first physicians to receive the support of the MRC for neurological research. His 1920 research project at the London Hospital focused on nerve injuries, and the subject was one that dominated his research interests throughout his professional career.

With war declared in 1939, Riddoch initially found himself in an Emergency Medical Services (EMS) unit at Chase Farm Hospital, which was the site to which the Neurological Department of the London Hospital had been evacuated. He eventually accepted a commission as brigadier general and 'devoted himself to the organisation of the Army neurological service'.[72] One obituarist, failing to note Riddoch's many administrative commitments to the MRC, observed that by 1938 Riddoch held administrative posts in the army, the Emergency Medical Services, and the Ministry of Pensions. He added:

> The development of centres for the treatment of wounds of the brain, spine, and peripheral nerves proved to be an essential part of the medical war effort, but the part Dr Riddoch played in insisting on the need for these centres and in guiding their development may have to some extent been forgotten. His tireless round of visits to those special centres was of great value in developing the remarkably high standard of treatment which was achieved, and this has often been acknowledged by the surgeons in charge of these special units.[73]

The account underreports: in a 1944 letter to Russell Brain, Riddoch acknowledge that his army and Emergency Medical Services work 'is not slackening and it well may increase'.[74] Most of his obituarists agree that his commitment to these posts quickly turned to overexertion.[75] Between 1938 and 1947, Riddoch balanced a large private practice, teaching and hospital practice at three hospitals, as well as all his government positions.[76] Testifying to these efforts are records in the National Archives. From 1938 until 1947, Riddoch's name appears everywhere in files pertaining to neurological subjects. His correspondence for the Ministry of Health, the Ministry of Pensions, and the MRC was voluminous. The number of different committees in which his name appears is equally impressive. It was these many-sided commitments and his intensity in completing the work he took on that led E. D. Adrian to eulogise him in *The Times*: 'His responsibilities were too great to be set aside for care of his own health and he worked to the end with the same courage which he inspired in his patients. He was a man of great ability, great personal charm, and great integrity.'[77]

In many ways, George Riddoch was responsible for initiating and maintaining the standards of treatment in all twenty-five brain, spine, and nerve injuries centres that emerged throughout Britain between 1940 and 1945. He also continually reminded physicians and administrators in those centres of the broader neurological research agenda. It was Riddoch who pointed out the problems created by the Ministry of Health's original refusal to recognise neurologists officially.

In a 1941 letter to the secretary of the Emergency Medical Services, Francis Fraser, Riddoch noted that neurologists were encountering a number of administrative difficulties, chiefly because government ministries – Health and Pensions – did not recognise their role. This fact had allowed a myth to flourish in nerve injuries centres that neurological research and treatment requirements for the MRC research project fell into second place in priority to the demands made by orthopaedic surgeons or the general edicts of hospital administrators:

> In regard to the Neurologist at each of the Centres in England, I think it would be helpful it they were officially recognised by the E.M.S. as acting in that capacity. As you know, each centre is officially in charge of an orthopaedic surgeon who does not always pass on information to the neurological colleague, and official recognition I think would ease matters. It would also be helpful if communications in regard to treatment and management were sent to the Neurologist at each Centre as well as the orthopaedic surgeon.[78]

The duties of neurologists and orthopaedic surgeons were similar and therefore deserving of equal recognition and status. A compromise, Riddoch suggested, between both workers was always required. Both workers had more control than hospital administrators commonly admitted.[79] The Ministry of Health baulked. It was reluctant because 'there are administrative objections to the official recognition of the Neurologists.'[80] What the basis for these objections was is not now clear. However, shortly after Riddoch made his complaint, Ministry of Health policy changed. Neurologists became appointed specialists.[81] Gordon Holmes, then neurological representative on the Emergency Medical Services Hospital Committee, received a letter indicating that fact: 'At the request of Dr Riddoch it has been suggested that...Medical Officers should be recognised as the Neurologists to the Peripheral Nerve Injury Centres.'[82] Holmes instantly saw Riddoch's achievement – another major national precedent had been set for the recognition of neurologists across Britain within government ministries.[83]

Measuring the outcome of that government recognition on neurology is harder to judge. As described in Chapter 2, among Walter Russell Brain's personal papers in the Royal College of Physicians is an undated report titled 'The Organization of Neurology in London after the War'.[84] Much in the source is worth analysing in the context of Riddoch's work. In the report's conclusions, Brain suggested several ways in which neurological services could be expanded across the country and proposed that the regionalisation of neurological services in Britain would be an exemplary means for organising services for all medical patients across the United Kingdom. He noted, for instance, that the policy of the Emergency Medical Services might be expanded by the Ministry of Health and made a permanent feature of future developments for neurology:

> The E.M.S. sector service has shown that it is possible to arrange a neurological unit for a Sector applying consultant service to all the hospitals, municipal, and voluntary, in that Sector even though the municipal hospitals belong to more than one authority, the Sector neurological service based upon a teaching hospital. In this way, a specialist service has become available to many patients who would otherwise have been admitted to hospitals where they would not normally be seen by a neurologist. Such a system as this could readily form the basis of a post-war organization, while perhaps

> ten or twelve sectors of the E.M.S. type would be needed for a neurological medical service, it would probably be impossible to have as many neurosurgical units and arrangements would have to be made whereby two or more sectors would be served by a single neurosurgical unit.[85]

It can be inferred without difficulty that Brain was referring in his report to the nerve injury centres being run by the Ministry of Health.[86] George Riddoch and Russell Brain had worked together in the neurological department at the London Hospital – indeed Riddoch was among those who recommended Brain to the London Hospital's permanent staff.[87] Riddoch's influence had actually led Brain to take up neurology.[88] Brain had administrative ambitions for neurology as well, and it is difficult to imagine that he was not in regular communication with Riddoch about developments in the Emergency Medical Services. However, because of the paucity of sources on this point, it is difficult to determine in what way either the existence of these new centres or Brain's report influenced the post-war organisation of neurological services. Both, however, may have greatly influenced the event that finally brought the members of the ABN back together in January 1944.[89]

Pragmatic choices in clinical neurology: the health service and neurologists

Although the members of the association did not meet throughout the war, it is clear that many were adopting new perspectives on politics and medical organisation. A new agenda for neurology was contrived partly by the ABN and partly by the Royal College of Physicians. On 29 January 1944, twenty-five members of the ABN convened 'to discuss questions on the teaching and practice of Neurology and the possible Official Grading of Neurologists in the future'.[90] At the close of the meeting six proposals had been adopted. Each would have substantial ramifications for neurology in the near future. The association's members voted that the Standing Joint Committee of the three Royal Colleges be asked to recognise the ABN 'as representing the specialty of neurology' in Britain. The Standing Joint Committee had been formed in 1933 between the

Royal College of Surgeons and the Royal College of Physicians to 'consider matters of common concern' in medicine and surgery.[91] Historian Rosemary Stevens described the Joint Committee as one of the first existing opportunities for specialists and consultants to enter debates on 'the sphere of national policy and planning'.[92] The decision of the members of the ABN to request this recognition was therefore a movement towards the national recognition of neurology as plans for the nationalisation of medicine advanced in government.

The association's members proposed that Charles Symonds should represent the association's interests on the Beveridge Committee, provided the Royal College of Physicians desired a formal representative. Neurologists were concerned that their financial interests and autonomy should be properly defended in pending debates on national health insurance.[93] They also unanimously recommended that psychiatrists and neurologists receive similar training, which should not commence 'until after one year's residence in Hospital after qualification'.[94] This training would be spread over four years. There would no 'Diploma in Neurology' because it was considered 'highly desirable that all neurologist specialists should possess a higher qualification in General Medicine, as the M.R.C.P., London'.[95] It was also planned that representatives of the Royal Medico-Psychological Association should be solicited to form a joint subcommittee with neurologists from the ABN to 'formulate a scheme for common basic training'.[96] These proposals marked a new era for British neurology. Such wilful political agitation would have been unthinkable for neurologists even ten years before.

Subsequent ABN meetings in 1944 and 1945 enhanced these developments. The council of the Royal Medico-Psychological Association agreed to meet with representatives from the ABN to discuss the training of neurologists and psychiatrists. The results of those discussions have not been located, although in 1944 the ABN minutes recommended: 'that the training and qualifications of specialists in neurology should be discussed at the Annual Meeting.'[97] At that time the ABN's council also recommended that 'The Royal College of Physicians be requested to set up a Committee to consider the training and qualifications of specialists in neurology.'[98] The Committee on Neurology was subsequently formed.[99]

Generally the years between 1944 and 1950 marked a period of increasing political participation by neurologists.[100] Their participation was often half-hearted. In 1947, when a committee for the Ministry of Health was investigating appropriate levels of remuneration for consultants and specialists, the ABN's minutes noted, 'It was decided to recommend to the committee that whatever terms were agreed for consulting general physicians should apply also to consulting neurologists.'[101] Although in the subsequent Ministry of Health report neurology was mentioned (only once) as a medical specialty, one possible effect of their apathy was a persisting conflation of neurology with general medical practice.[102] General medical culture continued to resist the idea of neurology as an independent specialty.

This inability to discriminate between neurology and general medicine had a curious consequence. The supposed crisis in British neurology which became evident to many in the 1950s, derived mainly from ambivalence about definitions. Neurology in the 1940s was thought to require knowledge of pathology, as well as an understanding of the connections between biology and physiology, and experience in numerous day-to-day general medical encounters. The result of these needs was that definitional ambiguity and relativism, as well as a pluralistic outlook, remained reigning hallmarks of neurological practice. Encounters with symptoms took many shapes. There were, for example, mental and physical signs of nervous diseases. None was necessarily the exclusive domain of neurology, but conditions combining many of those signs – e.g. cancers of the endocrine system – often required the best skills of a neurologist in diagnosis and prognosis.

Such an integrative approach required policymakers to have a special understanding of the field. Yet neurologists rarely communicated this aspect of their practice (or the value of the approach) to administrators and policymakers. The consequence was that neurologists continually highlighted commonalities between general medicine and neurology. It seems clear that this fact represented generational divisions: to the more senior figures the relationship between neurology and general medicine could not be disentangled. Younger neurologists experienced these challenges differently. Such accretion implied to policymakers and regional hospital authorities that general physicians with some neurological experience could handle neurological work. The outcome was that while some beds would be allocated in hospitals for neurological patients, few medical students were trained in neurology, and positions for neurologists were only created slowly in the 1950s.[103]

The Royal College of Physicians and the problem of neurology

In 1944 the council of the ABN proposed that the Royal College of Physicians form a Committee on Neurology. The likely stimulus was the 1944 report of the Inter-Departmental Committee on Medical Schools (known as the Goodenough Report), which completely ignored neurology.[104] The first meeting of the Royal College Committee on Neurology convened in December 1944.[105]

Members of the first Committee on Neurology mirrored the council of the ABN in 1944. Stanley Barnes, from Birmingham and then president of the ABN, was the first chairman of this committee. He was assisted by Lord Moran (then president of the Royal College of Physicians), Anthony Feiling, James Godwin Greenfield, and Philip Cloake (all of these members, save Moran, were on the ABN's council). There was also George Riddoch, Russell Brain, Aubrey Lewis (1900–75) representing psychiatry, Denis Brinton, Swithin Meadows (1902–93), Samuel Nevin, Harold Boldero (1889–1960), and John Elkington (1904–63).[106]

Initially the committee's remit was the training of neurologists. The committee was also to provide an explanation for neurology's relationship with general medicine and psychiatry.[107] The committee members recognised early on that there were tendencies to use consultant and specialist as synonyms, but their understanding was complex: 'It was generally agreed that the term "consultant" denoted a higher status than the term "specialist" but the Committee were of the opinion that it would not be necessary for this distinction in grade to be made in the subject of neurology.'[108] The neurologist thus remained the embodiment of the generalist-specialist practitioner; always a consultant and not a specialist. Though the title 'consultant' bridged the gap between specialist and generalist, it emphasised a status-conscious distinction implied by the neurologist-physician category.

In retrospect, that distinction appears somewhat artificial. But at the time the committee considered two categories seriously: '(1) the consultant neurologist who confined himself to neurology (2) the consultant neurologist who combined the work with general medicine.'[109] This unsurprising continuation of ambiguities from the past, though a realistic assessment of the conditions of the present, shows how many members of this committee could not envision how transformed social healthcare in Britain would be in the near future.

Ten years later, much would be different, but in 1944 the neurologists, though threatened by a new social order, had not yet overturned older priorities for the new ones that nationalisation would soon create.

Their first report, submitted to the members of the ABN and the Royal College of Physicians in 1945, described the differences and similarities between neurology and psychiatry, emphasised the closeness of neurology to general medicine, and offered guidelines for the training of the neurologist.[110] The members of the committee rejected a special Diploma in Neurology averring that the MRCP was the lowest qualification any neurologist should possess. Finally, recommendations were offered regarding the organisation of neurological services outside London. Among the aims they advocated was establishing 'an active neurological department in all medical teaching centres and in such other centres of population as may be considered necessary to cover the needs of the country'.[111] The constant reminders that neurology and general medicine could be united and that general physicians with training in neurology could provide neurological services placed a strong limit on the language of the report.[112] Yet the report was practical in its aspirations. If there were not enough neurologists now, then general physicians would be required to treat patients with nervous diseases. Yet the authors insisted that the lack of neurological centres and neurologists was a problem the state needed to resolve in short order. In sum, the report was the most concise programmatic statement ever issued on the state of neurology in Britain.

The report's message, however, could have been easily misinterpreted. One failing of the report was that it never explained what neurologists did and why their practice was important. The only justification given for neurology was historical:

> Neurology was one of the first medical specialties to be recognised and to be accorded a status of its own. During an important period in the history of medicine it was the most active growing edge of the subject and formed an ideal point for the entry of the scientific method into clinical medicine.[113]

There can be no doubt that this historical claim was significant from the committee's perspective, but it should be appreciated that non-neurologists might have viewed the claim differently. Was it implying that the important period in medical history was now over? Was the claim contending that because neurology had done so much for medicine in the past, it merited support now; or was it suggesting there would be future contributions no less significant than those of the past? Moreover, there was no sense of what new scientific and clinical research was promising or what was immediately relevant to neurological practice. Adding to this dilemma was the report's conciliatory stance towards psychiatry and general medicine. On one hand, psychiatry and neurology were close because 'each is concerned with the function of the brain.'[114] On the other hand, 'neurology remains a part...of general medicine.'[115] Any reader – lay or medical – could be forgiven for wondering what then was necessary about neurology per se.[116] Obviously this lack of clarity was not the intention of the committee, but the outcome was damaging – a fact later reflected in meetings of the committee and the actions it and the ABN took to counteract it in the 1950s.

The council of the ABN during the early 1950s was not particularly adept at handling the apparent political crisis. Two years after the National Health Service had been established, a critical investigation carried out by the Ministry of Health explored how the consultant medical service could be expanded throughout Britain.[117] The investigation ultimately placed neurology and cardiology's special relationship to general medicine into perspective: 'General physicians will...need to undertake some neurological and cardiological work.'[118] Thus, while neurologists and cardiologists would be required in regional centres, the investigation found that 'it is undesirable that general medicine should be so rigidly sub-divided that all the cardiological or neurological work becomes concentrated in the hands of consultants engaged only in those subjects.'[119] The investigation was not hostile to neurological specialisation per se, but neither did it hold out hope for a rapid structural change. 'There are not yet enough neurologists to provide a complete neurological service, and it will be necessary at first to make use of physicians who do not restrict their practice entirely to this specialty.'[120] Neurological departments still did not exist in most of the regional centres and 'such a comprehensive arrangement is not likely to be feasible for some years.'[121] There were not enough beds for neurological patients, and consequently 'patients admitted to hospital with nervous diseases cannot be directly under the care of a neurologist' and would be in the care of a general physician 'with a special interest in neurology'.[122] There were too few neurologists, almost no neurological departments, and neurological beds were located in general medical wards. The unintended consequence of claiming that neurology and general medicine were closely aligned was that the claim had allowed top-down pressure at both national and regional levels to flourish and drive neurologists into general medical positions.[123] Overall, the Ministry of Health recognised the problem as a national one but offered few solutions to what was a local problem. In fact, regional hospital boards preferred these circumstances; they effectively meant that patients were treated but that there was no need to form a neurological department.[124]

The ABN left this situation unchallenged until 1953. Between 1950 and 1955 the only significant move it took was to ask that all International Neurological Congress planning committees recognise the association as officially representing neurology in Britain.[125] The Committee on Neurology, at the request of Russell Brain, reconvened in 1953. Its new terms of reference were: 'the training of specialists in neurology, the conditions of recognition as a consultant in Neurology', and 'any other matters of importance to the development and welfare of neurology'.[126] Its report on the position of neurology was published in 1954 and was far more strongly worded than its 1945 predecessor.[127] A neurologist, the report stated clearly, was:

> a trained physician with a higher qualification in medicine who has received the necessary special training and experience in neurology and proposes thereafter to devote himself to that specialty. This definition *does not include* those general physicians who have gained some experience in neurology in the course of their training in general medicine and who include an interest in neurology as part of their general medical practice.[128]

This definition was essentially a corrective to the misinterpretation of the role of the general physician with an interest in neurology. Noting that medical specialisation remained 'controversial' and 'difficult' and that many felt it undesirable, the report claimed:

> Echoes of this controversy can be heard in the present context and the view is held by some in influential positions that in the provinces it is better, on the whole, that the neurology should be done by

> general physicians and that both the practice and teaching of general medicine might be impoverished by the appointment of more neurologists.[129]

The committee was not complacent. Circumstances, it claimed, were now 'worse' under the National Health Services than they had been in 1945.[130] They were worse, not because neurology was unnecessary, but because the government and the regional hospital boards for reasons of 'financial stringency' had committed themselves to an anti-progressive alliance 'contrary to the best interests of the Health Service'.[131] It was recommended that active neurological departments be immediately established 'in all medical teaching centres and in such other centres of population as may be considered necessary to cover the needs of the country'.[132] Moreover, no neurosurgical centre should be established without positions for neurologists. The report ended with a polemical blow:

> [The] Committee desires to draw attention to the serious long-term effects of the policy at presented adopted in the Health Service in relation to neurology. After the war, relying on the promised expansion of the consultant services and being aware of the need for more consultant neurologists, a considerable number of ex-service graduates undertook and completed their training as neurologists. Of these, only 15 per cent. have been able to find reasonable employment...in this country. At least five have emigrated. Promising graduates now regard the prospects as so discouraging that they are becoming increasingly reluctant to enter a branch of medicine in which this country is pre-eminent.[133]

There was no pluralism in the report. Nor was there relativist phrasing. Clinical neurology was constructed as an absolute clinical specialty. It was independent from both general medicine and psychiatry. The National Health Service was wasting talent by not offering opportunities for young graduates. In so doing, it was undermining the long-term quality of its neurological service. British neurology had led the world in the 1930s. That distinction was being systematically dismantled by government policies.

Such strongly worded language was not greeted with much enthusiasm. Members of the Comitia of the Royal College of

Physicians thought the case had been 'exaggerated'.[134] In a general committee discussion, one member, wondering what neurologists actually did, tactlessly pointed out that neurology's problem was not its specialisation but its inabilities. 'If they looked at the work done by the present neurologist, they would find that his time was completely taken up with a very long waiting list in outpatients, with chronic epileptics and similar cases, most of whom he cannot help at all.'[135] Another more constructively suggested that the problem was mainly financial. However, a third member stressed that the crisis was neither economic nor political. The trouble was a social one within the profession of medicine. The regional boards were not reluctant to hire neurologists. Instead the medical advice they received neglected neurologists. 'His impression was that many physicians would not welcome neurologists. They would rather have another general physician with a special interest in neurology.'[136]

These complaints show that while the 1954 report was controversial, it had succeeded in highlighting a new set of questions and eliciting a general response.[137] The council of the ABN, agreeing with the language of the report, formed a subcommittee 'to consider the status of Neurology in the National Health Service and to advise the Council on any action to be taken'.[138] By 1955, the Joint Consultants Committee (a body Rosemary Stevens described as giving 'leaders of the profession...more control of the future of doctors than had ever been given') had agreed to support the ABN and the mission of rapidly expanding neurological services.[139] It also advocated the creation of a post in the Ministry of Health for the 'appointment of a Consultant Advisor in Neurology'.[140] Importantly, informal discussion had made it clear 'that the Ministry were aware of the problem' of neurology 'and were most anxious to help in the creation of new posts'.[141] By 1958, Russell Brain, his tenure as president of the Royal College of Physicians recently completed, was appointed, 'Advisor in Neurology to the Ministry of Health as a result of Representations by the Association'.[142] In 1959, when the World Federation of Neurology was founded, the ABN was recognised by it as the official body 'speaking on behalf of Great Britain in neurological matters'.[143] All further influence of the Neurological Section of the Royal Society of Medicine ended in 1960, the same year that Russell Brain became the ABN president.[144] Political and social control of neurology was now entirely vested in the ABN.

The work of research

How were these organisational activities reflected in neurological research? Despite ongoing reports of investigations at ABN meetings and work at the MRC Clinical Neurological Research Unit at Queen Square, it is clear that the period from 1935 to 1955 was a challenging one for neurologists. The direction that clinical investigations should follow was somewhat uncertain and many neurologists experienced this uncertainty as evidence that the field was in decline. The 1950s, as historian Gordon Shepherd has observed, were revolutionary in the neurosciences, but many of those innovations became important for neurologists only in the decades that followed.[145] Edward Arnold Carmichael, for one, appears to have exemplified this challenge. A telling anecdote appears in his obituary:

> After the war [Carmichael] felt that the methods he and his collaborators had developed previously for studying autonomic responses had passed the peak of the usefulness. Rather than trying to revise these methods or learn new techniques, he decided that the best contribution he could make would be by providing facilities for younger people and encouraging them in following their own line of interest. In this policy he was a complete antithesis to the 'director' and he refused steadfastly to allow his name to be put on any paper unless he had taken a major share in the work leading to it. Advice, criticism, and occasional nudge were all just part of his job. So perhaps it was natural that he should be nicknamed affectionately 'the Boss'.[146]

Carmichael's attitude should not be interpreted as complacency. He occupied a central position in particularly ambiguous circumstances, circumstances that can be better illustrated by tracing views about the future direction of neurology. In 1933, the year the ABN formed, Francis Walshe observed that a central feature of neurology was its variety of scientific questions worthy of investigating and the methods that might be deployed in so doing:

> Neurology makes a strong appeal to men of many interests and diverse temperaments. The man with a flair for clinical medicine finds no branch of the subject that offers him more fascinating

> exercises; for the pathologist, the nervous system is a rich mine of problems awaiting discovery and solution; for the biochemist, it offers a new world scarcely yet explored, while for the experimental physiologist, it has been the scene of some of his greatest triumphs.[147]

But, as Walshe went on to observe, neurology was also dependent upon its special – semiological – method. The neurologist had to possess a profound practical training. It took time to train the neurologist in this way.

> However wide and deep may be the individual's knowledge of the anatomy, physiology or pathology of the nervous system, however cunning his hand and judgment in surgical technique, he is not and cannot become a neurologist in the full sense of this word until he is conversant with the phenomena and natural history of diseases of the nervous system and is the master of the clinical method.[148]

The clinical neurological researcher was thus profoundly ambitious. He or she needed to understand the principles of clinical practice and develop a wide knowledge of the methods used in a variety of the sciences. Walshe's view might have made sense in the 1930s, a time when more students were entering neurology and more opportunities for employment became available. But with the war and a subsequently lacklustre government policy regarding the specialty, such a position created structural impediments to generational transfer in neurology, a fact exaggerated when some students emigrated to America.

For reasons such as these, Edward Arnold Carmichael's wait-and-see attitude can be seen as rather wise, but his attitude speaks also to why so many neurologists articulated a sense of decline in the 1950s about their field's institutional status and lack of original research, even at a time when the field was represented institutionally and politically better than it had ever been before.[149] Nowhere was the contradiction between neurologists' perceptions about their work and its new institutional circumstances more sharply delineated than at a meeting to consider 'The Future of Neurology', held at the offices of the MRC in 1960. The meeting began with the view that neurology was in decline. In the minutes from the discussion, the neurologists followed their typical course by defining neurology in their usual broad fashion: neurology ranged 'from physiology on the one hand, through neurochemistry, clinical neurology and neurosurgery, to psychiatry and psychology at the other extreme'.[150] The supposed 'crisis' of neurological research, everyone concluded, was that little original research was being conducted at all. It was supposedly a management crisis, and a solution was immediately evident:

> It was agreed that the central problem was to bring together different scientific disciplines having a bearing on neurology. This could be done in several ways (a) by training clinicians in a separate discipline (e.g. biochemistry or immunology), (b) by bringing persons within other disciplines into close contact with neurologists and neuropathologists, (c) by grouping relevant University departments or research units.[151]

In point of fact, the meeting had started with a conclusion built upon faulty premises. When, following the meeting, the secretary of the MRC, Harold Himsworth (1905–93), conducted an internal audit to discover exactly how much neurological research the MRC had been supporting, the results were surprising. Despite the claim that little or no original research was being conducted, the internal audit found that research that would have qualified as neurological had received grants totalling approximately £317,000 between 1955 and 1960.[152] In a revealing letter to Russell Brain, Himsworth wrote, 'I also was startled when I saw the very large number of people at so many different centres who were interested in neurological research, and the inferences from this are rather disturbing...I think that everybody was rather taken aback by the evidence of the large number of people at work and the implications of this.'[153] Clearly a substantial disconnection existed between what clinical neurologists believed was being done in research and what was actually being conducted throughout the country, a point that had even eluded the officers of the MRC.

There are, of course, several reasons why this disconnection existed. Firstly, the definition that had been offered for neurology would likely have led to a wide audit of MRC funding. The second, more significant, point is that the neurologists had been caught off-guard by one of the chief features of their successful specialisation: namely that the acquisition of a monopoly over training in an area of medical practice rapidly limited options for basic and clinical research. Through their emphasis on clinical practice, neurologists had begun limiting themselves. The nervous system, however, being highly productive for scientific study, continued to be investigated by workers with only limited interests in clinical questions. In other words, the field was being taken over by basic scientists – in America these workers would eventually be called neuroscientists, an umbrella occupation that ironically captured all of those broad aspects that neurologists aggrandised in their past and in their present. Basic scientists had 'colonised' scientific neurology.

In subsequent decades, neurologists would be forced to recolonise the neurosciences. That mission was not really successful until the 1980s, at which point a new generation of clinicians, benefiting from rapidly improving imaging technologies and pharmacology, had also absorbed the methods of physiology, immunology, genetics, electron-microscopy, biochemistry, ethology, and transgenics. They incorporated these methods into a clinical research paradigm that used reductive approaches to answer larger questions about mental and nervous diseases. In their quest in the last decades of the twentieth century to recolonise the basic sciences, neurologists were aided by two important facts: their knowledge and practice found ready patrons in the pharmaceutical world. At the same time the dreaded diseases of old age were chronic disorders of the nervous system – Parkinson's and Alzheimer's. And the number of patients with these conditions increased as life expectancy trends in the West pushed ever closer to an average of eighty years for men and women.

The world of ordinary work

Thus far this chapter has focused on specialisation as a top-down project and its focus on research and science has likewise been from an elite perspective. But it is worth asking finally how these professional gains and concerns were experienced by clinicians less proximate to the power structures of their field. The formation of the National Health Service had led to the creation of a regionalised health service. Within that organisation regional hospital boards wielded enormous power. While the 1950s and 1960s were a period of professional gains for neurologists, the regional hospital boards remained largely conservative in their attitude towards the specialty. In a telling minute to the 1952 Royal College of Physicians Committee on Neurology,

George Edward Godber, then Deputy Chief Medical Officer to the Ministry of Health, offered an explanation:

> there was no chance so far as he saw of a single neurologist being appointed in any area outside the teaching centres, because the Regional Hospital Boards, all said without exception that if they needed a neurologist, they would appoint a general physician who would handle the neurology or if a specialist in neurological diseases was required they would appoint a surgeon. The reason for this was a double one: (1) they did not think of neurology as an exacting branch of medicine, and (2) with their very limited budget they would rather kill two birds with a single stone.[154]

What were the implications for the neurologists who worked beyond London or, for that matter, senior registrars in neurology hoping for a position? A few letters from the 1950s offer a picture of the labour of the ordinary neurologist. In one, Nathaniel Alcock, a neurologist in Devon and Cornwall, described his appointment as originating with the National Health Service in 1948. Creating a specialist service from scratch for a scattered population necessitated both great travel and an effort to keep a time-consuming outpatient service because 'to give these up' would be to give up 'the only link with the general practitioner'. Alcock observed that the work was far more than he could handle. He was dependent upon local general practitioners with some training in neurology and relied as well on a mixed service from psychiatrists. There was no local neurosurgeon, and he also observed that radiology services were inadequate.[155] Another neurologist, Philip Buckley, described his experiences as military provincial consultant in the Chesterford area and as a physician working with the North-Eastern Hospital Board. One problem he observed was that many patients had for so long been poorly treated that they were profoundly time consuming when he finally encountered them. He also noted that there was no replacement for him for holidays or for sickness. He ended:

> I hope the foregoing have given you a picture of a provincial Consultant Neurological Practice as it has been developed under the N. H. S. It is essentially clinical, based on experience and careful personal attention to detail, but incapable of finally diagnosing or

> healing the most difficult cases which require to be sent elsewhere. Residence in the area saves much time and enormously improves the quality and promptitude of the services given to patients at the cost of isolation and inevitable out-of-dateness in the Consultant.... The great advantage to the patients of having their Consultant live amongst them might in the future be combined with the 'further education' of the Consultant by means of 'Regional Centres' in which he would take part in the more elaborate investigation of his peripherally-collected cases. The 'Central' Consultants would then also learn of many things of interest which now never came to light.[156]

The issues of isolation were many. Living with the patients decreased the time spent travelling, and obligations to travel long distances was a complaint recorded by many.[157] Several also noted in letters that they were without any assistants who could aid them during vacations, sickness, or when they were, as A. M. Stewart-Wallace remarked, subpoenaed, which caused 'great inconvenience'. He added: 'This applies also to days or afternoons off to attend scientific meetings, congresses, post graduate lectures etc. This is a serious interference with keeping up to date.'[158] The situation was partially administrative, as John Penman observed:

> Until 1952, I used to take a fortnight's holiday a year and ask some neurological friend to act as a locum tenens during it. In February 1952 I was officially asked to state by March 1st when I proposed to take leave that summer, 'to enable continuity of specialist services to be preserved'. I stated several periods totaling five weeks and did not take any steps to provide a neurological locum tenens. Nor, as it turned out, did anyone else. The patients waited till I returned from holidays, when I made up the arrears. I have once been ill for one week, and again the patients waited.[159]

By 1960 most regional medical centres and teaching hospitals had neurology departments. The number of neurologists remained small (one neurologist per million population), as did the number of senior registrars in the field. But many of those departments that had been staffed by self-identified general physicians who practised some neurology were beginning to change in their composition. By 1965 a Royal College of Physicians report published by the Committee on Neurology could state emphatically that such physicians were 'outmoded'.[160] But the experience of that transformation exacted a cost on those first physicians who ventured beyond the major medical centres. The specialisation of medicine has never been as smooth a process as historians and sociologists have described, not as it was experienced by medical administrators and least of all for those whose opportunity for labour situated them in the middle of the process.

Conclusion

By the 1970s clinical neurology was a medical specialty in Britain. Not only were there self-identified neurologists, but government, hospital administrators, universities, professional organisations, and general practitioners recognised neurologists as a significant membership of the medical profession. But their successes within the modern structures of medicine had come with certain costs. Specialisation, sensible as it may be for administration and management, is not without burden. The labour involved in making a specialty, and the experience of a worker in the midst of a specialisation process, is not without consequence individually or collectively. Yet there are still other senses in which specialisation has an alienating influence. The creativity of scientific research, the pursuit of discovery for its own sake, and the formulation of novel hypotheses are all at risk. It is difficult to imagine that the creative genius of a John Hughlings Jackson or the Renaissance sensibilities of a Henry Head would be as appreciated today. Knowledge, research, and practice are, after all, supposed to be evidence based, paradigm or market driven, and practical. The specialist, of course, has economic position, but the creation of limitations has implications for the experience of work nonetheless. So too does it possess implications for the patient – implications that are well known. Somehow the world of medical specialisation came to be hailed as an unmitigated good, a necessity in times when human knowledge has so surpassed any one of us. Such platitudes should give pause. Who was the figure in the past who knew precisely everything stipulated by this understanding of knowledge? On the contrary, something special was lost in work with the rise of a preference for a management model of medicine that divided it into ever more divisions. That loss is as worthy of contemplation as is the writing of an historical record examining how the specialised ethos advanced and won.

• 5 •

The integrative legacy of contemporary specialists in neurology

Introduction

This book has traced the emergence of both neurology and medical specialisation by exploring the way in which physicians as well as scientists across two centuries understood and engaged with the novel idea and social phenomenon represented by specialisation and accordingly became neurologists. It is clear that physicians aspired to generalist competence and acumen throughout much of the period under investigation in this study. These physicians routinely fashioned themselves as Renaissance figures and as medicine's elite consultants. More than a few were patrician in their outlook and sensibilities.

To these physicians, the phenomenon of specialisation appeared an incomprehensible approach to medicine. For them, the human body –in health and illness – was an indivisible entity. They thus disapproved of the tendency of younger doctors to seek acclaim and fortune through the pursuit of narrow knowledge to the cost of their overall awareness and skill.

Nor were neurologists' concerns necessarily impractical ones: many recognised that the general practitioners they were responsible for training in medical schools would rarely have the luxury of so narrow an identity for their labour in house calls, provincial clinics, or general hospital wards. Moreover, they were aware that many of the great discoveries of medical science had been made by those who had cultivated their skills of observation, tempered them by experimentation, and were provided with the intellectual wherewithal to compare their results with medical theory. Much of this culture began changing administratively after the First World War. By the 1960s, neurologists could be found across the United Kingdom – but even then in small numbers relative to other groups of specialists.[1]

Yet in filling out the narrative of how and when physicians became neurologists in Britain, some final words should be added about the transformation that accompanied the rise of the independent specialty. Who were the neurologists? Were there any noteworthy developments in their work in the period after the 1960s? Were they able to maintain their integrative identity with the rise of specialised medicine? Did the neurologists' unique path to specialisation leave a marked legacy in the historiography of neurology? And finally, how might the neurologists' integrative identity have contributed to the rise of a postmodern culture preoccupied with the brain and the nerves?

To begin to answer these questions, it is necessary first to mention a few important trends in neurology then and now, and secondly to explore how neurologists' tendencies to possess and aggrandise the integrative perspective left them with a marked legacy of ambivalence towards specialised knowledge. In turn, that ambivalence created difficulties and problems in interpreting the history of neurology and neuroscience but also created opportunities for workers in other arenas to engage in the construction of the neuroculture that became so evident in the years after the 1990s.

Contemporary neurology

In the last three decades of the twentieth century, the number of British neurologists grew steadily. Although never rivalling, for example, the United States in terms of neurologists per capita, neurologists on the eve of the new millennium were approaching one neurologist per 200,000 of population in the United Kingdom and seeking to move towards one per 100,000.[2] The field was also more diverse. Neurology had long been dominated by men, but by the 1950s women had begun working in the field and were being recognised for their contributions. When interviewed about their early experiences in neurology, women who entered neurology in the 1960s recalled stories of male physicians evincing surprise at dinner parties that women could in fact become neurologists. Such attitudes had largely vanished from professional life by the twenty-first century.[3]

Accompanying these trends were other noteworthy institutional phenomena. Prior to the twentieth century, physicians with interests in nervous and mental diseases had been restricted largely to specialist hospitals. In the interwar years, a marked period of institutionalisation began, and the number of departments and academic neurology positions increased dramatically. Thus by the 1970s neurologists worked in neurology departments, held neurology professorships, and were readily found in large hospitals across the country.[4] The number of in-patient beds dedicated to neurological patients increased similarly, and at the same time neurological and neuroscientific research took place in sites across more of the country. In perhaps a great sign of the health and vitality of the specialty, new competitors such as Newcastle vied with London, the traditional seat of British neurology, in claims to be Britain's centre of neurology training, research, and treatment.[5]

After the 1950s, British neurologists also began showing increasing confidence in their ability to address questions of wider political and cultural import. German-born and Oxford-based neurologist Ludwig Guttman, for example, organised the first major international sporting competition for disabled people in 1960. By aiding the formation of the Paralympics, Guttmann was one of those leaders introducing a profound and global cultural change in public perceptions of the abilities and aspirations for those whom people in a different era had regarded as cripples.[6] In the same year, British neurologists also began advocating aggressively for changes in British boxing standards to reduce head injuries and concussions. These debates, which became prominent in the lay and medical press, were eventually taken up in the House of Lords and elicited controversy in some quarters.[7] These early signs of political mobilisation, controversial as they could be, saw perhaps their most significant moment when neurologist Christopher Pallis elaborated the brain death criteria, the burden of proof considered necessary for claiming that a patient's brain functions had ceased, which thereby permitted organ extraction for donation.[8] The philosophical and theological significance of such work and the controversies it subsequently engendered both established the brave new medical world of biomedical technology and elevated neurological signs over other physiological functions, which thereby collapsed the miracles of human sentience and life together.

A profound scientific and technical transformation was also under way. Immunology, cellular and molecular biology, and pharmacology had completely transformed neurological understanding of a myriad of neuropsychiatric and neurological disorders. In the first decades of the twentieth century, physicians with interests in nervous and mental diseases had been able only to speculate about the aetiology of a myriad of disorders. In the case of some – for example, Alzheimer's disease – the characteristic symptomatology and sometimes the gross morbid pathology of the diseases had been described.[9] Yet no one could have predicted that the very disease classifications that arose out of morbid pathology, statistics, and history taking would become one impediment to understanding nervous and mental diseases at the molecular level.[10] For, at cellular and molecular levels, many disease entities that presented with a perhaps two or three classical variations in the patient were found to have multiple and often profoundly different genetic and biochemical causes.[11] There were, too, parallel and persistent questions about the evolutionary characteristics of mental disorders such as bipolar conditions, autism, and the schizophrenias.[12] If such conditions had genetic origins, then how could such conditions persist in populations? Could it be that such mental pathologies conferred fitness to the population as a whole?[13] Thus, even as the reality of drug treatments for these conditions emerged, the implications of treating them became significant. Such questions collided with growing social and cultural tendencies to call attention to the social construction of numerous diseases, leading some commentators to question the very reality of diseases (especially mental ones) and others to reflect upon the limits of biomedical knowledge.[14] Indeed, the discovery of prions seemingly underscored those limits by appearing to overturn established dogmas of disease causation and the universal constancy of diseases – the ABN initiated a study of Creutzfeld-Jakob's disease in 1970.[15]

Neurologists and neuroscientists, of course, were not the only ones experiencing these changes – they influenced the whole of medicine and science, especially in the last three decades of the twentieth century. Accompanying these changes was another profound transformation, one that marked in a significant way the longevity of the semiological status of the clinical neurology exam. The rise of scanning technologies made the formerly invisible confines of the patient's nervous system startlingly observable to neurologists, neurosurgeons, ophthalmologists, and psychiatrists. Indeed, with the rise of functional imaging, evolutionary psychologists, behavioural psychiatrists, and neurologists saw a potential solution to neurology's hard problems – the question of mind and brain, holism and the cortical localisation of function, and dualism or monism –in the making.[16] The cost, however, for such technologies was prohibitive and the National Health Service was slow to acquire them. In 1974, for example, Bryan Matthews commented in a letter to Richard Doll, Regius Professor of Medicine at Oxford, that the 'capital cost' for installing an electromagnetic imaging scanner, 'is, I believe, of the order of £100,000'.[17] Doll responded that it 'was a bitter disappointment to me to hear that the Department of Health is unable to provide an earmarked sum from central sources to enable us to buy the apparatus'.[18] Circumstances in the United States, by contrast, were different.

Indeed, by far the most significant change for British neurology after the Second World War was the emergence of major governmental support for science and medicine in the United States. Although there was evidence of growing scientific and technological prowess there from the time of the First World War, the emergence of government patronage for scientific and medical research in the post-Second World War period had a significant impact in terms of both the production of neurobiological knowledge and also the administrative and institutional structure of post-war neurology and neuroscience in America.[19] Thus, in a dramatic reversal from the interwar period, not only did neurologists increasingly complete postgraduate training in the United States but many who trained in Britain – e.g. Derek Denny-Brown – also eventually took jobs there.[20] British universities, too, sometimes sought to recruit famous American neurologists to lead neurology departments. Although the position eventually went to W. Bryan Matthews, Richard Doll had for example in 1969 initially proposed Gilbert Glaser, a founder of Yale School of Medicine's Department of Neurology, as a potential recruit for Oxford's professorship in neurology.[21] These trends continued apace in the 1980s and into the 1990s, the so-called 'Decade of the Brain', as well. These patterns were perhaps responsible for the development of a transnational – or perhaps a highly Americanised – ideal of neurology as a specialty, which was poorly reflected in the overall organisation of British medicine. Such an ideal gave rise to the widespread (i.e. not just British) idea that the development of British neurological services lagged behind that found elsewhere, such as in France, Italy or the United States.

These widespread perceptions about the validity of specialisation, however, were far from universal. General physicians and professors of medicine continued to stymie efforts to address the allegedly dismal status of neurological services in Britain. Even in the 1980s one physician set off a firestorm of controversy in the *British Medical Journal* by arguing that neurology failed when it became an exclusionary activity. Wanted, he argued, were physicians with rich and wide backgrounds in a variety of specialty areas. He quoted one correspondent:

> Those who train postgraduates will have to come to terms with reality. By this I mean at the end of a training programme a specialist doctor should be equipped to provide the type of medical service which the National Health Service requires of him. To the department concerned and for the doctor who is being trained. If, however, the 'product' at the end of the line is a very specialised graduate who has been trained in excessive numbers for the needs of the service, this amounts to a kind of bad planning or thoughtlessness which can only lead to frustration for those fully trained doctors who cannot find employment.[22]

In other words, he was arguing for what had been the case for most of Britain for the previous century. The gentleman generalist, the philosopher neurologist, the courtly patrician, the Renaissance figure – it seems that the integrative spectre of neurology would forever haunt medical modernity's grandest project in Britain.

Medical modernity and the integrative spirit of neurology

Specialisation and subspecialisation could well be understood to have been the major modernising processes that influenced neurology. But, of course, specialisation was not a phenomenon restricted to medicine alone. It was an economic and cultural process, one easily identifiable in industry, professions, universities, and military and political institutions. People who studied the process, and contended with it, typically construed it as natural and inevitable, a law of economics, a product of technological progress, and a sign of progressive modernity. Specialisation was a synonym for progress. More specialisation was assumed good, necessary, and in any case unavoidable. Many sociologists and historians thought they had discovered the pattern and secrets of the process, mastered its details, and perfectly understood the identity-making mechanics of its disciplinary and inter-professional disputes.

As this study has endeavoured to elaborate, however, studies of specialisation have largely ignored the different modes of understandings that specialisation only slowly and incompletely replaced. Put succinctly, people had first to apprehend and value the specialisation phenomenon before they could become specialists. So too did there need to be practical value to the specialisation phenomenon, both for its producers and also for its consumers. The value of specialisation, at least for British neurologists and the health consumers of British neurology, was apparently ephemeral enough that few physicians were concerned to make the occupational distinction in the nineteenth century and even through to the interwar period of the twentieth.

The process of medical specialisation evidently originated in Victorian Britain, Napoleonic era France, Germany prior to unification, and antebellum America. In Britain, specialist hospitals began appearing from the beginning of the nineteenth century. Yet, the British were largely ambivalent about the process. Consultants regularly denigrated it throughout the last four decades of that century.[23] The formation of the Royal Society of Medicine marked the highpoint of consultant protests against specialisation. Such critiques, if more resigned in tone, continued unabated into the interwar period. It seems clear that the emergence of specialisation was routinely checked by the fact that general practitioners and general physicians continued to provide a wide range of diagnostic and therapeutic services. Neurology in Britain was highly indicative of this reality.

It may well be tempting to analyse such resistance as evidence of widespread, qualified acceptance of specialisation. It might also be tempting to ascribe a peculiar historical novelty to the British situation and describe specialisation there as backward and thus against the prevailing long-term trends of modernising societies that were naturally producing specialties and subspecialties. Both views ignore, however, the fact that while there were specialists, they were comparatively rare figures – everywhere. In Britain, that fact was magnified by the generalist aspirations popular in British medical culture. That there were specialist societies and specialist journals, and that there was specialist knowledge as well, does not imply that people necessarily possessed a monopoly on specialist practices or even thought such a monopoly desirable. On the contrary, often those few who might retrospectively be called the founders of specialties communicated their knowledge to young doctors in training who would become the next generation's general practitioners and general physicians. The hospitals, by and large, remained generalist institutions. The formation of specialist wards and departments in any of the hospitals was always a fraught, controversial, and expensive process. But even the existence of those departments and wards again did not necessarily imply any distancing from the realities of general medicine. In short, much energy has been spent exploring the specialisation phenomenon without equal consideration of the professional and patient context in which the process occurred.

Put succinctly, there was nothing natural about specialisation. It did not occur because scientific knowledge became too large for individuals to grasp. Technologies did not create the social phenomenon. Market forces did not inexorably produce it. Rather, and for a variety of reasons, specialisation emerged as an organisational and administrative logic that triumphed largely in the post-First World War period. It was an ideal that brought with it a variety of potent rhetorical devices, which often proved productive of a variety of practitioner monopolies. It streamlined opportunities for funding and billing. It simplified and reified medical work. It provided clinical practitioners and their organisations identities. It provided patients a choice between physicians with specialised skills and expertise and physicians with general competence. It gave bureaucrats a means of organising the population's access to healthcare. It provided a structure for medical research in the university and it provided medical educators a means of organising the medical curriculum in a digestible way.

All of the social benefits from specialisation could never really counteract the implicit contradictions the phenomenon also created. The case of British neurology makes those contradictions unusually explicit. The most obvious one was when and where the process should stop. Why would neurologists be called neurologists, when they could be called – as some few sometimes self-identified – electrologists, syphilogists or epileptologists?[24] Reductive biomedicine invited physicians and scientists to contemplate the seemingly unlimited specialisation of medicine: a physician could become a neurologist; a neurologist could become a specialist in headaches; a headache specialist could focus on migraines; a migraine specialist could focus on faulty second messenger systems. There was always a smaller, narrower area for inquiry and practice.

Many neurologists worried about the implications of these reductive revolutions in science for holistic neurological practice, clinical method, and perhaps even discerning medical judgement. Even in the early years of the twenty-first century, neurologist John Walton could stress his 'view that the skills of clinical history-taking and examination and assessment of the whole patient, and not solely of the nervous system, remain the cornerstones of clinical neurology and practice'.[25] In other words, even as specialisation emerged, there were countervailing determinants and tendencies. In medicine, that reality was manifested most clearly in the body of the patient, but science, too, trended away from the administrative disciplinary structures that emerged in modernity and shifted back towards the more general model of the university, the interdisciplinary collaborative structure, the research institute, and perhaps also even towards an entrepreneurial research environment.[26]

Another seeming contradiction, one observed by sociologist Andrew Abbott, was that specialisation and discipline formation invariably invited an idea of conflict between occupational groups. At a superficial level, that certainly seems to be the case for neurology, in Britain and beyond. Emergent groups – psychiatry, neurology, neuropsychiatry, and clinical psychology – appear to have fought with each other for diagnostic, therapeutic, and institutional monopolies across the twentieth century. But how often were the conflicts 'real', and how often were they exaggerated by charismatic individuals seeking to assert a new role for themselves or for the purposes of telling good stories?[27] Putting it differently, were circumstances surrounding the condition of the shell-shocked patient really the result of contrasting medical views of those patients between groups (i.e. psychiatrists and neurologists), or were they the result of a conflict between indecisive public opinion and state exigencies and economic realities?[28] It is self-evidently true that if public sympathies and state policy had determined differently, then neurologists and psychiatrists would have determined differently as well.

Secondly, it is probably truer to observe that very few figures in the nineteenth and early twentieth centuries fell neatly into any of occupational categories in medicine – and when they did, they were usually individuals with axes to grind or a means of instigating polemics that became the primary sources that later historians and sociologists evidenced as proof of jurisdictional conflicts. Rarer was the individual with position, power, and time actually to instantiate such conflicts, and even rarer still was the individual who truly wished to do so. Indeed in Britain, the consultants actively drew upon gentlemanly modes of science and practised patrician values to dissolve many putative communities of specialists in favour of the wider community of physicians and scientists. The formation of the Royal Society of Medicine was just one powerful example, and another was the Association of Physicians. Indeed, interwar British neurologists called attention to both those organisations as embodying a different system of values directly in conflict with the institutional and administrative direction of the hospitals, the military, philanthropy, and alternative approaches internationally. [29]

In other words, in order to see conflicts between groups, commentators imposed retrospective categories on the past that accorded with the alleged reality of those categories in the present. In terms of ordering tributaries to British neurology's intellectual watersheds, perhaps such activities made sense. But as, for example, an explanation for why there were few neurologists in Britain in the 1950s and 1960s, such an activity could not really offer much in the way of an explanation. Indeed, quite strangely, by magnifying and delineating the achievements of past luminaries as neurological ones, British neurologists experienced a sense of decline in the 1950s and after – at a time when arguably the institutionalisation and proliferation of opportunities for employment as neurologists were better than they had ever been nationally.[30] The tendency to retrospectively reconstruct past specialties made it easier for sociologists, historians, and practitioners to demonstrate conflicts between the groups, but at least in the case of neurology such retrospective reconstructions failed to explain the various and anomalous experiences clearly reflected in mountains of primary and secondary sources – through to the present.

The emergent identity of British neurologists

Over the two centuries, hundreds – perhaps thousands – of individuals with interests in the nervous system made contributions to its science and medicine in Britain alone. At some point, some of those people began describing themselves as neurologists and they also began referring to their predecessors as neurologists. Part of the creation of the specialty demanded the formation of an historically transcendent community. In this sense, once neurology existed, then it had always existed. Yet such historicity was an act of reification. In past worlds where there were no neurologists, twentieth-century practitioners of neurology as well as professional historians and sociologists made an effort to locate, define, and ultimately describe past figures as neurologists. In other words, there was an intentional decision to overlook features of their lives and careers that contested easy categorisation and a view of knowledge and practice that was ultimately presentist.

Consider the obituaries of the British neurologists. Establishing which obituaries to examine involves significant conceits. On its face, membership in a neurological society would seemingly be one of the more appropriate means for establishing a common identity. But what does membership in more than one specialty society imply? Many physicians with interests in the nervous system belonged to more than one scientific and medical society. Membership of a society can be construed only as membership of a society; in no way does it establish clearly a specialist identity. The obituaries of members of the Neurological Society of the United Kingdom, the Neurological Section of the Royal Society of Medicine, and even those who were early members of the ABN reflect this fact.

In the nineteenth century, most of the obituaries occupied one or two pages of the *British Medical Journal* or the *Lancet*, or a column's worth in *The Times*. In the pages of hospital magazines and gazettes as well as academic journals, the death notices were frequently longer, including appreciations from friends, colleagues, and former pupils. For those illustrious enough to have become Fellows of the Royal Society, obituary notices could span fifty pages or more. These nineteenth-century obituaries conveyed the multiplicities of a life lived – ancestry, education, places of work, military service, involvement in religion and politics and scientific and leisure societies, hobbies, and marriage and family.

By contrast, in the twentieth century, obituaries shortened, became less expository, and focused more on career and education. Family and private life became largely insignificant. The tone became clipped and concise. The copy devoted to celebration was wholly reduced, and even the accuracy of the details sometimes suspect. In these later obituaries it is also noteworthy that work in scientific and clinical realms affiliated with the nervous system became increasingly definite and delimited, rendering acts of career identification easier for obituarists. Exemplary perhaps of this trend is the fact that while the word 'neurologist' appeared uncommonly and with little pomp at the close of the nineteenth century, in the interwar period and subsequently the term became common.[31] More typically, obituarists used phrases like 'physician in mental and nervous diseases', 'physician with a special interest in neurology' or 'physician in nervous diseases'. Moreover, they almost always contrived a picture of the deceased's dispositions and habits as that of a broadminded generalist, a gentleman scientist, and perhaps even a courtly 'patrician'.[32]

This generational transience of identity left an indelible mark in obituaries. Obituarists in the late nineteenth century and throughout much of the twentieth routinely observed multiple occupational identities. Only a very few claimed the deceased as a 'neurologist'. More typical was a broader representation. The president of the Royal College of Physicians of Dublin, Francis Carmichael Purser (1876–1934), had maintained, for example, 'his practice as a general physician' despite his 'special interest in neurology'.[33] Ronald Grey Gordon of Bath held eclectic interests in neurology, hydrology, child guidance, and psychiatry, and his *Lancet* obituarist identified further interests in hysterical and rheumatic conditions.[34] Gordon's obituary in the *British Medical Journal* memorialised this as a pleasing 'manysidedness'.[35] Conrad Meredyth Hinds Howell (1877–1960) was remembered as being 'primarily a neurologist' but his obituarist observed, 'he was also a general physician of wider knowledge and experience'.[36]

When such rhetoric appeared, it was usually critical of contemporary culture and nostalgic for a lost past.[37] It tended to downplay specialist interests while emphasising generalist acumen. The obituary of Donald Elms Core, for example, recorded that, 'in a world of bustle and hurry Core belonged to the old-world type of physician who believed in the pre-eminence of his own disciple of medicine over others, in a manner worthy of the seventeenth and eighteenth century'.[38] In what way Core had emulated such manners and customs in his Manchester practice is left untold.[39] It seems clear, however, that Core's obituarist intended it to communicate values medical men should emulate. Similar themes appear as late as Edwin Bramwell's 1952 obituary. His obituarist described Bramwell as being 'at his best in his clinical neurological demonstrations', but noted that he had possessed 'all of the qualities of a great physician, with an old-fashioned courtly demeanour much to be admired in these strenuous days'.[40] The obituarist assumed the universality of these values.

Such claims were hardly just rhetorical grandstanding. They captured real misgivings about the increasingly specialised and bureaucratised nature of twentieth-century British medicine and science. Moreover, most of the deceased physicians, as their obituaries revealed, did not work as exclusive specialists. They worked in a variety of spaces, from general hospitals and teaching hospitals to provincial clinics or private practices in London on Wimpole Street and Harley Street.

For them, a general medical outlook had not only been necessary but was also redemptive and educational. Thus, many, as for instance Edwin Bramwell, expressed apprehension, sometimes privately and sometimes publicly, about the development of a neurological specialty.[41] In the lifetime of workers like Bramwell, younger workers had come to conceive of clinical neurology as underrepresented within hospital medicine. For practitioners of an older generation, that view was completely illogical because neurological cases made up so many of those cases seen in general practice.

This seeming amalgam of identities – in actuality an identity at once more complex and nuanced than might now be assumed – reveals how embedded was neurological practice in general medical culture and general practice. The amalgam also makes clear that the medical culture and these identities were continually changing, generation by generation, obituary by obituary. Thus, increasingly, physicians whose careers had flourished or begun in the interwar period came to identify themselves with a sphere of specialised practice called neurology. By the last quarter of the twentieth century an increasing number of obituarists remembered them as neurologists only.[42] In their modes of production, obituaries testify to changes only by recognising a familiar absence – the deceased has departed; the deceased's world continued. Obituaries were testimonies to both worlds. And they thus reveal at once an emergent and at the same time complicated identity for the makers of the science and medicine of the nervous system.

The retrospective reconstruction of neurological identity

If obituaries – even those drawn from membership lists of neurological societies – demonstrate an emergent identity for British neurologists, then it is worthwhile studying the ways past historians also dealt with the challenge this represented. Consider an important and often-cited work in the historiography of neurology – *The Founders of Neurology*, first published in 1953 and re-edited and published in a second edition in 1970.

The idea for the volume originated in 1949 at the Fourth International Neurological Congress, which was held in Paris. At this event there was a historical exhibit celebrating the great men of neurology,[43] from which the first edition ultimately resulted. The final product was a prosopography comprising 133 biographical sketches, each penned by living authors who could bring alive their firsthand knowledge of the 'founders'. Fascinatingly, however, although the 1970 edition had increased in size from 133 to 146 individuals, twenty-one figures included in the first edition were omitted from the latter. The authors involved in producing the second edition thus provided in total thirty-five new biographical sketches.[44] In other words, in less than seventeen years, twenty-one individuals previously deemed 'founders' ceased to be so regarded.

What had happened? The context of the two volumes is important. The editors were Americans, although any number of authors and 'founders' were from Britain. In the early 1950s, an attitude of internationalism was pervasive. By the early 1970s, American political and cultural discourse had shifted towards a pluralism coloured by Cold War nationalism. Thus, in the first edition, Webb Haymaker wrote: 'that the history of neurology cannot be divorced from its pursuit and that scientific achievement knows no national boundary'.[45] By 1970, however, the editors admitted that the selection of individuals as 'founders' might breed controversy: 'Our selection and our compromises will no doubt be subject to criticism on many counts, as selections must be. Some men, some discoverers, may loom larger on San Francisco Bay than they do say, on the banks of the Meskva, the Thames, the Seine, or the Danube, and vice versa.'[46]

Revisions for the 1970 edition necessitated answering many questions. The first question was obvious: what, in fact, was neurology? The 1953 edition had dealt with this problem by categorising contributions in terms of academic disciplines and a select group of medical specialties – neuroanatomy, neuropathology, clinical neurology, and neurosurgery. The second edition ultimately emulated that pattern, but the editors added three new categories, including neuroanatomists born before 1850, neurochemistry, and neurohistory.

Establishing and arranging these categories was no simple matter. In numerous letters, Haymaker and Schiller discussed various options, suggesting initially that the volume be arranged around centuries – figures before 1900 and figures after 1900.[47] They ultimately abandoned this approach for two reasons. Firstly, it presented no logical framework for dealing with individuals whose worked spanned both centuries, although Francis Schiller believed the 'dividing line between the 2 parts or centuries was near [Santiago Ramón y] Cajal', presumably a reference to Cajal's formulation of the neuronal cell theory.[48] Secondly, there seemed to be no adequate means of categorising the occupations of those born before 1900. Haymaker wrote to Schiller, 'In regard to arrangement, those before 1900: wouldn't it be better to list them chronologically as any one of them could be two or three things? For those after 1900: anatomists, physiologists, etc.' This concern about categories was also raised by William McMenemy, then pathologist at the National Hospital, London, who wrote in mid-October 1968 to Haymaker, 'in spite of the great stature of Henry Dale and his work on acetyl choline we seldom think of him as a neurologist.'[49]

Another equally complex question raised by the 1970 edition was what really constituted a 'founder'? Haymaker and Schiller had been discussing this problem since June of 1967. Then Schiller had sent a note to Haymaker suggesting omissions and new additions. 'Here is a very preliminary note on Founder. Deletions suggested because the claim for "Foundership" of "neurology" may seem exaggerated.' In the same letter he wrote, 'suggested additions, real Founder's they!'[50] Part of Haymaker and Schiller's concern arose from the peculiar way candidates were nominated for the volume. In a letter to Haymaker, Schiller worried that certain contributors had picked founders because of their personalities alone.[51] The question of who constituted a 'founder' was not merely one for the editors. In September of 1968, David Bodian, director of the Department of Anatomy at Johns Hopkins University, wrote to Haymaker that the 'concept of Founders seems to me to be a troublesome one, especially when "more recent" names are concerned'. Despite this, Bodian felt able to recommend Ross Harrison and Karl Lashley, to which Haymaker responded in the margins when he forwarded Bodian's letter to Schiller, 'can [Lashley] be considered a neurologist?'[52] The point, however, is that both questions – What is neurology? What is a founder? – were obviously linked in the 1970 edition.

One answer to both was provided in the final draft of the preface: 'Who...we continued to ask ourselves, was a Founder, and not merely a Refiner?' They continued a little later in the preface, to 'approximate the 1953 format we have, reluctantly, eliminated a sizable number of previous names, for reasons of economy, and on the grounds – history being a fickle mistress – that some contributions seemed less resilient to the in-roads of time.'[53] In a 1967 letter to Haymaker, Schiller noted that the contributions of such British neurologists as William John Adie and Frederich Mott seemed 'ephemeral'. He deemed others of greater importance. 'Why not one from the 17th century?' he asked, referring to Thomas Willis (1621–75), the father, he claimed, of neurology and also British neurology. For him, Charles Sherrington was an obvious addition as well.[54]

Other reasons for why individuals might have been omitted from the second edition can be suggested by analysing their biographies in the first edition. There is no reason to think that individuals were taken out of *The Founders* out of nationalistic prejudices – although the figures removed tended to be from Eastern Europe, Italy, Austria, and the United Kingdom. Yet a pattern does emerge in terms of their occupational categories, with fifteen clinicians being removed. In comparison, no neurosurgeons were deleted, and only one neurophysiologist, two neuropathologists, and three neuroanatomists were excised.

Why were clinical neurologists the most likely to be removed? Firstly, Haymaker and Schiller tended to remove founders with professional and research experience in nervous *and* mental diseases. Although this affected all of the volume's categories, clinical neurologists were particularly vulnerable because many – not just British founders – worked with mental patients.[55] Haymaker and Schiller, moreover, seem to have been uneasy about accepting 'founders' whose contributions did not appear self-evidently neurological in 1970. Hence, William John Adie (1886–1935), a British clinician whose major work had been closely affiliated with ophthalmology, was removed.[56] Similarly, others were renowned as institution builders, i.e. their careers had been defined more from their efforts to build the field of neurology than from their original research. George Riddoch's contemporaries, for example, would have been familiar with his studies of peripheral nerves, but they would likely have seen his greatest achievements on behalf of neurology in his administrative efforts to acquire government patronage for British neurology. Those accomplishments, which were highly regarded in the years leading up to 1953, might have been forgotten or deemed unimportant by 1970.[57]

The final product of Haymaker and Schiller's labours appeared in 1970. It subsequently sold 2,836 copies.[58] There was never any discussion of a third edition, although some comparable works appeared in related fields like paediatric neurology and neurosurgery. In many respects, some patterns do emerge. The second edition focused more on individuals we might loosely label as knowledge-makers – there was less emphasis on institution builders. Similarly, Haymaker and Schiller generally avoided figures whose research and practice could be associated with psychiatry, while many of the new figures included in the second edition were from a much earlier era. In the 1953 edition, neurology had appeared as an eclectic, modern field. In the 1970 edition, the editors forcefully reconstructed the specialty. Neurology so formed appeared more limited in its intellectual scope and ambitions and historically older in terms of its actual foundation. Thus, like the obituaries of members of neurological societies, the 1970 edition implied that neurology and 'founders' of neurology embraced a heterogeneous set of occupational interests. But in vast contrast to the obituaries, the 1970 edition argued for a long history. Although obituaries of neurologists might well have been regarded as a mere century old, the editors retrospectively reified past work into the neurological specialty. In this way, neurology was retrospectively reconstructed.

Integrative identities and specialisation

There were many shared creative elements producing this history of neurology, many of which were a product of neurology's emergence within general medicine in Britain. Neurologists had come to possess an all-encompassing and heterogeneous knowledge. In 1923, for example, one author stated, 'we do not know when the term "neurologist" came into vogue, nor for that matter can we define the limits of his specialty, but we have always supposed it concerns the totality of the problems presented by the nervous system in health and disease.'[59] Who would have been excluded from such a holistic definition?

Nowhere were these views more clearly expressed, however, than by Walter Russell Brain in a 1958 address to the Royal College of Physicians of Edinburgh entitled 'Neurology: Past, Present and Future'. Brain began his lecture with the question: 'What is neurology?'

> The subtitle of the journal *Brain* is 'A Journal of Neurology,' and the scope of that journal may therefore be taken as a useful index of the scope of neurology. Any volume...contains articles on the physiology, anatomy, and biochemistry of the nervous system, on neuropathology, on the psychological and psychiatric aspects of nervous disorders, and on clinical neurology, including neurosurgery. In the most comprehensive sense, then, neurology comprises all aspects of the normal and abnormal functioning of the nervous system. In one important respect neurology differs from all other branches of physiology and of medicine: it is concerned with that part of the human organism which is most distinctly human, and it is therefore unique among branches of medicine in the extent of its contributions to scientific knowledge beyond the scope of animal physiology, through its study of the neural basis of all the psychological and physiological functions of man.[60]

Brain took as self-evident that the contribution of clinical neurology and neurologists to general medicine, psychiatry, physiology, and pathology, as well as other subjects, existed because all contributed in some way to neurological knowledge. The relationships between these fields he saw as reciprocal. Furthermore the diversity and complexity of neurology were signs that progress had been made; the social process of medical specialisation had led to a profound growth in knowledge. 'What I have said well illustrates,' Brain asserted, 'the rich contribution specialisation has made to medicine.' Specialisation had spawned an accumulation of knowledge that had invigorated the status and productivity of neurology, and therefore medicine. Brain cautioned, however, 'far from knowing more and more about less and less, the specialist, like every one of his colleagues in medicine, needs to know more and more about more and more.'

Integration, he elaborated, remained the neurologist's highest calling; it was the neurologist's most difficult charge:

> If we ask what part neurology is to play...the answer begins to emerge from our survey of the scope of the subject. Neurology plays a part in physiology, psychology, psychiatry, pathology, bacteriology, medicine, surgery, and no doubt other disciplines, and all of these in their turn have a contribution to make to neurology. What, then, is the role of the neurological physician? The fact that he alone is

> commonly called a neurologist surely reflects his key position in relation to neurology. The process of integration...is more likely to be successful if there is an integrator; and the neurologist, though he cannot possibly be an expert in all these fields, is the person most fitted by training, experience, and opportunity to be a nodal point in the relations of neurology.[61]

The neurologist's function was to work at the centre of overlapping spheres of clinical and scientific knowledge. The neurologist embodied the cooperative labourer, a practitioner at the centre of medicine and science's many divisions. Neurologists, through the proclivities of their training, knowledge, and expertise, were prepared to act in a tacit operational mode that manufactured commensurability between the multiple ways of believing and knowing in various arenas of science and medicine. For Brain, this was what differentiated the neurologist occupationally from the general physician who treated patients with nervous diseases. Some believed, he observed, that because general physicians saw patients with nervous diseases, the general physician was a kind of neurologist; or, alternatively, because neurologists saw patients with nervous diseases (i.e. systemic disorders), they were a kind of general physician. Neither view, according to Brain, properly categorised the neurologist's role. The neurologist's importance derived from the nature of his or her practice. Defining the neurologist meant firstly recognising that his or her practitioner space was defined by idiomatic rules that adopted as standard the neurologist's all-encompassing view, desire to integrate forms of knowledge, and continual efforts to consolidate and construct bridges between academic and clinical worlds. This was practice seemingly of an indefinable type and unlike other medical specialties that limited their views to succinct areas of knowledge, practice, or technical interventions. In short, neurology for Russell Brain was a specialty defined by its lack of limitations.

This integrative legacy never vanished from neurology. Although neurology was transformed over the nineteenth and twentieth century in various ways with changes in medicine's overall social and political structure, certain continuities in neurological practice remained. Neurology in the 1870s and 1880s was broadly defined; and some practitioners, as evidence shows, clearly would understand it that way even in the 1970s and 1980s. From the point of view of neurology's many practitioners at any point during those years, the scope of the subject's practices made professionalisation around a defined, delimited, or demarcated jurisdiction impossible.[62] In historical writing, especially, neurology was thus depicted as a vast subject studied throughout the ages.[63] This view of neurology was one that elite figures with interests in the nervous system and its diseases intentionally and unintentionally produced and reproduced. Moreover, it was one consciously and unselfconsciously cultivated and organised by students of neurology seeking to emulate their teachers.

In the nineteenth century, the term neurologist, rarely used, was a label that might be pinned on any physician – just like other descriptors such as scientist, musician, writer, or teacher. The physician of nervous diseases saw little distinction between mental and nervous diseases. As past chapters have elaborated, central to the practice of these physicians was a belief in the unity of medicine, and therefore the necessity of a broad practical outlook. The physician of nervous diseases before the First World War could not be a specialist; he or she was a general physician of wide learning and knowledge. The scientific neurologist before the First World War, though sometimes medically qualified, might just as easily be described now as a physiologist, anatomist, or pathologist.[64] Thus, the physiologist Charles Sherrington was as much a neurologist as the clinician Samuel Alexander Kinnier Wilson. Retrospectively, the vagaries of this definition allowed anyone to be included within the sphere of neurological practice; likewise, it permitted rather arbitrary reasons for exclusion. What was key to this characterisation was that it allowed for a personal self-fashioning that placed greater emphasis on individual autonomy, achievement, and self-determination.

Contemporaries perceived knowledge 'founders' as makers of their own destinies – inexhaustible and able to create knowledge through their own intellectual capacity. The belief in these qualities was reproduced in subsequent generations of neurologists. Indeed, it was one of several social dispositions underlying the habits of the emergent field. Another disposition, no less important, was continual adherence to the view that general medicine and neurology were inseparable. Thus for each new generation of students, neurology's definition remained broad in the occupational sense and was perceived as being delimited only by individual ability. To be described as a neurologist was to be recognised for producing and reproducing the dispositions of a particular scholarly habitus, which, though truly unique to the twentieth century, was depicted as allegedly commonplace among scholars in all historical periods.[65]

All three neurological societies in the period between 1860 and 1960 shared these continuities, but they were ones regularly challenged by external circumstances beyond the control of the emergent community. The Neurological Society of the United Kingdom, which derived from several contexts – including the emergence of medical specialties like ophthalmology and a nineteenth-century legacy of psychiatric practices – was founded upon broad and general principles. It never adopted a vision of itself as a specialist society per se but rather was embedded in a generalist medical culture and operated as a society comprising medical generalists, concerned only with establishing the clinical and scientific principles governing the nervous system.

Nevertheless, with the emergence of numerous specialties at the turn of the century, British medical elites in London – many were members of the Neurological Society – found themselves dissatisfied with medicine's fragmenting structure. Arguing that excessive specialisation should be curtailed, they formed the Royal Society of Medicine in 1907 to defend the unity of medicine. Members of the Neurological Society of the United Kingdom favoured this defence of general medical practice. They voted to dissolve their society and become the Neurological Section of the Royal Society of Medicine.

In practice the meetings of the Neurological Section between 1907 and 1914 were little different from those of its predecessor. Moreover, there was little effort to move the section's membership towards a new ethos of specialised practice. Rather, the habits of the section's members mirrored those of the Royal Society of Medicine more generally. They were not inclined towards specialist practice and, like many Edwardian physicians, typically held prejudices against such practice. Although members of the Neurological Section were interested in the science and clinical study of the nervous system, most were no less interested in general medicine. Indeed, some of the section's more illustrious members were presidents of various sections of the Royal Society of Medicine. Few saw the need for special neurological departments in hospitals of medical schools, and most viewed the development of such departments as impractical and ill conceived: what mattered was that medical students develop a wide view of clinical practice. Those few students who would pursue further training in nervous diseases at one of the three specialist nerve hospitals understood that their careers would invariably lead them to a consultant's position in one of the larger London or provincial hospitals.[66] There, though they might see patients with nervous and mental diseases, it was likely they would be treating patients with other medical conditions as well.

For a time the disposition favouring generalist medical practice prevailed in twentieth-century Britain. Furthermore, this general disposition aligned with a perception of the nervous system as a broad, all-encompassing object of study. However, the First World War prompted several important social transformations in medicine. Among these were changes in practitioner self-perception matching a new social and political order promoting and constituting (and in some cases demanding) the rationalisation of medical practice. The effects, though not immediate, were palpable in many arenas, including neurology. Whereas before the war consultant general physicians were the norm in British hospitals and private practice, the early 1920s saw the rapid creation of many specialist departments, including departments of nervous diseases and neurology. Lectureships in the subject were created as well, and a host of outpatient neurology clinics were also formed. Funds from the state and philanthropy suffused the field in unprecedented fashion, introducing new institutions and funding older ones, which assumed new rational structures. Early on in the interwar period, younger members of the Section of Neurology, most of them fresh from their military medical service, became self-described neurologists, while some older members adopted iconoclastic roles and called for reforms in the political and social structure of the field. Both groups in the interwar period began to be more restricted in their practice: the patients they treated increasingly suffered from organic conditions and clinical neurological research tended to focus less on functional conditions and more on biological and physiological studies of the nervous system. Although most practitioners continued to laud the ideals of general practice, the practices of neurology were moving in the opposite, specialist, direction. Nevertheless, though special neurologic practice was becoming normative in ways never before seen in Britain, neurology retained atavistic features. Its practices even in the late-1950s embraced a continuous self-perception. Neurology, broad and unlimited, required at once the profoundest understanding of the clinical examination as well as the ability to integrate separate spheres of knowledge in ways that no other group of medical workers could.

It is clear from many of their pronouncements to various audiences – public, legal, and professional – that British neurologists throughout the later decades of the twentieth century believed they required no professional jurisdictions per se, at least in so far as the nervous system was concerned. However, this very lack of jurisdiction made neurology difficult to administer effectively. For example, it is difficult to see how government agencies like the Ministry of Health or the MRC could manage a field that claimed work and knowledge of all fields so long as they pertained in some way to the nervous system. Administrative units like these, as well as hospitals and universities, in the 1950s and after, had to create formal barriers or classifiers to distinguish the work of the neurologist from other medical professionals, especially since various closely aligned occupational groups such as general physicians, psychiatrists, rehabilitative specialists, and neurosurgeons claimed neurological territory as well.

For these practical administrative purposes, neurology became increasingly restricted to biological and physiological idioms in its research from the 1930s onwards. At the level of pedagogy, understanding of clinical-pathology, rigorous clinical examination, and understanding of scientific research methods remained the hallmarks of neurological training. Increasingly, however, interest in cognitive aspects of the nervous system, embodied in the work of psychology, psychopathology, or psychiatry became restricted to those fields alone (although limited training and discussions on these subjects continued in neurology).[67] These structural realities led many neurologists in the 1950s and after to the conclusion – startling to them – that various other agents were defining neurology's practices. These agents included the state, other medical specialties and scientific disciplines, and hospital and university administrators. Consequently these agents, intentionally and unintentionally, introduced limitations into a field that was perceived by its leaders (and practitioners) to be justly and rightly unrestricted in its focus. In this sense, all of the benefits of the rationalisation of medicine, the funding of research, and the growth of workers in neurology that had accompanied the emergence of neurology, were tempered by another reality of modern life. Neurology, to some, was beginning to look as if it might just be another medical job.

Was this to become the status of neurology? For older neurologists in the period after the Second World War the question was not rhetorical. They, unlike younger workers in the field, remembered a time when things seemed different in medicine. Nor was theirs mere nostalgia for a lost world or imagined past: it was a profound recognition that social rationalisation had resulted in new forms of autonomy but also the loss of older forms. Neurologists, in accepting the evolving and pragmatic institutional, political, and practical definitions necessary for their occupational recognition, had relinquished the advantages of definitional ambiguity.

The rise of neuroculture

> Hug me till you drug me, honey;
> Kiss me till I'm in a coma:
> Hug me, honey, snuggly bunny;
> Love's as good as *soma*.[68]

'The functions of the central nervous system are not a palimpsest, where a new text is written over an earlier manuscript, partly erased,' argued Henry Head in 1918, observing in addition that, 'the more primitive activities have been profoundly modified by the advent of new centres, which utilise some of the faculties originally possessed by the older mechanism. In many cases the higher function could not be exercised without the existence of these lower powers which it dominates and controls.'[69] In this way was the link between evolution and neurology established. The integrative ideal which emerged in the late nineteenth century combined anatomy, physiology, pathology, and evolution with neurology. Pathological states became the means for grasping not only the patient's history but humanity's history as well.[70] Yet the metaphor of the palimpsest was an evocative choice, conjuring as it did at once the power of the retrospective imagination in neurology and hinting at the same time towards a larger cultural narrative that would always supposedly be indelible and permanent in the human nervous system.

It was only in the late 1970s that the power of this integrative idol manifested. It was a period, historian Paul Forman has observed, that began embracing a culture that worshiped technology, multidisciplinarity, and entrepreneurialism.[71] At precisely this moment of cultural conjuncture, at the moment when neuropharmacology, scanning technologies, and biomolecular science also began to give very real shape to neuroscience and neurobiology and began as well to vest neurology with wholly new understandings of the nerves in sickness and in health, neuroculture began to reframe human self-understanding.[72] 'The fundamental justification', as authors of a report for the US National Academy of Sciences for *Manpower in Basic Neurologic and Communicative Sciences* put it, 'is that basic insights into neuroscience constitute one of the major scientific achievements of contemporary civilization.'[73] Neurology's long legacy of definitional ambiguity, the propensity of its practitioners for generality, their obvious interests in psychiatry and physiology, and their long history of engaging evolutionary theory had thus served up the feast of arguments, tropes, and rhetorical devices that would feed the appetites of the 'cerebral subject' and the Huxlian 'neurochemical self'.[74]

In short, after the Second World War, people figuratively became their brains. They dreamed of and then manufactured extended minds. They used neuroscience to question personhood, behavioural economics, animal-hood, gender, diversity, and even to recast 'man as machine metaphors' into new forms. Mind became a digital product of matter; the brain became a computer; the nerves – picking up on an old refrain – became cyber-networks. Snails made manifest the mechanisms of memory. Florescent proteins embedded addiction into the reductive substance of the cell membrane. The brain became a cultural refrain. And many educated people believed it, and many uneducated and young people practised reiterating it. The brain was its own justification. It was civilisation.

Any number of figures in the history of science and medicine could be claimed to have constructed this neurologic metanarrative. Given its claims to historical transcendence, it is easy to imagine as well that any number of figures could be reconstructed in hindsight as the heroes who constructed this new cultural understanding. Yet it was the neurologists who made this world. Indeed, it was the Jacksonian ideal that would ultimately underpin the emergent logic of neuroculture. It was the neurologists, among the physicians, who were most 'fully engaged in the philosophical status of man'.[75] And while that story was not solely a British one, it was nevertheless the British neurologists who resisted the inexorable trends of rational modernity, of progressive administration, and who held on to the promise of generality and catholicity, and defended a world of Newtons and Darwins and a tradition of Jacksons and Sherringtons against a world of normal science and its would-be tradition of scriveners.

What then was the 'neuro' in neurology as the British neurologists understood it? If it was a tradition of generalism and integration, and hero worship too, then it was also a powerful and transformative cultural discourse. It was one that borrowed heavily from artistic and literary currents even as it transformed those movements. It was a discourse that saw in the action of disease a new understanding of the living subject, being, and knowing. It drew heavily upon evolutionary theory. And it eventually reforged the essence of humanity into a story of gene regulation, neurotransmitters, membrane physiology, nerve impulses and synaptic transmission. Accordingly sleep, pleasure, pain, memory, language, even fighting and fleeing, became the stuff of central nervous system organisation and limbic systems. It was, in other words, a particular strand of British neurology that provided neuroculture with its essential shape, integrative social structure, and, alas, also laid the foundations for the now-emergent hegemony of the brain and nerves.

Notes

Foreword

1 Gordon Holmes, *The National Hospital, Queen Square, 1860–1948* (Edinburgh: Livingstone, 1954).
2 Ibid., p. 34.
3 V. A. McKusick, 'A 60-year Tale of Spots, Maps, and Genes', *Annual Review of Genomics and Human Genetics* 7:1 (2006), 1–27.

Introduction

1 Michael Bliss, *Harvey Cushing: A Life in Surgery* (New York: Oxford University Press, 2005), p. 496; Montreal Neurological Institute, *Neurological Biographies and Addresses: Foundation Volume Published for the Staff, to Commemorate the Opening of the Montreal Neurological Institute of McGill University* (London: Oxford University Press, 1936), pp. 1–25.
2 Edwin Bramwell Papers, Carnoustie, Scotland, Private Collection (hereafter Bramwell Papers), Letter from Harvey Cushing to Edwin Bramwell, 1 September 1934.
3 Private Collection, Letter from Edwin Bramwell to Harvey Cushing, 14 September 1934.
4 The sources on neurology's intellectual history are extensive. Among the best are: Owsei Temkin, *The Falling Sickness: A History of Epilepsy from the Greeks to the Beginnings of Modern Neurology* (Baltimore: Johns Hopkins University Press, 1971); Robert M. Young, *Mind, Brain, and Adaptation in the Nineteenth Century* (New York: Oxford University Press, 1990); Anne Harrington, *Medicine, Mind, and the Double Brain: A Study in Nineteenth-Century Thought* (Princeton: Princeton University Press, 1987); Roger Smith, *Inhibition: History and Meaning in the Sciences of the Brain and Mind* (London: Free Association Books, 1992); L. Stephen Jacyna, *Lost Words: Narratives of Language and the Brain, 1825–1926* (Princeton: Princeton University Press, 2000).

5 Fernando Vidal, *The Sciences of the Soul: The Early Modern Origins of Psychology*, trans. Saskia Brown (Chicago and London: University of Chicago Press, 2011), pp. 346–50.

6 Thomas Neville Bonner, *Medical Education in Britain, France, Germany, and the United States, 1750–1945* (Baltimore and London: Johns Hopkins University Press, 1995); Arthur S. Link (ed.), *Fifty Years of American Neurology: An Historical Perspective* (Winston-Salem, NC: Stratford Books, 1998); Jacalyn Duffin, *History of Medicine: A Scandalously Short Introduction* (Toronto and London: University of Toronto Press, 1999); Stanley Finger, *Origins of Neuroscience: A History of Explorations into Brain Function* (New York: Oxford University Press, 2001); Stanley Finger, Francois Boller, and Kenneth L. Tyler (eds), *History of Neurology* (Edinburgh and New York: Elsevier, 2010).

7 George Rosen, *The Specialization of Medicine with Particular Reference to Ophthalmology* (New York: Froben Press, 1944); Hans-Heinz Eulner, *Die Entwicklung der medizinischen Specizlfächer an den Universitäten des deutschen Sprachgebietes* (Stuttgart: Ferdinand Enke Verlag, 1970); Rosemary Stevens, *Medical Practice in Modern England: The Impact of Specialization and State Medicine* (New Haven: Yale University Press, 1966); Andrew Abbott, *The System of the Professions: An Essay on the Division of Expert Labor* (Chicago: University of Chicago Press, 1988); George Weisz, *Divide and Conquer: A Comparative History of Specialization* (Oxford: Oxford University Press, 2006).

8 M. Jeanne Peterson, *The Medical Profession in Mid-Victorian London* (Berkley, Los Angeles, and London: University of California Press, 1978).

9 Christopher Lawrence, 'Incommunicable Knowledge: Science, Technology and the Clinical Art in Britain, 1850–1914', *Journal of Contemporary History* 20:4 (1985), 502–20.

10 There is a wide literature here, for example: Kapil Raj, *Relocating Modern Science: Circulation and the Construction of Knowledge in South Asia and Europe, 1650–1900* (Basingstoke: Palgrave Macmillan, 2007); Susan Gross Solomon (ed.), *Doing Medicine Together: Germany and Russia between the Wars* (Toronto and London: University of Toronto Press, 2006); Peter Galison, *Image and Logic: A Material Culture of Microphysics* (Chicago: University of Chicago Press, 1997).

11 There is an anecdote, no doubt apocryphal, that goes something like this: one day a neurologist on the eve of his retirement met an historian of long acquaintance. The historian tells the neurologist that he, too, is about to retire and then asks the neurologist what he plans do with his newfound time for leisure. Without hesitation, the

neurologist says that he has decided to take up history. To which the historian replies, 'That's funny, I plan on taking up neurology.' The sources on neurology's intellectual history are extensive. Some of the best are: Temkin, *The Falling Sickness*; Young, *Mind, Brain, and Adaptation in the Nineteenth Century*; Harrington, *Medicine, Mind, and the Double Brain*; Smith, *Inhibition*; Jacyna, *Lost Words*.

12 This problem has long been recognised. See F. Clifford Rose, 'Historiography: An Introduction', *Journal of the History of Neurosciences* 11 (2002), 35–7; Helge Kragh, 'Problems and Challenges in the Historical Study of the Neurosciences', *Journal of the History of Neurosciences* 11 (2002), 55–62; Ellen Dwyer, 'Toward New Narratives of Twentieth-Century Medicine', *Bulletin of the History of Medicine* 74 (2000), 786–93, especially 788.

13 See, for instance, F. Clifford Rose (ed.), *Twentieth-Century Neurology: The British Contribution* (London and River Edge, NJ: World Scientific Publishing Company, 2002); F. Clifford Rose (ed.), *A Short History of British Neurology: The British Contribution, 1660–1910* (Butterworth-Heinemann, 1999); L. Stephen Jacyna, *Medicine and Modernism: A Biography of Henry Head* (London and Brookfield, VT: Pickering & Chatto, 2008); Macdonald Critchley and Eileen A. Critchley, *John Hughlings Jackson: Father of English Neurology* (New York: Oxford University Press, 1998); Edwin Clarke and L. Stephen Jacyna, *Nineteenth-Century Origins of Neuroscientific Concepts* (Berkley: University of California Press, 1992); Finger, *Origins of Neuroscience*.

14 Gordon M. Shepherd, *Creating Modern Neuroscience: The Revolutionary 1950s* (New York and Oxford: Oxford University Press, 2010); Warwick Anderson, *The Collector of Lost Souls: Turning Kuru Scientists into Whitemen* (Baltimore: Johns Hopkins University Press, 2008); Jesse F. Ballenger, *Self, Senility, and Alzheimer's Disease in Modern America: A History* (Baltimore: Johns Hopkins University Press, 2006); Jacques Philippon and Jacques Poirier, *Joseph Babinski: A Biography* (New York: Oxford University Press, 2009); Robert Laureno, *Raymond Adams: A Life of Mind and Muscle* (New York: Oxford University Press, 2009); Lewis P. Rowland, *The Legacy of Tracy J. Putnam and H. Houston Merritt: Modern Neurology in the United States* (New York: Oxford University Press, 2008); Christopher Goetz, Michel Bonduelle, and Toby Gelfand, *Charcot: Constructing Neurology* (New York and London: Oxford University Press, 1995); Russell N. DeJong, *A History of American Neurology* (New York: Raven Press, 1982).

15 Parallel and important works include: Elizabeth Green Musselman, *Nervous Conditions: Science and the Body Politic in Early Industrial*

Britain (Albany, NY: State University of New York Press, 2006); George Rousseau, *Nervous Acts: Essays on Literature and Sensibility* (Houndmills and Basingstoke: Palgrave Macmillan, 2005); Jacyna, *Lost Words*.

16 Leonard George Guthrie, *Contributions to the Study of Precocity in Children: The History of Neurology. The Fitzpatrick Lectures on the History of Medicine, Delivered at the Royal College of Physicians in the Years 1907 and 1908* (London: E. G. Millar, 1921), pp. 71–160; see also Roy Porter, *The Greatest Benefit to Mankind: A Medical History of Humanity* (New York and London: W. W. Norton, 1997).

17 George Saliba, *Islamic Science and the Making of the European Renaissance* (Cambridge, MA, and London: MIT Press, 2011), pp. 233–55.

18 Erwin H. Ackernecht, *Medicine at the Paris Hospital* (Baltimore: Johns Hopkins University Press, 1967); Owsei Temkin, *The Double Face of Janus and Other Essays in the History of Medicine* (Baltimore: Johns Hopkins University Press, 1977).

19 H. Floris Cohen, *The Scientific Revolution: An Historiographical Inquiry* (Chicago: University of Chicago Press, 1994), pp. 39–40.

20 Herbert Butterfield, *The Origins of Modern Science* (New York: Free Press, 1957); see also Ernst Mayr, 'When is Historiography Whiggish', *Journal of the History of Ideas* 51:2 (1990), 301–9. Mayr's critique of the charge that some histories are Whiggish bears on this story. Mayr claimed that the distinction between a developmental history of science and a social history of science should be made, and he argued that the charge of Whiggishness in the historiography of science was often faulty. A social history of science, he argued, might not be concerned with scientific progress, but a developmental history always would be. This volume seeks some middle ground between Mayr's contentions and fruitful approaches in the social and cultural history of science. It is possible to recognise that some contributions to science and medicine have withstood the test of time and to argue that the social and cultural context of those contributions made progress both possible and perhaps had little to do with the development of scientific and medical knowledge. Where possible, this volume describes trends in neurological knowledge and trends in the social and cultural context of medicine which influenced the specialisation of neurology overtly and accidently.

21 Anon., 'The Harveian Oration', *The Times* (20 October 1902), 10.

22 Cohen, *The Scientific Revolution*, p. 112.

23 Edwin Clarke and C. D. O'Malley, *The Human Brain and Spinal Cord: A Historical Study Illustrated by Writings from Antiquity to the Twentieth Century* (San Francisco: Norman Publishers, 1996).

24 Walther Riese, 'An Outline of a History of Ideas in Neurology', *Bulletin of the History of Medicine* 23:2 (1949), 111–36; Roy Porter, *Flesh in the Age of Reason* (New York and London: W. W. Norton and Co., 2003); Rousseau, *Nervous Acts*; Robert L. Martensen, *The Brain Takes Shape: An Early History* (Oxford and New York: Oxford University Press, 2004); Charles Sherrington, *The Endeavour of Jean Fernel: With a List of the Editions of his Writings* (Cambridge: Cambridge University Press, 1946); Edward George Tandy Liddell, *The Discovery of Reflexes* (Oxford: Clarendon Press, 1960).

25 M. Neuburger, *Die historische Entwicklung der experimentellen Gehern und Rüchenmarks-physiologie vor Flourens* (Stuttgart: Ferdinand Enke, 1897); Jules Soury, *Le système nerveux central, structure et fonctions, histoire critique des théories et des doctrines* (Paris: Georges Carré et C. Naud, 1889); Guthrie, *Contributions to the Study of Precocity in Children*, pp. 71–160; Fielding H. Garrison, 'History of Neurology', in Charles L. Dana (ed.), *Text-Book of Nervous Diseases: For the Use of Students and Practitioners of Medicine*, 10th ed. (New York: William Wood and Co., 1925), pp. xv–liii.

26 Daniel Kevles and Gerald Geison, 'The Experimental Life Sciences in the Twentieth Century,' *Osiris* 10 (1995), 97–121, especially 101–7.

27 William Feindel, 'Thomas Willis...The Founder of Neurology', *Canadian Medical Association Journal* 87 (1962), 289–6; Hansruedi Isler, *Thomas Willis, 1621–1675: Doctor and Scientist* (New York and London, 1968), pp. 101–2; William Feindel, 'The Beginning of Neurology: Thomas Willis and his Circle of Friends', in Rose (ed.), *A Short History of British Neurology*, pp. 1–18; Robert Martensen 'When the Brain Came out of the Skull: Thomas Willis (1621–1675), Anatomical Technique and the Formation of the "Cerebral Body" in Seventeenth-Century England', in Rose (ed.), *A Short History of British Neurology*, pp. 129–44.

28 For example: George Thomson, *Syllabus. Pointing out Every Part of the Human System* (London: Hughs, 1739), pp. 123–33; Richard Brookes, *An Introduction to Physic and Surgery* (London: J. Newbury, 1754), pp. 177–83; John Aitken, *Principles of anatomy and physiology* (London, J. Murray, 1786), pp. 1–23.

29 Roger Cooter, *The Cultural Meaning of Popular Science: Phrenology and the Organisation of Consent in Nineteenth-Century Britain* (Cambridge: Cambridge University Press, 1985).

30 John Coghill, 'Lectures on the Structure and Relations of the Nervous System at the Periphery, including the Neurology of the Organs of Special Sense', *Lancet* (1859), 279–81.

31 Thomas Pope, 'A Matter of Fact View of the Use of Mercury in Disease', *British Medical Journal* 1 (1861), 76.

32 George Beard, 'Editorial', *Archives of Electrology and Neurology: A Journal of Electro-Therapeutics and Nervous Diseases*, 1 (1874), 116–21.

33 See, for example, Mervyn Eadie, *The Flowering of a Waratah: The History of the Australian Neurology and of the Australian Association of Neurologists* (Eastleigh: John Libby, 2000), pp. 41–51; Howard Kushner, *A Cursing Brain: The Histories of Tourette's Syndrome* (Cambridge, MA, and London: Harvard University Press, 1999), p. 235, fn. 21.

34 Kevles and Geison, 'The Experimental Life Sciences in the Twentieth Century', 101–7.

35 Andrew Wear, *Knowledge and Practice in English Medicine, 1550–1680* (Cambridge: Cambridge University Press, 2000); also see Andrew Wear (ed.), *Medicine in Society: Historical Essays* (Cambridge: Cambridge University Press, 1992).

36 Mark S. R. Jenner and Patrick Wallis (eds), *Medicine and the Market in England and its Colonies, c. 1450–c. 1850* (Basingstoke: Palgrave Macmillan, 2007); Harry Whitaker, C. U. M. Smith, and Stanley Finger (eds), *Brain, Mind and Medicine: Essays in Eighteenth-Century Neuroscience* (New York: Springer, 2007); Karen Buckle, 'The Culture of Oculists in England, 1660–1740' (MA dissertation, University of York, 2005); Wear, *Knowledge and Practice.*

37 Stephen Jacyna, 'Medicine in Transformation, 1800–1849', in W. F. Bynum, Anne Hardy, Stephen Jacyna, Christopher Lawrence, and E. M. Tansey (eds), *The Western Medical Tradition, 1800–2000* (Cambridge: Cambridge University Press, 2006); also see the classic articles by N. D. Jewson, 'Medical Knowledge and the Patronage System in 18th-Century England', *Sociology* 8 (1974), 369–85; and 'The Disappearance of the Sick-Man from Medical Cosmology, 1770–1870', *Sociology* 10 (1976), 225–44.

38 Weisz, *Divide and Conquer*, p. 18; also see Toby Gelfand, *Professionalizing Modern Medicine: Paris Surgeons and Medical Science and Institutions in the 18th Century* (Westport, CT: Greenwood Press, 1980); Ackernecht, *Medicine in the Paris Hospital.*

39 Xavier Bichat, *Physiological Researches on Life and Death*, trans. F. Gold (London: Longman, Hurst, Rees, Orme and Brown, n.d.) first quote on p. 265, second on p. 260.

40 Philippe Pinel, *A Treatise on Insanity in which Are Contained the Principles of a New and More Practical Nosology of Maniacal Disorders than Has Yet Been Offered to the Public*, trans. D. D. Davis (Sheffield: W. Todd, 1806), pp. 2–3; also see Andrew Scull, *Social Order/Mental Disorder: Anglo-American Psychiatry in Historical Perspective* (Berkeley: University of California Press, 1989), p. 81.

41 Jan Goldstein, *Console and Classify: The French Psychiatric Profession in the Nineteenth Century* (Cambridge: Cambridge University Press, 1987), pp. 47–60 and pp. 149–51.

42 Michael Brown, *Performing Medicine: Medical Culture and Identity in Provincial England, c. 1760–1850* (Manchester: Manchester University Press, 2011); Anne Digby, *The Evolution of British General Practice, 1850–1948* (New York: Oxford University Press, 1999); Anne Digby, *Making a Medical Living: Doctors and Patients in the English Market for Medicine, 1720–1911* (Cambridge: Cambridge University Press, 1994); Irvine Loudon, *Medical Care and the General Practitioner, 1750–1850* (Oxford: Clarendon Press, 1986).

43 S. W. F. Holloway, 'Medical Education in England, 1830-1858', *History* 49 (1964), 299–324; A. H. T. Robb-Smith, 'Medical Education at Oxford and Cambridge Prior to 1850', in F. N. L. Poynter (ed.), *The Evolution of Medical Education in Britain* (London: Pitman Medical Publishing, 1966), pp. 51–2 and also p. 59.

44 J. R. Ellis, 'The Growth of Science and the Reform of the Curriculum', in Poynter (ed.), *The Evolution of Medical Education in Britain*, p. 156.

45 Weisz, *Divide and Conquer*, pp. 28–34.

46 Charles Newman, 'The Rise of Specialism and Postgraduate Education', in Poynter (ed.), *The Evolution of Medical Education in Britain*, pp. 169–91, pp. 173–5.

47 Buckle, 'The Culture of Oculists in England, 1660–1740'.

48 George Cheyne, *The English Malady or a Treatise of Nervous Diseases of All Kinds as Spleen, Vapours, Lowness of Spirits, Hypochondriacal, and Hysterical Distempers, etc.* (London: Strathan, 1733), pp. 6–7, pp. 10–11, pp. 60–5, pp. 111–18.

49 Lawrence, 'The Nervous System and Society in the Scottish Enlightenment', in Barry Barnes and Steven Shapin (eds), *Natural Order: Historical Studies of Scientific Culture* (London: Sage, 1979), pp. 23–31.

50 Rousseau, *Nervous Acts*; Guenter B. Risse, 'Medicine in the Age of Enlightenment', in Wear (ed.), *Medicine in Society*, pp. 149–95.

51 As any modern reader of Jane Austen or Wilkie Collins can readily observe, women – their bodies and minds – bore the brunt of these social and cultural anxieties. See Roy Porter, 'Madness and its Institutions', in Wear (ed.), *Medicine in Society*, pp. 277–301; Janet Oppenheim, *'Shattered Nerves': Doctors, Patients, and Depression in Victorian England* (New York: Oxford University Press, 1991), pp. 181–232; Elaine Showalter, *The Female Malady: Women, Madness, and English Culture, 1830-1980* (New York: Pantheon Books, 1985); Dona L. Davis and Setha M. Low (eds), *Gender, Health, and Illness:*

The Case of Nerves (New York: Hemisphere, 1989); Evelyn Ender, *Sexing the Mind: Nineteenth-Century Fictions of Hysteria* (Ithaca, NY: Cornell University Press, 1995), pp. 1–66. But women were not alone. Some claimed male genius vulnerable as well. As historian Janet Browne has noted, Charles Darwin's illnesses – his depression, fatigue, and hypochondria – might well be such an instance. Janet Browne, 'I Could Have Retched All Night: Charles Darwin and his Body', in Christopher Lawrence and Steven Shapin (eds), *Science Incarnate: Historical Embodiments of Natural Knowledge* (Chicago and London: University of Chicago Press, 1998), pp. 240–80.

52 Martensen, *The Brain Takes Shape*, pp. 175–213; Alan Richardson, *British Romanticism and the Science of the Mind* (Cambridge: Cambridge University Press, 2001), pp. 39–65; Lawrence, 'The Nervous System and Society in the Scottish Enlightenment', pp. 19–40; Eric J. Engstrom, *Clinical Psychiatry in Imperial Germany: A History of Psychiatric Practice* (Ithaca, NY, and London: Cornell University Press, 2003), pp. 58–61.

53 Bakken Library and Museum, Minneapolis, MN (hereafter Bakken Library), John Buddle Blyth, 'The Dependence of the Animal and Organic Functions on Nervous Influence; and the Identity of the Latter with Electricity' (MD dissertation, Edinburgh University, 1839), p. 8.

54 Whitaker, Smith, and Finger (eds), *Brain, Mind, and Medicine*, pp. 13–14; Lawrence C. McHenry, *Garrison's History of Neurology* (Charles C. Thomas, 1969), p. 71.

55 Marchello Pera, *The Ambiguous Frog: The Galvani-Volta Controversy on Animal Electricity* (Princeton: Princeton University Press, 1992).

56 L. S. Jacyna, 'Galvanic Influences: Themes in the Early History of British Animal Electricity', in Marco Bresadola and Giuliano Pancaldi (eds), *Luigi Galvani: International Workshop Proceedings* (Bologna: Centro Internazionale per la Storia della Università e della Scienza, 1999), p. 184.

57 Alison Winter, *Mesmerized: Powers of Mind in Victorian Britain* (Chicago and London: University of Chicago Press, 1998); Cooter, *The Cultural Meaning of Popular Science.*

58 *Liverpool Mercury* (8 May 1846).

59 Charles Bell, 'Reprint of the "Idea of a New Anatomy of the Brain"', *Journal of Anatomy and Physiology* 3:1 (1868), 147–82, 153.

60 For an excellent digest of Bell's place in British science and medicine, see Carin Berkowitz, 'Medical Science as Pedagogy in Early Nineteenth-Century Britain: Charles Bell and the Politics of London Medical Reform' (PhD dissertation, Cornell University, 2010).

61 David M. Vess, *Medical Revolution in France, 1789–1796* (Gainesville: University Presses of Florida, 1975), pp. 185–93.

62 Christopher Lawrence, *Medicine in the Making of Modern Britain, 1700–1920* (London and New York: Routledge, 1994), pp. 27–36.

63 Bynum, Hardy, Jacyna, Lawrence, and Tansey (eds), *The Western Medical Tradition, 1800 to 2000*, pp. 53–64, 120–3; also see Shepherd, *Creating Modern Neuroscience*, pp. 100–10; Engstrom, *Clinical Psychiatry in Imperial Germany*, pp. 88–120.

64 Bell, 'Reprint of the "Idea of a New Anatomy of the Brain"', p. 156.

65 Henry Harris, *The Birth of the Cell* (New Haven: Yale University Press, 1999); Richard Rapport, *Nerve Endings: The Discovery of the Synapse. The Quest to Find How Brain Cells Communicate* (New York and London: St Edmundsbury Press, 2005), pp. 82–93 and 114–29; Robert Bentley Todd and William Bowman, *The Physiological Anatomy and Physiology of Man* (Philadelphia: Blanchard and Lea, 1857), pp. 194–5.

66 W. F. Bynum, *Science and the Practice of Medicine in the Nineteenth Century* (New York: Cambridge University Press, 1994), p. 124; of course, the reflex was another matter. See Engstrom, *Clinical Psychiatry in Imperial Germany*, pp. 58–60.

67 Thomas Laycock, 'On the Reflex Function of the Brain: A Correction of Dates', *British Medical Journal* (1874), 705–6.

68 Stephen Jay Gould, *The Mismeasure of Man* (London and New York: W. W. Norton, 1981); Janet Browne, *Charles Darwin: A Biography. Volume 1: Voyaging* (Princeton: Princeton University Press, 1995), pp. 167–340; also see Steven Shapin, 'History of Science and its Sociological Reconstructions', *History of Science* 198:20 (1982), 157–211.

69 Smith, *Inhibition*, pp. 27–65; also see Daniel Pick, *Faces of Degeneration: A European Disorder, c. 1848–c. 1918* (Cambridge: Cambridge University Press: 1989).

70 Marijke Gijswjt-Hofstra and Roy Porter (eds), *Cultures of Neurasthenia: From Beard to the First World War* (Amsterdam: Rodopi, 2001).

71 L. Stephen Jacyna, 'Somatic Theories of Mind and the Interest of Medicine in Britain, 1850–1879', *Medical History* 26:3 (1982), 233–58.

72 George K. York and David A. Steinberg, *An Introduction to the Life and Work of John Hughlings Jackson with a Catalogue Raisonné of his Writings* (London: Wellcome Trust Centre for the History of Medicine at UCL, 2006), pp. 9–19; Gerald L. Geison, '"Divided We Stand": Physiologists and Clinicians in the American Context', in Martha Vogel and Charles E. Rosenberg (eds), *The Therapeutic Revolution: Essays in the Social History of Medicine* (Philadelphia: University of Pennsylvania Press, 1979), pp. 67–90.

73 Kurt Danziger, *Constructing the Subject: Historical Origins of Psychological Research* (Cambridge: Cambridge University Press, 1994).

74 Engstrom, *Clinical Psychiatry in Imperial Germany*, pp. 98–102.

75 Jacyna, *Lost Words*, pp. 81–141; Liddell, *The Discovery of Reflexes*, pp. 44–97; Julius Althaus, *The Functions of the Brain: A Popular Essay* (London: Longmans and Co., 1880), pp. 5–44; William Gowers, *Diseases of the Nervous System* (Philadelphia: B. Plackston Son and Co., 1899); James Purves Stewart, *The Diagnoses of Nervous Diseases* (London: Edward Arnold, 1906).

76 Consider the variety of subjects addressed: Charles Denison, 'The Influence of the Climate of Colorado on the Nervous System', *Archives of Electricity and Neurology* 1 (1874), 179–93; L. Duncan Bulkley, 'The Relations of the Nervous System to Diseases of the Skin', *Archives of Electricity and Neurology* 1 (1874), 242–68; John Hughlings Jackson, 'Ophthalmology and Diseases of the Nervous System', *Transactions of the Opthalmological Society of the United Kingdom* 6 (1886), 1–22; Shadworth Hodgson, 'The Philosophical Relations of Neurology', *Brain* 14 (1891), 1–17; J. S. Bristowe, 'On the Nature and Relations of Mind and Brain', *Brain* 14 (1891), 18–34; William Gowers, 'The Designation of Musical Notes in Science and Medicine', *Review of Neurology and Psychiatry* 1 (1903), 228–33; Leonard J. Kidd, 'Lachrymal Reflexes: Pressure-Sensibility of Head and Neck: And the Squeezed-Tongue Sensation', *Review of Neurology and Psychiatry* 7 (1909), 167–80.

77 These efforts seem common in the Anglo-American world. Circumstances are less clear for Europe. See, for instance, Anne Hardy, 'Poliomyelitis and the Neurologists: The View from England, 1896–1966', *Bulletin of the History of Medicine* 71:2 (1997), 249–72; Kenton Kroker, 'Epidemic Encephalitis and American Neurology, 1919–1940', *Bulletin of the History of Medicine* 78:1 (2004), 108–47.

78 See, for example, Christopher Crenner, *Private Practice: In the Early Twentieth-Century Medical Office of Dr Richard Cabot* (Baltimore: Johns Hopkins University Press, 2005), pp. 137–88; Engstrom, *Clinical Psychiatry in Imperial Germany*, pp. 16–50.

79 See, for example, Samuel Wilks, *A Memoir: On the New Discoveries or New Observations Made During the Time he Was a Teacher at Guy's Hospital* (London: Adlard and Son, 1911); Humphrey Rolleston, *Life of Sir Clifford Allbutt* (London: Macmillan and Co., 1929); M. E. Broadbent (ed.), *The Life of Sir William Broadbent*, (London: John Murray, 1909), pp. 228–33.

80 Chandak Sengoopta, 'A Mob of Incoherent Symptoms? Neurasthenia in British Medical Discourse, 1860–1920', in Gijswijt-Hofstra

and Porter (eds), *Cultures of Neurasthenia*, p. 107; Critchley and Critchley, *John Hughlings Jackson*, ch. 18; Anon., 'The Story of "Brain": Complimentary Dinner to Dr Head', *British Medical Journal* 2 (1924), 880–1; see also Nikolas S. Rose, *The Psychological Complex: Psychology, Politics and society in England, 1869–1939* (London: Routledge, 1985), p. 4.

81 William R. Gowers, 'Reports: Pathological', *Mind* 1:4 (1876), 552–4; William R. Gowers, 'Clinical and Physiological Researches on the Nervous System: On the Localisation of Movements in the Brain', *Mind* 1:1 (1876), 125–7; James Sully, 'Dr Hughlings Jackson on Morbid Affections of Speech', *Mind* 5:17 (1880), 105–11; also see Jacyna, 'Somatic Theories of Mind and the Interest of Medicine in Britain', 233–58, especially 257.

82 The most relevant literature on neurological journals and societies is for those in America. See, John Burnham, 'The Founding of the Archives of Neurology and Psychiatry; or, What Was Wrong with the Journal of Nervous and Mental Disease?', *Journal of the History of Medicine and Allied Sciences* 34 (1981), 310–24; also see DeJong, *A History of American Neurology*, pp. 139–44. I sought circulation information for *Brain*, *Review of Neurology and Psychiatry*, *Archives of Neurology and Psychopathology*, and *Mind*. The only information I located was for *Brain*, which had 273 subscribers in 1905.

83 Alexander Bruce, 'Preliminary Statement', *Review of Neurology and Psychiatry* 1 (1903), 1–2.

84 The classic work on specialisation is Rosen, *The Specialization of Medicine*. For related and important literature see Abbott, *The System of Professions*; and John Burnham, *How the Idea of Profession Changed the Writing of Medical History* (London: Wellcome Institute for the History of Medicine, 1998).

85 The classic study is Stevens, *Medical Practice in Modern England*.

86 See, for example, Engstrom, *Clinical Psychiatry in Imperial Germany*; Roger Cooter, *Surgery and Society in Peace and War: Orthopaedics and the Organization of Modern Medicine, 1880–1948* (London: Macmillan, 1993); Goldstein, *Console and Classify*; W. Bruce Fye, *American Cardiology: The History of a Specialty and its College* (Baltimore: Johns Hopkins University Press, 1996); Glenn Gritzer and Arnold Arluke, *The Making of Rehabilitation: A Political Economy of Medical Specialization* (Berkeley: University of California Press, 1985).

87 See Rosen, *Specialization of Medicine*; Eulner, *Die Entwicklung der medizinischen Specizlfächer*, Stevens, *Medical Practice in Modern England*, Weisz, *Divide and Conquer*.

88 Anon., 'Specialism in Medicine', *The Times* (11 October 1910), 7.

89 Anon., letter to the editor, *The Times* (12 August 1886), 12.

90 S. Leonard Simpson, 'Specialization', *British Medical Journal* (1949), 368.

91 Important exceptions can found in the following analyses: Christopher Lawrence, 'Still Incommunicable: Clinical Holists and Medical Knowledge in Interwar Britain', in Christopher Lawrence and George Weisz (eds), *Greater than the Parts: Holism in Biomedicine, 1920–1950* (Oxford and New York: Oxford University Press, 1998); Weisz, *Divide and Conquer*; Paul Starr, *The Social Transformation of American Medicine* (New York: Basic Books, 1982), pp. 76–7; Arleen Marcia Tuchman, *Science, Medicine, and the State in Germany: The Case of Baden, 1815–1971* (Oxford: Oxford University Press, 1993), pp. 120–5; Roger Cooter and Steve Sturdy, 'Science, Scientific Management, and the Transformation of Medicine in Britain c. 1870–1950', *History of Science* 36 (1998), 421–66.

92 Weisz, *Divide and Conquer*, pp. 210–13.

93 Thomas Hobbes, *Leviathan, or The Matter, Forme, and Power of a Common-Wealth* (London: Andrew Crooke, at the Green Dragon in St Pauls Church-yard, 1651), p. 1. See: http://archive.org/stream/hobbesleviathan00hobbuoft#page/n35/mode/2up (accessed on 6 July 2012); Fabio de Sio, 'Leviathan and the Soft Animal: Medical Humanism and the Invertebrate Models for Higher Nervous Functions, 1950s–90s', *Medical History* 55:3 (2011), 369–74.

94 Jean-Jacques Rousseau, *The Social Contract* (Ware: Wordsworth Editions, 1998), p. 89.

95 Laura Salisbury and Andrew Shail (eds), *Neurology and Modernity: A Cultural History of Nervous Systems, 1800–1950* (Basingstoke: Palgrave Macmillan, 2010); Musselman, *Nervous Conditions*; Rousseau, *Nervous Acts*; Lawrence, 'The Nervous System and Society in the Scottish Enlightenment'.

96 Martensen, *The Brain Takes Shape*, pp. 175–213; also see Richardson, *British Romanticism and the Science of the Mind*.

97 Shepherd, *Creating Modern Neuroscience*; Jack Pressman, *Last Resort: Psychosurgery and the Limits of Medicine* (Cambridge: Cambridge University Press, 1998); Nathan G. Hale, *The Rise and Crisis of Psychoanalysis in the United States: Freud and the Americans, 1917–1985* (New York: Oxford University Press, 1995); Gerald A. Grob, *From Asylum to Community: Mental Health Policy in Modern America* (Princeton: Princeton University Press, 1991); Danziger, *Constructing the Subject*; Rose, *The Psychological Complex*; Gerald A. Grob, *Mental Illness and American Society, 1875–1940* (Princeton: Princeton University Press, 1983).

98 Young, *Mind, Brain, and Adaptation in the Nineteenth Century*; Harrington, *Medicine, Mind, and the Double Brain*; Jacyna, *Lost Words*.

99 Anne Stiles, *Popular Brain Science in the Late Nineteenth Century* (Cambridge: Cambridge University Press, 2012); James Kennaway, *Bad Vibrations: The History of the Idea of Music as a Cause of Disease* (Farnham: Ashgate, 2012).

100 See, for instance, Winter, *Mesmerized*.

101 Weisz, *Divide and Conquer*, pp. xi–xxx.

102 This is a point that is largely absent from William F. Bynum, 'The Nervous Patient in 18th- and 19th-Century Britain: The Psychiatric Origins of British Neurology', in William Bynum, Roy Porter, and Michael Shepard (eds), *The Anatomy of Madness: Essays in the History of Psychiatry*, 1990), pp. 89–102.

103 Clarke and Jacyna, *Nineteenth-Century Origins of Neuroscientific Concepts*; Susan Leigh Star, *Regions of the Mind: Brain Research and the Quest for Scientific Certainty* (Stanford: Stanford University Press, 1989).

104 A point excellently made by Musselman, *Nervous Conditions*.

105 Weisz, *Divide and Conquer*, pp. 28–34; also see Francis Fraser, 'The Rise of Specialism and the Special Hospitals' in F. N. L. Poynter (ed.), *The Evolution of Hospitals in Britain* (London: Pitman Medical Publishing, 1964), pp. 179–80.

106 Cooter and Sturdy, 'Science, Scientific Management, and the Transformation of Medicine in Britain', 424.

107 Stevens, *Medical Practice in Modern England*, p. 28.

108 Digby, *Making a Medical Living*, p. 34.

109 Thomas Laycock, 'On the Prevalence of Nervous Diseases Arrest of the Urine', *Lancet* (1840), 608.

110 Quoted in James Taylor, 'The Ophthalmological Observations of Hughlings Jackson and their Bearing on Nervous and Other Diseases', *Brain* 38 (1915), 395.

111 William Hale-White, *Great Doctors of the Nineteenth Century* (London: Edward Arnold, 1935), pp. 246–67, especially 258.

112 Brian Abel-Smith, *The Hospitals, 1800–1948: A Study in Social Administration in England and Wales* (London: Heinemann, 1964).

113 Florence Nightingale, *Notes on Nursing* (New York: Dover Publications, 1969), pp. 37–44.

114 Newman, 'The Rise of Specialism and Postgraduate Education', pp. 173–5.

115 Stevens, *Medical Practice in Modern England*, p. 27.

116 Fraser, 'The Rise of Specialism and the Special Hospitals', pp. 169–85.

117 Stevens, *Medical Practice in Modern England*, p. 33.

118 Wellcome Library, London (hereafter WL), GC/83/13 Minute Books QS1.859/6G, 30-04-1862.
119 The best up-to-date summaries appear in Ann Scott, Mervyn Eadie, and Andrew Lees, *William Richard Gowers, 1845–1915* (Oxford: Oxford University Press, 2012), pp. 81–97; Michael J. Aminoff, *Brown Séquard: An Improbable Genius who Transformed Medicine* (Oxford: Oxford University Press, 2011), pp. 97–120.
120 It is noteworthy that in the same period physician Wilhelm Griesinger in Germany endeavoured to facilitate similar reforms for somatic psychiatry by the creation of urban psychiatric clinics. Yet, in Britain, the responsible agents were the Victorian middle classes and not medical practitioners. Engstrom, *Clinical Psychiatry in Imperial Germany*, pp. 85–7.
121 Anon., 'The Scope of Neurology in Hospital Practice', *Journal of Neurology and Psychopathology* 3:10 (1922), 168.
122 Stevens, *Medical Practice in Modern England*, pp. 31–41.
123 Broadbent (ed.), *The Life of Sir William Broadbent*, pp. 92–3, quote on p. 297.
124 Oppenheim, *'Shattered Nerves'*, pp. 1–62; Stevens, *Medical Practice in Modern England*, pp. 39–41.
125 Bonnie Ellen Blustein, *Preserve your Love for Science: Life of William A Hammond, American Neurologist* (Cambridge: Cambridge University Press, 1991); Andrew Oliff, 'History and Development of Neurology as a Distinct Specialty in America', *Journal of Civil War Medicine* 3 (1999), 33–41.
126 Bonnie Ellen Blustein, 'New York Neurologists and the Specialization of American medicine', *Bulletin of the History of Medicine* 53 (1979), 170–83; Douglas Lanska, T. A. Chumura, and Christopher Goetz, 'Part 1: The History of 19th-Century Neurology and the American Neurological Association', *Annals of Neurology* 53 (2003), S2–S26; Rosemary Stevens, *American Medicine and the Public Interest: A History of Specialization* (London: University of California Press, 1998).
127 William Welch, 'S. Weir Mitchell: Physician and Man of Science', in *S. Weir Mitchell, M.D., LL.D, F.R.S., 1829–1914: Memorial Addresses and Resolutions* (Philadelphia: College of Physicians of Philadelphia, 1914), pp. 97–127; Charles W. Burr, *The S. Weir Mitchell Oration. S. Weir Mitchell: Physician, Man of Science, Man of Letters, Man of Affairs* (Philadelphia, The College, 1920); S. Weir Mitchell, *The Complete Poems* (New York: Century, 1914); S. Weir Mitchell, *Constance Trescot: A Novel* (New York: Century Co., 1905); S. Weir Mitchell, *A Comedy of Conscience* (New York: Century Co., 1903).
128 See how Michael Denning, *The Cultural Front: The Laboring of*

American Culture in the Twentieth Century (London and New York: Verso, 1996), pp. 27–8 and throughout explores the notion of generational time.

129 Quoted in McHenry, *Garrison's History of Neurology*, pp. 254–7; for a discussion of Charcot's chair see Goetz, Bonduelle, and Gelfand, *Charcot: Constructing Neurology*, pp. 222–31; Engstrom, *Clinical Psychiatry in Imperial German*, pp. 123–7.

130 Mark Micale, *Approaching Hysteria: Disease and its Interpretations* (Princeton: Princeton University Press, 1995).

131 Jean M. Charcot, *Lectures on the Diseases of the Nervous System* (New York: Hafner Publishing Co., 1962), p. iii.

132 York and Steinberg, *An Introduction to the Life and Work of John Hughlings Jackson*, pp. 10–18.

133 Peter Koehler, 'The Evolution of British Neurology in Comparison with Other Countries', in Rose (ed.), *A Short History of Neurology*, pp. 58–74.

134 Bynum, 'The Nervous Patient in 18th- and 19th-Century Britain', pp. 89–102; likewise, Joan Jacobs Brumberg, *Fasting Girls: The History of Anorexia Nervosa* (New York: Vintage Books, 2000), pp. 100–228; Micale, *Approaching Hysteria*, pp. 7–98; for the case of America, see Ballenger, *Self, Senility, and Alzheimer's Disease in Modern America*.

135 John E. Senior, 'Rationalising Electrotherapy in Neurology, 1860–1920' (PhD dissertation, Oxford University, 1994).

136 The substantial primary and secondary literature on medical and professional societies deserves recognition here. Examples include: Samuel Miller, *A Brief Retrospect of the Eighteenth Century. Volume 1 of 3: A Sketch of the Revolutions and Improvements in Science, Arts, and Literature During that Period* (London: Elllerton and Byworth, 1805), pp. 99–106; James Gray and A. M. McFarlan, 'The Royal Medical Society of Edinburgh', in D'Arcy Power (ed.), *British Medical Societies* (London: Medical Press, 1939), pp. 12–19; Steven Shapin, 'The Royal Society of Edinburgh: A Study of the Social Context of Hanoverian Science' (PhD dissertation, University of Pennsylvania, 1971); R. J. Morris, 'Clubs, Societies, and Associations', in F. M. L. Thompson (ed.), *The Cambridge Social History of Britain, 1750–1950. Volume 3: Social Agencies and Institutions* (Cambridge: Cambridge University Press, 1990), pp. 395–443; Jacqueline Jenkinson, 'The Role of Medical Societies in the Rise of the Scottish Medical Profession, 1730–1939', *Social History of Medicine* 4 (1991), pp. 253–75.

137 David Williams, 'RSM 1907: The Acceptance of Specialization', *Journal of the Royal Society of Medicine* 93 (2000), 642–5; Penelope Hunting, *The History of the Royal Society of Medicine* (London: Royal Society of Medicine Press, 2001).

138 These remarks are made with the caveat that these changes did not represent 'progress' but rather 'necessity'. See Roger Cooter and Steve Sturdy, 'Of War, Medicine, and Modernity: Introduction', in Roger Cooter, Mark Harrison, and Steve Sturdy (eds), *War, Medicine, and Modernity* (Stroud: Sutton, 1998), pp. 2–7. The appeal to progress in knowledge through war research was made by neurologists, especially in America. See, for instance, Percival Bailey, 'The Present State of American Neurology', *Journal of Neuropathology and Experimental Neurology* 1 (1942), 111–13.

139 Stephen T. Casper, 'Atlantic Conjunctures in Anglo-American Neurology: Lewis H. Weed and Johns Hopkins Neurology, 1917–1942', *Bulletin of the History of Medicine* 82 (2008), 646–71.

140 See, for instance, Bernard Sachs, 'Presidential Address', in *Proceedings of the First International Neurological Congress, Berne (Switzerland), August 31 to September 4, 1931* (Berne: Stämpfli, 1932), pp. 17–18; John Fulton, 'Arnold Klebs and Harvey Cushing at the 1st International Neurological Congress at Berne in 1931', *Bulletin of the History of Medicine* 8 (1940), 332–54.

141 Macdonald Critchley, undated address [c. 1985]; Council Minutes of the Association of British Neurologists, Volume 1, Archives of the Association of British Neurologists, London.

142 Stephen T. Casper, '"Then Why Not an Association of British Neurologists?" British Neurologists and the Founding of an Elite Medical Society', *Annals of Clinical Neuroscience and Rehabilitation* 7 (2007), 16–17; Peter Robinson, *The History of the Association at the 50th Anniversary Meeting, 4th November 1983* (Winchester: Peter Robinson, 1985).

143 Royal College of Physicians, *Interim Report of the Committee on Neurology* (London: Harrison & Sons, 1954).

144 Michael Foucault, *The Birth of the Clinic* (London: Routledge, 2000), p. 198.

145 Note that while I am endorsing rather strongly here arguments and observations made by Fernando Vidal, I am also contrasting my own sense of the chronology with his. See Fernando Vidal, 'Brainhood, Anthropological Figure of Modernity', *History of the Human Sciences* 22:1 (2009), 15–36 and, compare, for example, with Shepherd, *Creating Modern Neuroscience*, pp. 3–14 and pp. 235–6. In this, I am perhaps also entering into a rather longer-standing debate between intellectual and social history, as exemplified by Kevles and Geison, 'The Experimental Life Sciences in the Twentieth Century', 101; and Clarke and Jacyna, *Nineteenth-Century Origins of Neuroscientific Concepts*, p. 1.

Chapter 1

1 William MacCormac and George Henry Makins, 'Discussion on the Localization of Function in the *Cortex Cerebri*', *Transactions of the International Medical Congress* (London: J. W. Klockman, 1881), pp. 237–48; the best study of Ferrier's early career is Michael Anthony Finn, 'The West Riding Lunatic Asylum and the Making of the Modern Brain Sciences in the Nineteenth Century (PhD dissertation, University of Leeds, 2012), especially chs 3–4.
2 Ibid., ch. 5.
3 David Ferrier, *The Functions of the Brain* (London: Smith, 1876), quote on p. v, but see pp. 126–7 and 256 for illustrations of Jackson's influence on his thought.
4 David Millett, 'Illustrating a Revolution: An Unrecognized Contribution to the "Golden Era" of Cerebral Localisation', *Notes and Records of the Royal Society* 52 (1998), 292–3.
5 David Ferrier, 'Localisation of Function in the Brain', *Proceedings of the Royal Society* 22 (1874), 229–32; see also David Ferrier, 'Experiments on the Brain of Monkeys – First Series', *Proceedings of the Royal Society* 23 (1875), 409–32; and David Ferrier, 'The Croonian Lecture: Experiments on the Brain of Monkeys – Second Series', *Transaction of the Royal Society of London* 165 (1875), 433–88.
6 Bynum, 'The Nervous Patient in 18th- and 19th-Century Britain', pp. 115–27.
7 George Rosen's classic essay on specialisation invites this conclusion. 'The significance of the relation between ophthalmology and internal medicine, especially neurology, was recognized very soon.' Rosen offers as evidence the following statement of Hughlings Jackson in 1863: 'I write as a physician, and not as an ophthalmologist. I have studied ophthalmic medicine merely as a help to the study of diseases of the Nervous System. I look at the fundus of the eye, in cerebral cases, when there is even slight failure of sight, in order to ascertain the caliber of the retinal vessels, and the supply of blood to the optic disc, as evidenced by their greater coloration.' Rosen, *The Specialisation of Medicine*, p. 22.
8 Context is provided in: Jenkinson, 'The Role of Medical Societies in the Rise of the Scottish Medical Profession'.
9 'Rules', *Transactions of the Ophthalmological Society of the United Kingdom* (hereafter *Trans.*) 1 (1880–81), xxvii–xxx.
10 'Bye-Laws Concerning Communications', *Trans.* 1 (1880–81), xxx.
11 'Report of the Committee on Colour Blindness', *Trans.* 2 (1882), 191; 'The Prevention of Blindness from Opthalmia Neunatorum', *Trans.* 4 (1884), 32–5.

12 William Bowman, 'Inaugural Address at the First Meeting of the Society on 23 June 1880', *Trans.* 1 (1880–81), 1–5 and specifically 4; on Bowman's patronage to the society see: Jonathan Hutchinson, 'Introductory Address at the Opening Meeting of the Session 1883–84, October 11th, 1883', *Trans.* 4 (1884), 1–13.
13 William Bowman, 'Address by the President at the First Annual Meeting, 6 July 1881', *Trans.* 1 (1880–81), 228.
14 John Hughlings Jackson, 'On the Eye Symptoms in Locomotor Ataxy', *Trans.* 1 (1881–82), 139–54; John Hughlings Jackson, 'On the Relation between the Movements of Objects and the Rotation of the Eyes', *Trans.* 2 (1882), 213–17.
15 John Hughlings Jackson, 'On Ocular Movements, with Vertigo, Produced by Pressure on a Diseased Ear', *Trans.* 3 (1883–84), 261–4.
16 Anon., 'Eye Symptoms in Diseases of the Spinal Cord', *Trans.* 3 (1882–83), 190–228.
17 Anon., 'XII. Affections of Muscular and Nervous Systems', *Trans.* 4 (1884), 300–15.
18 Jackson, 'Ophthalmology and Diseases of the Nervous System'.
19 Taylor, 'The Opthalmological Observations of Hughlings Jackson', 392.
20 On Jackson's theories of devolution see, David Steinberg, 'What Modern Neuroscience Can Learn from Hughlings Jackson', in Rose (ed.), *A Short History of Neurology*, pp. 165–77; Oppenheim, *Shattered Nerves*, pp. 274–5.
21 Jackson specifically mentioned Herbert Spencer. See Jackson, 'Ophthalmology and Diseases of the Nervous System', fn., p. 2; the classic work describing the influence of Spencer in the mind and brain sciences is Robert J. Richards, *Darwin and the Emergence of Evolutionary Theories of Mind and Behavior* (Chicago: University of Chicago Press, 1987), pp. 157–294.
22 Jackson, 'Ophthalmology and Diseases of the Nervous System', 1.
23 Ibid., 1–2.
24 Ibid., 2.
25 Ibid.
26 Ibid., 16–17.
27 Ibid., 22.
28 Samuel Greenblatt, 'The Major Influences on the Early Life and Works of John Hughlings Jackson', *Bulletin of the History of Medicine*, 39:4 (1965), 346–76; also see Janet Browne, *Charles Darwin: The Power of Place* (Princeton: Alfred A. Knopf, 2002), vol. 2, ch. 1.
29 On Herbert Spencer see: Mark Francis, 'Herbert Spencer and the Mid-Victorian Scientists', *Annual Review of the Australasian Association for the History, Philosophy, and Social Studies of Science*,

4 (1986), 2–21; David Oldroyd, *Darwinian Impacts: An Introduction to the Darwinian Revolution* (Milton Keynes: Open University Press, 1983), pp. 204–11.

30 P. H. Schurr, 'Outline of the History of the Section of Neurology of the Royal Society of Medicine', *Journal of the Royal Society of Medicine* 78:2 (1985), 146–8, 147.

31 'Officers and Council for the Session 1888–89', *Trans.* 7 (1889).

32 Rosen, *The Specialization of Medicine*, p. 3.

33 Humphrey Davy Rolleston, *The Right Honourable Sir Thomas Clifford Allbutt* (London: Macmillan and Co., 1929), pp. 56–9.

34 William Gowers, *A Manual and Atlas of Medical Ophthalmoscopy* (London: J. & A. Churchill, 1879).

35 John Hughlings Jackson, 'Value of the Ophthalmoscope in the Investigation and Treatment of Diseases of the Brain', *Lancet* (1880), 906.

36 See Royal Society of Medicine Archives, London (hereafter RSMA), NS/A/1 Neurological Society Minute Book, 1898–1907, which includes reports, letter regarding amalgamation of medical societies and names and addresses of members (hereafter NS/A/1, Minutes), vol. 1, p. 1.

37 Critchley and Critchley, *John Hughlings Jackson*, ch. 18.

38 RSMA, NS/A/1, Minutes, vol. 1, p. 1.

39 RSMA, NS/A/2, Letter from Thomas Buzzard to Leonard Guthrie, 29 January 1908.

40 Ibid.

41 Burnham, 'The Founding of the Archives of Neurology and Psychiatry', 323.

42 In fact, both the proceedings of the Neurological Society and announcements of special lectures occasionally appeared in *Lancet* from 1888 until 1905. See, for instance: 'Neurological Society of London', *Lancet* (1888), 325–6; 'Neurological Society: Presidential Address on Heredity in Neurosis', *Lancet* (1897), 178–9; 'Neurological Society: The Presidential Address', *Lancet* (1898), 16.

43 RSMA, NS/A/1, Minutes, vol. 1, p. 5.

44 RSMA, NS/A/1, Minutes, vol. 1, pp. 12a, 12–13.

45 RSMA, NS/F/1, Memorandum of Agreement between the Neurological Society and Messrs Macmillan & Co.

46 The strain on the society's budget was tremendous. See, for example, RSMA, NS/A/1, Minutes, vol. 1, p. 27.

47 RSMA, NS/A/1, Minutes, vol. 1, p. 13.

48 'The Proceedings of the Neurological Society from its foundation to the year 1893', *Brain* 17 (1894), 19–24.

49 RSMA, NS/A/1, Minutes, vol. 1, p. 4.

50 RSMA, NS/A/1, Minutes, vol. 1, p. 16.

51 RSMA, NS/E/1. No biographical information has emerged for either woman.

52 RSMA, NS/A/2, Neurological Society Minute Book, 1898–1907, vol. 2, no page numbers given; includes reports, letter reamalgamation of medical societies and names and addresses of members(hereafter NS/A/2), Minutes of 111th Meeting.

53 RSMA, NS/A/2, Neurological Society of London, Draft Report of Council for 1902, 22 January 1903.

54 Alan Mason Chesney Medical Archives of Johns Hopkins Medical Institutions, Baltimore, Adolf Meyer Papers (hereafter Adolf Meyer Papers), 11/405/1, Neurological Society of London, Letter from C. E. Beevor to Adolf Meyer, 8 June 1897.

55 Adolf Meyer Papers, 11/405/1, Neurological Society of London, Letter from C. E. Beevor to Adolf Meyer, 29 September 1897.

56 The difference between the number of applications to the society and its total membership can be explained by attrition. Neurological Society of London, Report of Council, 17 December, 1889, pp. 1–2; Copy of Treasurer's Balance Sheet for 1890, pp. 47–9; Neurological Society of London (insert p. 68) Report of Council, 19 January, 1893; Neurological Society of London (insert p. 71) Report of Council, 25 January 1894; Neurological Society of London (insert p. 80) Report of Council, 25 January 1895; Neurological Society of London, Report of Council, 14 January 1897; Neurological Society of London, Report of Council (undated, but c. 1898); RSMA, NS/B/2 Neurological Society of London, Report of Council, 6 February 1902, pp. 1–6; RSMA, NS/B/2, Neurological Society of London, Draft Report of Council for 1902, 22 January 1903, pp. 1–3; NS/B/2 Neurological Society of United Kingdom, Report of the Council for 1903, 4 February 1904, pp. 1–3; Neurological Society of the United Kingdom, Report of the Council for 1905, 1 February 1906, pp. 1–4; NS/B/2, Neurological Society of the United Kingdom, Report of the Council for 1906, 21 February 1907, pp. 1–4.

57 RSMA, NS/D/1, Neurological Society Attendance Book. There were obvious exceptions to this rule. Members from an Oxbridge circle attended frequently.

58 RSMA, NS/D/1, Neurological Society Attendance Book, 1886–98.

59 RSMA, NS/A/1, Minutes, vol. 1, p. 6.

60 RSMA, NS/A/1, Minutes, vol. 1, p. 8.

61 RSMA, NS/A/2, Minutes, vol. 2, 61st Meeting, 2 March 1899; This was the first extra-metropolitan meeting of the society, but it was not envisioned in the same light as the meeting in Edinburgh in 1903; the best description of Rivers' research and its connection to neurology,

physical anthropology, and psychology is: George W. Stocking, *After Tyler: British Social Anthropology, 1888–1951* (Madison: University of Wisconsin Press, 1995), chs 4–5.

62 RSMA, NS/A/2, Minutes, vol. 2, 79th Meeting of the Neurological Society of London.

63 RSMA, NS/A/2, E. A. Schafer to W. S. Coleman, 22 January 1903.

64 RSMA, NS/D/2, Neurological Society Attendance Book, 1898–1907.

65 RSMA, NS/F/1, Fred Batten to Members of Neurological Society, 11 January 1905.

66 RSMA, NS/F/1, Neurological Society of the United Kingdom, p. 1.

67 RSMA, NS/F/1, Programme of Meeting of the Neurological Society of the United Kingdom, 24 June 1905.

68 RSMA, NS/F/1, Menu (three pages), 24 June 1905.

69 RSMA, NS/F/1, Names of Extra-Metropolitan Members who have accepted.

70 Power (ed.), *British Medical Societies*, p. vii.

71 RSMA, NS/A/1, Report of the Council, 25 January 1894.

72 RSMA, NS/A/2 Report of the Council, 14 January 1897.

73 RSMA, NS/A/2, Neurological Society of the United Kingdom, 113rd Meeting, 30 March 1905, pp. 2–3.

74 Ibid., pp. 3–4.

75 Ibid.

76 This showmanship was not restricted to clinical meetings only. See by way of illustration Thomas Buzzard's presidential lecture of 1890. Thomas Buzzard, 'On the Simulation of Hysteria by Organic Disease of the Nervous System', *Brain* 13 (1890), 1–44.

77 Such debates were frequent. For example, see: D. Hack Tuke, 'Imperative Ideas', *Brain* 17, (1894), 179–97 and the subsequent debate, 'On Imperative Ideas, Being a discussion on Dr Hack Tuke's Paper', *Brain* 18 (1895), 318–51.

78 For example, see the presidential address of John Batty Tuke, 'The Relation of the Lunacy Laws to the Treatment of Insanity', *Brain* 28 (1905), 1–12.

79 RSMA, NS/A/1, Neurological Society Report, 25 January 1894; E. A. Shäfer, 'The Nerve Cell Considered as the Basis of Neurology', *Brain* 16 (1893), 134–69.

80 RSMA, NS/A/2, Neurological Society Report, 14 January 1898.

81 RSMA, NS/A/2, Neurological Society Report, 1897.

82 Discussion about creating the lecture began in 1896. 'The Secretary read a letter from Dr [Walter] Coleman, which advocated the desirability of founding a lectureship in honour of Dr Hughlings Jackson. Dr Coleman pointed out a precedent existed in the [Bowman] lectureship founded by the Ophthalmological Society

during the lifetime of Sir W. Bowman.' RSMA, NS/A/1, Minutes, vol. 1, 47th Meeting, 19 March 1896.

83 RSMA, NS/A/1, Minutes, vol. 1, 47th Meeting, 19 March 1896.

84 RSMA, NS/A/2, Neurological Society Report, 14 January 1897.

85 RSMA, NS/A/2, Neurological Society Report, 1898.

86 All of these lectures were published in *Brain*, with the odd exception of the first one by Jackson.

87 RSMA, NS/A/2, The Neurological Society of the United Kingdom Circular, 28 May 1907.

88 The subject of medical societies, however, has a rich literature. See, for example, Jenkinson, 'The Role of Medical Societies in the Rise of the Scottish Medical Profession', 253–75.

89 James Crichton-Browne, *Victorian Jottings, from an Old Commonplace Book* (London: Etchells & Macdonald, 1926), pp. 36–7; Herbert Hutchinson (ed.), *Jonathan Hutchinson, Life and Letters* (London: W. Heinemann, 1946), p. 217; York and Steinberg, *An Introduction to the Life and Work of John Hughlings Jackson*, p. 4.

90 For example, see Thomas Laycock, *Mind and Brain: Or, The Correlations of Consciousness and Organization; Systemically Investigated and Applied to Philosophy, Mental Science, and Practice* (New York: Appleton, 1869).

91 F. E. James, 'The Life and Work of Thomas Laycock, 1812–1876' (PhD dissertation, University of London, 1995), pp. 360–72.

92 Stephen T. Casper, 'Idioms of Practice: British Neurology, 1880–1960' (PhD dissertation, University College London, 2006), pp. 131–53, 381–3.

93 York and Steinberg, *An Introduction to the Life and Work of John Hughlings Jackson*.

94 Gerald L. Geison, *Michael Foster and the Cambridge School of Physiology: The Scientific Enterprise in Late Victorian Society* (Princeton: Princeton University Press, 1978), pp. 5–6; Casper, 'The Idioms of Practice', pp. 381–3.

95 Terrie Romano, *Making Medicine Scientific: John Burdon Sanderson and the Culture of Victorian Science* (Balimore: Johns Hopkins University Press, 2002).

96 Ruth Barton, '"An Influential Set of Chaps": The X-Club and Royal Society Politics, 1864–85', *British Journal for the History of Science* 23 (1990), 53–4.

97 We might also link George Romanes and Charles Darwin to the X-Club; Romanes proposed ten individuals for Fellowship, while Charles Darwin proposed two. On Carpenter and Busk, see Browne, *Charles Darwin: A Biography. Volume 2*, p. 137.

98 Holmes, *The National Hospital*, pp. 1–26.

99 Ibid.

100 Michael J. Aminoff, *Brown-Séquard: An Improbable Genius who Transformed Medicine* (New York: Oxford University Press, 2010), pp. 124–34.

101 Geison, 'Divided We Stand'.

102 Anon., 'John Robert Lord, C.B.E., M.D., F.R.C.P.Ed', *British Medical Journal*, 2 (1931), 363–5, 365.

103 Abbott, *The System of the Professions*, pp. 285–318.

104 'Proceedings of the Neurological Society', *Brain* 28 (1905), 609.

105 Ibid.

106 His case study is of psychiatry and neurology in America. Abbott, *The System of the Professions*, ch. 9.

107 Rousseau, *Nervous Acts*.

108 David Millett, 'Wiring the Brain: From the Excitable Cortex to the EEG, 1870–1940' (PhD dissertation, University of Chicago, 1998), pp. 11–12.

109 Dorothy Ross (ed.), *Modernist Impulses in the Human Sciences, 1870–1930* (Baltimore and London: Johns Hopkins University Press, 1994).

110 Weisz, *Divide and Conquer*, p. 36.

111 Nor was he alone in having been a president of the Royal College of Surgeons. Jonathan Hutchinson was elected president in 1889 and Rickman John Godlee in 1911.

112 William Osler, 'Internal Medicine as a Vocation', in William Osler (ed.), *Aequanimitas: With Other Addresses to Medical Students, Nurses, and Practitioners of Medicine* (London: H. K. Lewis & Co., 1946), p. 133 but see pp. 133–45.

113 Nor need this be seen as a systematic approach to medicine, or even a holistic view of the body. It had practical implications. One of the important revelations of Ock-Joo Cho Kim's dissertation was that Harvey Cushing perceived neurosurgery as a process of integration between systemic problems of the body and technical interventions. If Cushing's approach was specialist, the scientific practices he utilised were philosophically generalist, and it was in the generalist practice that the practical implications emerged. Ock-Joo Cho Kim, 'The Integration of Science with the Healing Art: Harvey Cushing's Development of Neurosurgery, 1896–1912' (PhD dissertation, University of Minnesota, 1998).

114 Marc Berg, 'Turning a Practice into a Science: Reconceptualizing Postwar Medical Practice', *Social Studies of Science* 25:3 (1995), 437–76, 465.

115 RSMA, NS, 'Union of Medical Societies: Report of the Executive Committee as Amended and Adopted at the Meeting of the General

Committee of Representatives of the Societies, Held on July 19th, 1905'.

116 Weisz, *Divide and Conquer*, pp. 41–3, 176, 223.

117 RSMA, NS/A/2, Report of the Council for 1906, 21 February 1907.

118 Weisz, *Divide and Conquer* p. 207, notes that other specialties found similar solutions, which actually unified fields in the Royal Society of Medicine. Thus, obstetrics and gynaecology aggregated together. That neurology and psychiatry were not is interesting, and it is important to note that the Section of Psychiatry was only formed in 1912.

119 Editorial, 'International Neurological Congress, Berne', *Journal of Neurology and Psychopathology* 21:45 (1931), 66–8.

Chapter 2

1 Edwin Bramwell Papers, Transcript 'Neurology', 25 April 1933.

2 Williams, 'RSM 1907'; Hunting, *The History of the Royal Society of Medicine.*

3 Stevens, *Medical Practice*, quote on p. 51, also see p. 31.

4 Weisz, *Divide and Conquer*, p. 41.

5 All of the observations recorded here may be made by scrutiny of the *Proceedings of the Royal Society of Medicine.* As part of this project, the author has constructed a bibliography of the Section of Neurology of the Royal Society of Medicine for the years 1907 to 1965 which informs this analysis.

6 Publishing become a significant issue for the Neurological Section in the interwar period for two reasons. The Royal Society of Medicine held a copyright over its proceedings, and during the Anglo-American Neurological Conference of 1927 special permission was required from the editorial committee of the Royal Society of Medicine for the American Neurological Association to print abstracts of the meeting. Second, to pay for burgeoning publishing costs, the editorial committee regularly requested increases in the society's membership charges, diminishing their already limited exclusivity. See RMSA, K73, Minutes of the Royal Society of Medicine Neurological Section Council (hereafter Council Minutes), 28 October 1920, p. 172. Macdonald Critchley complained about this in Archive of the Association of British Neurologists, London (hereafter AABN), '50th Anniversary Dinner Party of the Association of British Neurologists,' folder 'Origins' (c. 1983), p. 5.

7 RSMA, NS/A/2, Report of the Council for 1906, 21 February 1907.

8 WL, PP/HEA/D4/19 Box 7 1905–22, Letter from Henry Head to Ruth Mayhew 1904.

9 For example, WL, PP/HEA/D4/19 Box 7 1905–22, Letter from Henry to Ruth, 19 May 1907; 20 May 1907; 29 August 1909; 13 March 1915; 7 April 1916.
10 See the *Proceedings of the Royal Society of Medicine* throughout 1907–60 for the joint discussions. Note that these discussions were published separately from the proceedings of individual sections.
11 RSMA, K73, Council Minutes, 5 April 1916, p. 128.
12 Archives of the Royal College of Physicians, London (hereafter ARCP), Association of Physicians of Great Britain and Ireland (hereafter AP), 2434/100, Notes on the History of the Association by Dr Herringham, pp. 1–2.
13 Ibid., p. 1.
14 ARCP, AP, Minutes, vol. 1, MS 2428, 23 May 1907, p. 1.
15 Ibid.
16 Ibid., p. 2.
17 Ibid., p. 11.
18 The latter point was admitted later in this address. ARCP, AP, 2427/64, Annual Dinner, Whitsuntide, 1952; AP Misc. notes etc. including Presidential Address by Dr Arthur Gurney Yates at Annual Dinner.
19 Lawrence, 'Still Incommunicable', p. 96.
20 ARCP, AP, 'Membership Book' Rule 20, Association of Physicians of Great Britain and Ireland.
21 For example: ARCP, AP, Minutes, vol. 1, MS 2428, 18 April 1912, p. 81, 84, or 115.
22 Ibid., p. 6.
23 Ibid., p. 84.
24 Ibid.
25 Ibid., p. 329.
26 On creating the ornaments of respectability, see Keith Macdonald, 'Building Respectability', *Sociology* 23:1 (1989), 55–80.
27 ARCP, AP, 2427/64, Annual Dinner, Whitsuntide, 1952.
28 Ian Whitehead, 'The British Medical Office on the Western Front: The Training of Doctors for War', in Roger Cooter, Mark Harrison, and Steve Sturdy (eds) *Medicine and Modern Warfare* (Amsterdam: Rodupi, 1999), pp. 173–5; Modris Eksteins, *Rites of Spring: The Great War and the Birth of the Modern Age* (London: Bantam, 1989); Stephen Walshe, *Stravinsky: A Creative Spring Russia and France, 1882–1934* (London: Pimlico, 2002), especially pp. 256–7.
29 Arthur Marwick, *The Deluge: British Society and the First World War* (Palgrave Macmillian 2006).
30 Enid Bagnold, *A Diary Without Dates* (London: Virago, 1978).
31 James Joyce, *Ulysses* (London: Penguin Books, 2000), p. 777.

32 Arthur Marwick, *A History of the Modern British Isles, 1914–1999* (London: Blackwell, 2000), pp. 50–1.
33 George W. Pickering, 'Walter Russell Brain, First Baron Brain of Eynsham, 1895–1966', *Biographical Memoirs of Fellows of the Royal Society* 14 (1968), 61–82.
34 ARCP, Walter Russell Brain Papers (hereafter Brain Papers), W. Russell Brain, Diary, MS 3137.1–57, 3137.1–2.
35 Ibid.
36 ARCP, Brain Papers, W. Russell Brain, Autobiographical Notes by Lord Brain, MS 3174.6.
37 ARCP, Brain Papers, W. Russell Brain, Diary, MS 3137.1-57, 3137.19.
38 ARCP, Brain Papers, W. Russell Brain, Diary, MS 3137.1-57, 3137.25.
39 ARCP, Brain Papers, W. Russell Brain, Diary, MS 3137.1-57, 3137.26.
40 ARCP, Brain Papers, W. Russell Brain, Diary, MS 3137.1-57, 3137.61.
41 ARCP, Brain Papers, W. Russell Brain, Diary, MS 3137.1-57, 3137.87.
42 ARCP, Brain Papers, W. Russell Brain, Diary, MS 3137.1-57, 3137.124.
43 ARCP, Brain Papers, W. Russell Brain, Diary, MS 3137.1-57, 3137.126.
44 ARCP, Brain Papers, W. Russell Brain, Autobiographical Notes by Lord Brain, MS 3174.7.
45 ARCP, Brain Papers,W. Russell Brain, Diary, MS 3137.1-57, 3137.21.
46 ARCP, Brain Papers, W. Russell Brain, Diary, MS 3137.1-57, 3137.50.
47 ARCP, Brain Papers, W. Russell Brain, Diary, MS 3137.1-57, 3137.58.
48 ARCP, Brain Papers, W. Russell Brain, Diary, MS 3137.1-57, 3137.63–3137.64.
49 ARCP, Brain Papers, W. Russell Brain, Diary, MS 3137.1-57, 3137.18.
50 ARCP, Brain Papers, W. Russell Brain, Diary, MS 3137.1-57, 3137.22.
51 ARCP, Brain Papers, W. Russell Brain, Diary, MS 3137.1-57, 3137.27.
52 ARCP, Brain Papers, W. Russell Brain, Diary, MS 3137.1-57, 3137.30.
53 ARCP, Brain Papers, W. Russell Brain, Diary, MS 3137.1-57, 3137.40.
54 ARCP, Brain Papers, W. Russell Brain, Diary, MS 3137.1-57, 3137.119.
55 Special Collections, Brotherton Library, University of Leeds, Charles Symonds to Janet Poulton, 1 December 1917.
56 Helen Jones, *Health and Society in Twentieth-Century Britain* (London and New York: Longman, 1994), p. 50.
57 Joel Howell, '"Soldier's Heart": The Redefinition of Heart Disease and Specialty Formation in Early Twentieth-Century Great Britain', in William F. Bynum, Christopher Lawrence, and Vivian Nutton (eds), *The Emergence of Modern Cardiology* (London: Wellcome Institute Press, 1985), pp. 34–52; Cooter, *Surgery and Society in Peace and*

War; Weisz, *Divide and Conquer*, pp. 165–7; also see, Anne Hardy, *Health and Medicine in Britain since 1860* (New York: Palgrave, 2001), pp. 47–76.

58 D'Arcy Power, 'St. Bartholomew's and the War, 1914–1919', *St. Bartholomew's Hospital Reports*, 53 (1920), 12; Owen Richards, 'The Development of Casualty Clearing Stations', *Guy's Hospital Reports* 70 (1922), 121–2; Roger Cooter and Steve Sturdy, 'Of War, Medicine, and Modernity: Introduction', in Roger Cooter, Mark Harrison and Steve Sturdy, *War, Medicine and Modernity* (Stroud: Sutton, 1998), p. 2.

59 Weisz notes that it had a similar effect on cardiology, orthopaedics, and psychiatry. *Divide and Conquer*, p. xxxviii; also see, Anon., 'The Medical Call-up, War Committees and the New Situation, Need of Doctor Economy', *The Times* (24 April 1917), 3.

60 University College London (hereafter UCL) Special Archives and Collections Francis Walshe Papers (hereafter Francis Walshe Papers), Folder A4, MS ADD 301, Letter from Francis Walshe to Director General, 31 August 1915; Letter from War Office to Walshe, 20 June 1919.

61 UCL, Francis Walshe Papers, Folder A4, Letter from War Office to Francis Walshe, 22 September 1919.

62 Ben Shephard, *A War of Nerves: Soldiers and Psychiatrists, 1914–1994* (London: Pimlico, 2002), p. 17.

63 James Purves Stewart, *Sands of Time: Recollections of a Physician in Peace and War* (London: Hutchinson & Co., 1939), pp. 115–215.

64 Indeed, Jack Pressman argued that this ambiguity in America led to a merger between psychiatry and neurology which, when combined with Adolf Meyer's socio-psychobiological theories, created neuropsychiatry. Pressman, *Last Resort*, pp. 20–8.

65 T. J. Mitchell and G. M. Smith, *History of the Great War, Based on Official Documents: Medical Services, Casualties and Medical Statistics of the Great War* (London: HMSO, 1931), pp. 285–6.

66 Ibid., p. 280.

67 Ibid., p. 288.

68 Ibid., p. 115.

69 Eric Hobsbawm, *Age of Extremes: The Short Twentieth Century, 1914–1991* (London: Michael Joseph, 1994), p. 25; Ronald Blythe, *The Age of Illusion: England in the Twenties and Thirties, 1919–40* (Middlesex: Penguin, 1963), p. 11.

70 Part of this reorganisation of field medicine occurred because of novel disciplinary rhetoric being deployed by a small vocal group of proponents for medical specialisation. Pairings of war, i.e. war and increased specialisation, or war and epidemics, are always difficult

to pinpoint. The view taken here is that the widely held belief that specialised medicine was encouraged by the conditions of the war is uncritical. On similar issues, see Roger Cooter, 'Of War and Epidemics: Unnatural Couplings, Problematic Conceptions', *Social History of Medicine* 16:2 (2003), 283–302.

71 This was especially true in the American context. Theodore Weisenburg, 'The Military History of the American Neurological Association', *Archives of Neurology and Psychiatry* 1:1 (1919), 2.

72 Anon., 'W. J. Adie', *The Times* (20 March 1935), 16.

73 Macdonald Critchley, '1886–1935 William J. Adie', in Macdonald Critchley (ed.), *The Ventricle of Memory: Personal Recollections of Some Neurologists* (New York: Raven Press, 1990), pp. 3–4.

74 Anon., 'William John Adie, M.D.Ed., F.R.C.P.', *British Medical Journal* (1935), 624–5.

75 Anon., 'William John Adie, M.D.Edin., F.R.C.P.Lond.', *Lancet* (1935), 717.

76 Cf. Webb Haymaker, 'William John Adie, 1886–1935' in Webb Haymaker (ed.), *The Founders of Neurology: One Hundred and Thirty-Three Biographical Sketches Prepared for the Fourth International Neurological Congress in Paris* (Springfield, IL: Charles C. Thomas, 1953), p. 231.

77 British Red Cross, personal communication with the author, 23 July 2003, E/CAS/03/HP.

78 Ibid., British Red Cross Archive, Summary of Work for the Week Ending 30 September 1914.

79 Ibid., British Red Cross Archive, Summary of Work for the Week Ending 7 October 1914.

80 R. J. Minney, *The Two Pillars of Charing Cross: The Story of a Famous Hospital* (London: Cassell, 1967), pp. 174–5.

81 Bliss, *Harvey Cushing*, p. 292.

82 A. D. Macleod, 'Shell Shock, Gordon Holmes and the Great War', *Journal of the Royal Society of Medicine* 97 (2004), 86–9.

83 W. G. MacPherson, W. P. Herringham, T. R. Elliot, and A. Balfour, *History of the Great War, Based on Official Documents: Medical Services, Diseases of the War. Vol. 2: Including the Medical Aspects of Aviation and Gas Warfare, and Gas Poisoning in Tanks and Mines* (London, HMSO, 1923), p. 10.

84 Ibid.; Anon., 'Dr. C S Myers', *The Times* (14 October 1946), 7. For a discussion of Myers' 'fall from grace' and Holmes' involvement, see Shephard, *War of Nerves*, pp. 46–51.

85 Rockefeller Medical Library, Institute of Neurology, National Hospital, Queen Square.

Box: Gordon Holmes, undated notes.

86 Gordon Holmes, 'The Symptoms of Acute Cerebellar Injuries from Gunshot Wounds', *Brain* 40 (1917), 461–535; Gordon Holmes, 'Disturbances of Spatial Orientation and Visual Attention, with Loss of Stereoscopic Vision', *Archives of Neurology and Psychiatry* 1:4 (1919), 385–407; Gordon Holmes and W. Lister, 'Disturbances of Vision from Cerebral Lesions with Special Reference to the Cortical Representation of the Macula', *Brain* 39 (1917), 34–73; see also F. E. Lepore 'Harvey Cushing, Gordon Holmes, and the Neurological Lessons of World War I', *Archives of Neurology* 51(1994), 711–22.

87 Gordon Holmes, 'Foundation Lecture', in *Neurological Biographies and Addresses; Foundation Volume; Published for the Staff to Commemorate the Opening of the Montreal Neurological Institute of McGill University* (London: Oxford University Press, 1936), pp. 6–15, p. 7.

88 'F. Kennedy to I. Kennedy, October 1916 [Letter 43]', in Isabel Kennedy Butterfield (ed.), *The Making of a Neurologist: The Letters of Foster Kennedy M.D. F.R.S.Edin., 1884–1952 to his Wife* (Hatfield: Stellar Press, 1981), p. 60.

89 Ben Shephard, 'Shell-Shock on the Somme', *Royal United Services Institute Journal* 141:3 (1996), 51–6, especially 52–3; for a discussion of disciplinary practices, see Showalter, *The Female Malady*, pp. 175–80.

90 Harvey Cushing, *From a Surgeon's Journal, 1915–1918* (Boston: Little, Brown and Co., 1936), p. 57.

91 'F. Kennedy to I. Kennedy, September 1916 [Letter 42]' in Butterfield (ed.), *The Making of a Neurologist*, p. 59; Yale University Library, Manuscripts and Archives, the Harvey Williams Cushing Papers in the Yale University Library (hereafter Cushing Papers), Microfilm Series I, Box 36, 704, Microfilm Reel 30, Holmes, Gordon, 1915–1936, Letter from Cushing to Holmes, 24 May 1915.

92 The situation began to be remedied in 1918 by a course of lectures offered by Frederick Mott. These had the effect, however, of training general practitioners rather than neurologists. See Anon., 'Post-Graduate Teaching in Neurology' *British Medical Journal* (1918), 597.

93 Cushing, *From a Surgeon's Journal*, p. 357.

94 On this point, see Rose, *The Psychological Complex*, pp. 180–7.

95 Cushing, *From a Surgeon's Journal*, p. 357.

96 See Rose, *The Psychological Complex*, pp. 180–7.

97 Andrew Abbott has noted that in America in 1920, neurologists and psychiatrists were bound together based upon a loose agreement on this very point. It did not last long (if at all), and, shortly thereafter, psychiatrists separated. The agreement never existed in Britain. Abbott, *The System of Professions*, p. 300.

98 Macdonald Critchley, 'Gordon Holmes: The Man and the Neurologist', in Macdonald Critchley (ed.), *The Divine Banquet of the Brain and Other Essays* (New York: Raven Press, 1979), pp. 228–34; Shephard, *War of Nerves*, p. 49.

99 Mark Mazower, *Dark Continent: Europe's Twentieth Century* (New York: A. A. Knopf, 1999) p. 80.

100 Richard Lovell, remarking on the crisis, noted, for instance, that one problem was simply that, 'In Britain, five million men had to be reabsorbed into civilian life,' Richard Lovell, *Churchill's Doctor: A Biography of Lord Moran* (London: Royal Society of Medicine, 1992), p. 55.

101 Peter Leese, *Shell Shock: Traumatic Neurosis and the British Soldiers of the First World War* (Basingstoke: Palgrave Macmillan, 2002), pp. 2–4.

102 MacPherson, Herringham, Elliott, and Balfour, *History of the Great War*, pp. 40, 43–4.

103 For orthopaedics, see: Cooter, *Surgery and Society in Peace and War*; for neurosurgerym see G. J. Fraenkel, *Hugh Cairns: First Nuffield Professor of Surgery, University of Oxford* (Oxford: Oxford University Press, 2003).

104 Sidney Schwab, 'The Neurologic Dilemma', *Archives of Neurology and Psychiatry* 6:3 (1921), 255.

105 John Russell Silver, *History of the Treatment of Spinal Injuries* (New York: Kluwer Academic/Plenum Publishers, 2003), pp. 17–56; A similar case has been made for cardiology, see Hardy, *Health and Medicine*, p. 68.

106 'F. Kennedy to I. Kennedy, 17 June 1917 [Letter 45]', in Butterfield (ed.), *The Making of a Neurologist*, p. 59.

107 Exceptions include a study focusing on French neurologists by Marc Roudebush, 'A Battle of Nerves: Hysteria and its Treatment in France during World War I', in Mark S. Micale and Paul Lerner (eds), *Traumatic Pasts: History, Psychiatry, and Trauma in the Modern Age, 1870–1930* (Cambridge: Cambridge University Press, 2001), pp. 253–79. Also see comments in Shepherd, *A War of Nerves*.

108 The degenerative aspect of shell shock has also been explored to the nth degree and would warrant a bibliography. See Oppenheim, *Shattered Nerves*, pp. 141–80 for basic information; also see Showalter, *The Female Malady*, pp. 167–97; alternatively, see Pat Barker's 'Regeneration' trilogy for a fictional but grounded and completely enjoyable account.

109 UCL, Francis Walshe Papers, Folder A4, Letter from Walshe to Command, [undated, c. 23 November 1918].

110 A most explicit statement of one neurologist's prejudices appeared

in a 1911 meeting of the Section of Neurology. See Frederick Mott, 'Presidential Address: The Inborn Factors of Nervous and Mental Disease', *Proceedings of the Royal Society of Medicine* 5:2 (1911), 1–30, 1 and 29: 'Every neurologist recognises the importance of the inborn factor in the production of neuroses and psychoses, and in certain degenerative conditions of the nervous system, which Gowers has designated under the collective term abiotrophies.' Later he wrote, 'It has always struck me that Jews were, on account of their neurotic temperament, more liable to insanity than Christians.'

111 See, for example, the criticism against Freud's methods in Arthur Hurst, 'Psycho-analysis and War Neuroses', *Guy's Hospital Gazette* 31 (1917), 308–9.

112 Edward Shorter, *A History of Psychiatry: From the Era of the Asylum to the Age of Prozac*; (New York, John Wiley; 1997) see p. 42, and fn. 13; also see Hale, *The Rise and Crisis of Psychoanalysis in the United States*; John C. Burnham (ed), *After Freud Left: A Century of Psychoanalysis in America* (Chicago: University of Chicago Press, 2012).

113 Leese, *Shell Shock*, pp. 141–54.

114 Ted Bogacz, 'War Neurosis and Cultural Change in England, 1914–22: The Work of the War Office Committee of Enquiry into "Shell Shock"', *Journal of Contemporary History* 24:2 (1989), 227–56; Shephard, *A War of Nerves*, p. 152.

115 *Report of the War Office Committee of Enquiry into 'Shell-Shock'* (London: HSMO, 1922), pp. 4–6.

116 Ibid., p. 81.

117 Ibid., pp. 17–18.

118 Ibid., pp. 19–21, 23–8, 68–71, 74–5.

119 Ibid., pp. 38–9.

120 Ibid., p. 24.

121 Leese makes a similar point, see *Shell Shock*, pp. 159–68.

122 Ibid., 92-3.

123 Ted Bogacz, 'War Neurosis and Cultural Change in England, 1914-22', p. 228.

124 *Report of the War Office Committee of Enquiry into 'Shell-Shock'* (HSMO, 1922), pp. 160–89.

125 Ibid., p. 193.

126 One *Lancet* editorial commented polemically after the report: 'A change has come over neurology since the war; a war legacy which the pre-war neurologist might be pardoned for not, perhaps welcoming altogether without reserve...the study of functional nervous cases seems to be passing to some extent into the hands of a generation of self-styled "neurologists", not a few of whom – it may

be said without exaggeration and without offense – seem to act as though knowledge of the anatomy and physiology of the nervous system were immaterial, if not an actual hindrance.' Anon., 'Editorial: The Future of Neurology', *Lancet* (1923), 792–3.

127 Bogacz, 'War Neurosis and Cultural Change in England', 250.

128 Leese, *Shell Shock*, p. 155.

129 Thomas Graham Brown, for example, although he had held a position according to the report as a 'neurologist' in the British Salonica Force, was Professor of Physiology in the University of Wales. *Report of the War Office Committee of Enquiry into 'Shell-Shock'*, p. 213.

130 Anon., 'Post-Graduate Teaching in Neurology', 597.

131 London Hospital Archives, LH/X/145/2, Sir Henry Head, Notes by Donald Hunter, Physician to the London Hospital, Director of the Occupational Disease, see passage for 3 May 1919.

132 London Hospital Archives, Letter from Henry Head to Lord Knutsford, 8 January 1919 inserted between pp. 91 and 92 of LH/A/5/56, House Committee Minutes 1918, 22 July 1918 to 12 July 1920.

133 London Hospital Archives, LH/A/23/53. Among the relevant communications, see: Letter from Sydney Holland to Henry Head, 24 May 1919; Letter from Walter Fletcher to Sydney Holland, 27 May 1919; Letter from Anon. (presumably Sydney Holland) to Sir Walter Fletcher, 29 May 1919.

134 Henry Head, 'Presidential Address: Some Principles of Neurology', *Proceedings of the Royal Society of Medicine*, 12 (1918), 1–12, 1.

135 Ibid.

136 Ibid., 2.

137 Ibid., 7–8.

138 Ibid., 8.

139 Ibid.

140 Ibid., 9–10.

141 Ibid., 11–12.

142 London Hospital Archives, LH/A/23/53, Dr Head's Reply to Lord Knutsford, 20 January 1919.

143 RSMA, K73, Council Minutes, 18 December 1919, p. 160.

144 RSMA, K73, Council Minutes, 18 December 1919, p. 158; William Gowers, 'Special Sense Discharges in Organic Disease', *Proceedings of the Royal Society of Medicine* 3 (1909), 1–16.

145 RSMA, K73, Council Minutes, 28 October 1920, p. 174.

146 W. Aldren Turner, 'Presidential Address: The Influence of Psychogenic Factors in Nervous Disorders', *Proceedings of the Royal Society of Medicine* 13 (1919), 1–16.

147 E. Farquhar Buzzard, 'Case of Spastic Quadriplegia Following Injury

of the Spinal Cord in the Upper Cervical Region, Showing Certain Unusual Reflex Phenomenon', *Proceedings of the Royal Society of Medicine* 13 (1920), 44–7.

148 Alfred Carver, 'Some Biological Effects due to High Explosives', *Proceedings of the Royal Society of Medicine* 12 (1919), 36–51.

149 E. G. Fearnsides, *Proceedings of the Royal Society of Medicine* 11 (1918), 42–8; Henry Head, 'Shell Wound of Head, Right Temporal Region', *Proceedings of the Royal Society of Medicine* 13 (1920), 53.

150 Arthur Hurst, 'The Hysterical Element in Organic Disease and Injury of the Nervous System', *Proceedings of the Royal Society of Medicine* 12 (1919), 21–9.

151 George Riddoch, 'Case of Meningitis Circumscripta Serosa Following Bullet Wound of the Neck', *Proceedings of the Royal Society of Medicine* 13 (1919), 40–2; Percy Sargent, 'Some Lessons of the War Applied to Spinal Surgery', *Proceedings of the Royal Society of Medicine* 13 (1920), 17–27.

152 T. A. Ross, 'Certain Inter-Relations of Peace and War Neuroses', *Proceedings of the Royal Society of Medicine* 12 (1919), 13–20; R. G. Rows, Anxiety States', *Proceedings of the Royal Society of Medicine* 13 (1920), 61–6.

153 Francis Walshe, 'Forms of Peripheral Neuritis among Troops Serving in the Egyptian Expeditionary Force, 1915–1919', *Brain* 43 (1920): 74–85.

154 For a discussion see Anon., 'The Organic Aspect of Shell Shock', *Journal of Neurology and Psychopathology*, 2:5 (1921), 49–51.

155 Anon., 'Neurology in the War', *British Medical Journal* (1919), 790–1.

156 Edwin Bramwell Papers, Transcript, 'Neurology', 25 April 1933.

157 RSMA, K75, Minutes of the Royal Society of Medicine Neurological Section Meetings, 11 December 1919, p. 194.

158 ARCP, Brain Papers, W. Russell Brain, 'The Organization of Neurology in London After the War', n.d., but c. 1945.

159 Ibid.

160 Ibid.

161 Ibid.

162 Ibid.

163 National Archives, London (hereafter NA), MH 52/91, Frederick Menzies, Consultants Employed at General and Special Hospital, 1932, p. 18, London Medical Services, Appointments of Consultants and Specialists. When Frederick Menzies, the Medical Officer of Health for the London County Council, wrote a 1933 report on the appointment of specialists in the London County Council hospitals, he suggested each hospital acquire a: 'gynaecologist; ophthalmic surgeon; ear, nose and throat surgeon; orthopaedic surgeon;

dermatologist; pediatrist; urologist; radiologist; obstetrician; tuberculosis officer'. As for neurologists, Menzies thought them desirable, 'but as the amount of time for which he would be required is difficult to estimate, I suggest a panel of neurologists should be formed and their services should be utilised as required, and that they should be paid a fee of £2.12s.6d. per session.' NA, MH 52/91 London Medical Services, Appointments of Consultants and Specialists, Frederick Menzies, Committee Report by the Medical Officer of Health [1 February 1933].

164 ARCP, Brain Papers, W. Russell Brain, 'The Organisation of Neurology in London After the War'.

165 John Senior has shown the early connections between Armand de Wattville's Electricity Department at St Mary's Hospital and British neurology. John E. Senior, 'Meteorological Awakenings' in Eileen Magnello and Anne Hardy (eds), *The Road to Medical Statistics* (Amsterdam and New York: Rodopi, 2002), pp. 77-93; also see John E. Senior, 'Rationalising Electrotherapy in Neurology, 1860-1920' (PhD dissertation, Oxford University, 1994).

166 Anon., *St Mary's Hospital, a London Family of Six Hospitals a Medical School and an Institute of Research* (London: Newman Neame Limited, 1965), p. 34; E. A. Heaman, *St Mary's: The History of a London Teaching Hospital* (Montreal, Kingston, London, and Ithaca, NY: Liverpool University Press and McGill Queen's University Press, 2003), p. 108; Eric Nieman, 'Wilfred Harris (1869–1960): Pioneer of Neurology at St. Mary's Hospital', *St Mary's Gazette* 104:2 (1998), 733.

167 H. Campbell Thomson, *The Story of the Middlesex Hospital Medical School* (London: John Murray, 1935), pp. 102, 132–3.

168 Anon., 'Douglas McAlpine, M.D., Glasg., F.R.C.P.', *Lancet* (1981), 510.

169 Anon., 'William Johnson M.C., M.D. Lond., F.R.C.P.', *Lancet* (1949), 589.

170 H. C. Cameron, *Mr Guy's Hospital, 1726–1948* (London, New York, and Toronto: Longmans, Green and Co., 1954), pp. 359–60.

171 London Metropolitan Archives, H9/GY/A89/3, Guy's Hospital, Memorandum by Dr. Shaw upon Special Departments, 1913.

172 London Metropolitan Archives, H9/GY/A89/1, Guy's Hospital, Report of the Committee on Specialisms in Medicine and Surgery, 1908.

173 This comment is owed to interviews with Dr Michael O'Brien, formerly neurologist of Guy's Hospital.

174 Anon., 'Charles Putnam Symonds', *Lancet* (1978), 1389–90; Ian Mackensie, 'Symonds, Sir Charles Putnam (1890–1978)', *Oxford Dictionary of National Biography* (Oxford: Oxford University Press, 2004).

175 Anon., 'S. A. Kinnier Wilson, M.D., D.Sc.Edin., F.R.C.P.Lond.', *Lancet* (1937), 1253–4.

176 UCL, Francis Walshe Papers, Folder B1, Transcript, Francis Walshe, 'Pride and Prejudice: The Case for Specialism in Medicine,' *University College Hospital Magazine*, 41:2 [undated].

177 Anon., 'A. Feiling, B.A., M.D., F.R.C.P.', *British Medical Journal* (1975), 621.

178 Anon., 'George Hall, C.M.G., M.D.London., B.Sc.Durh., F.R.C.P., J.P.', *Lancet* (1955), 210.

179 Anon., 'H.G. Garland, T.D., M.D., F.R.C.P.', *British Medical Journal* (1967), 300.

180 Ray Cooper, *The Burden: Fifty Years of Clinical and Experimental Neuroscience at the Burden Neurological Institute* (Bristol: White Tree Books, 1989). The records of the Burden are: NA, FD 1/1426, Minutes of the Burden Neurological Clinic, 16 December 1938.

181 University of Birmingham, Special Collections Department, 'Report of the Committee Appointed to Consider Matters Connected with the Establishment of the Department of Neurology, 1947'.

182 S. T. Anning, *The General Infirmary at Leeds. Vol. 2: The Second Hundred Years, 1869–1965* (Edinburgh and London: E. & S. Livingston, 1966).

183 Ian Murray, *The Victoria Infirmary of Glasgow, History of a Voluntary Hospital, 1890–1948* (Glasgow: C. L. Wright, 1967), p. 65.

184 Loudon MacQueen and Archibald B. Kerr, *The Western Infirmary, 1874–1974: A Century of Service to Glasgow* (Glasgow and London: John Horn, 1974), p. 137.

185 Iain Levack and Hugh Dudley, *Aberdeen Royal Infirmary: The People's Hospital of the North-East* (London, Philadelphia, Toronto, Sydney, and Tokyo: Bailliere Tindall, 1992), pp. 154–7.

186 National Archives Scotland (hereafter NAS) HOS/1/6/W/ Hospital Services Development Western Region, Neurology and Neurosurgery, 1958–59.

187 Cushing Papers, Microfilm Series I, Box 24, 448, Microfilm Reel 21, Enclosure, 1931, Dott, Norman M. 1924–1938; a unit was eventually established along different lines: Martin Eastwood and Anne Jenkinson, *A History of the Western General Hospital: Craigleith Poorhouse, Military Hospital, and Modern Teaching Hospital* (Edinburgh: John Donald Publishers, 1995), p. 171.

188 Edwin Bramwell Papers, 'Edwin Bramwell Curriculum Vitae'.

189 'Russell, William Ritchie', in *Lives of the Fellows (Munk's Roll)* (London: Royal College of Physicians: 1985), vol. 7, pp. 514–15; Oxford University later appointed Ritchie Russell Lecturer in Neurology in 1949, and he eventually held the first Chair of Clinical

Neurology at the university, established in 1966. 'Dr Ritchie Russell', *The Times* (11 December 1980), 16.

190 NA, MH 96/1797, Welsh Regional Hospital Board, 1948–57.

191 NA MH 96/1797 Welsh Regional Hospital Board, 1948–57. By contrast, there were 2,519 domiciliary visits by neurologists in 1962 throughout the entire United Kingdom.

192 Denis Brinton, 'President's Address: The Development of Neurological Services under the NHS', *Proceedings of the Royal Society of Medicine* 53:261 (1960), 263.

193 I am borrowing methodologically here from Denning, *The Cultural Front*, pp. 27–8.

Chapter 3

1 Norman Howard-Jones, 'Fake!', *British Medical Journal* 284 (1982), 511.

2 For a full account, see: Stephen T Casper, 'Trust, Protocol, Gender, and Power in Interwar British Biomedical Research: Kathleen Chevassut and the "Germ" of Multiple Sclerosis', *Journal of the History of Medicine and Allied Sciences* 66:2 (2011), 180–215.

3 Royal Holloway University Library (hereafter RHUL), Kathleen Chevassut Papers, Folder BC AR200/1 1985, index card in file (last updated 1983); also see the later comments made in Folder BC AR200/1 1985, Letter from Grafton Elliot Smith to Tuke, 5 December 1929.

4 Carol Dyhouse, 'Driving Ambitions: Women in Pursuit of a Medical Education, 1890–1939', *Women's Historical Review* 7 (1998), 321–43, 337. The literature on the difficulties for women doctors in interwar London is extensive. See also Leah Leneman, 'Medical Women at War, 1914–1918', *Medical History* 38 (1994), 160–77; Carol Dyhouse, 'Women Students and the London Medical Schools, 1914–39: The Anatomy of a Masculine Culture', *Gender Hist*ory 10 (1998), 110–32; J. F. Geddes, 'The Doctors' Dilemma: Medical Women and the British Suffrage Movement', *Women's Historical Review* 18 (2009), 203–18.

5 Kathleen Chevassut, 'Glycolysis in Cerebro-spinal Fluid and Its Clinical Significance', *Quarterly Journal of Medicine* 21:104 (1927–28), 105.

6 Kathleen Chevassut, 'The Aetiology of Disseminated Sclerosis', *Lancet* (1930), 552–60; James Purves Stewart, 'A Specific Vaccine Treatment in Disseminated Sclerosis,' *Lancet* (1930), 560–4.

7 Edward Arnold Carmichael, 'The Aetiology of Disseminated Sclerosis: Some Criticisms of Recent Work, Especially with Regard to

"Spherula Insularis"', *Proceedings of the Royal Society of Medicine* 24 (1931), 591–606.

8 Edwin Bramwell Papers, Diary of Edwin Bramwell, 13 October 1934, vol. 1, pp. 40–1. According to Bramwell: 'I had thought that Stewart had abandoned the treatment of disseminated sclerosis by vaccines, but a few weeks ago I had a letter from Dr Ross Haddon of Hawick in which he told me that a patient of his, a lad of 20, was being treated by Purves Stewart for disseminated sclerosis with vaccines, and that the lad's mother, a Scottish minister's wife, in whose case I had diagnosed disseminated sclerosis, wanted to know whether I would advise her to go to London and have the same treatment? Ross Haddon enclosed copies of several letters from Purves Stewart to the doctor in London who had sent the lad to see him. In the first letter Purves Stewart narrated the facts of the case, and these on paper were suggestive, though not perhaps conclusive, of disseminated sclerosis. Finally he wrote on examining the cerebrospinal fluid, "we found a growth or culture and I have advised an autogenous vaccine which I have prepared and propose to give. I should like to see the patients again in three months." In a second letter he writes, "I have again examined the patient; the cerebrospinal fluid is now sterile and we may I think discontinue the vaccine". "It is important (I think these were his words) that I should see this patient again in six months". I wrote to Ross Haddon telling him that there was no published proof of the existence of the organism in the cerebrospinal fluid of disseminated sclerosis and that I did not advise the boy's mother to undergo the treatment. Further I asked Ross Haddon whether Purves Stewart was charging any fee for treating the lad for if he was not doing so I felt that Stewart had an excuse. Haddon replied that Stewart was charging the boy, a minister's son, fifteen guineas each time he went up to London.'

9 Katrina Gatley, 'When Book Medicine Meets Patient', Work-in-Progress Seminar, Wellcome Trust Centre for the History of Medicine at University College London, London, 17 May 2006.

10 Few scholars have examined the history of British neurology after 1920. An exception is: Peter Koehler, 'The Evolution of British Neurology in Comparison with Other Countries', in Rose (ed.), *A Short History of Neurology*, pp. 58–74.

11 Delia Gavrus, 'Men of Dreams and Men of Action: Neurologists, Neurosurgeons, and the Performance of Professional Identity, 1920–1950', *Bulletin of the History of Medicine* 85 (2011), 57–92.

12 For the full case study, see Casper, 'Atlantic conjunctures in Anglo-American Neurology.

13 Marwick, *A History of the Modern British Isles*, p. 63.

14 Ibid., p. 64.
15 P. M. Bennet, 'Great Doctors in English Literature: Sir Roderick Glossop', *British Medical Journal* (1983), 1962–4.
16 By far the most convincing explanation for this phenomenon generally is: Lawrence, 'Still Incommunicable, pp. 95–7. Also see Harry M. Marks, '"Until the Sun of Science...the True Apollo of Medicine Has Risen": Collective Investigation in Britain and America, 1880–1910', *Medical History* 50 (2006), 154–6.
17 John Pickstone, *Medicine and Industrial Society: A History of Hospital Development in Manchester and its Region, 1752–1946* (Manchester: Manchester University Press, 1985), p. 184.
18 My emphasis. Archibald Garrod, 'The Laboratory and the Ward', in *Contributions to Medical and Biological Research, Dedicated to Sir William Osler Bart., M.D., F.R.S. in Honour of his Seventieth Birthday, July 12, 1919 By His Pupils and Co-Workers* (New York: Paul B. Hoeber, 1919), vol. 1, pp. 59–69, p. 61.
19 Ibid., p. 61.
20 Ibid., p. 65; St Bartholomew's Hospital, where Garrod worked, like many others in 1919, did not have a department of nervous diseases or neurology. 'Sir Archibald E. Garrod, K.C.M.G., D.M., F.R.C.P., F.R.S., 1858–1936', *Saint Bartholomew's Hospital Reports* 69 (1936), 12–19.
21 The British government largely avoided funding scientific and medical research before the war. Only the National Physical Laboratory, founded in 1902, and the Imperial College of Science and Technology, established in 1907, qualified as national investments in science. In 1915, an advisory council to a committee of the Privy Council received grants for military scientific research. It is worth noting that from the 1880s on, the British government had been growing substantially in terms of new ministries. The Board of Agriculture, established in 1889, the Board of Education, set up in 1899, and the 1911 National Insurance Act were part of the shift towards larger government. Likewise, post-war Britain saw the Representation of the People Act of 1918, which shifted the country towards a democratic state. Robert Rhodes James, *The British Revolution: British Politics, 1880–1939* (London: Methuen & Co., 1976) , p. 357, p. 362, and p. 400; Mark Harrison, 'Medicine and the Management of Modern Warfare: An Introduction', in Roger Cooter, Mark Harrison and Steve Sturdy (eds), *Medicine and Modern Warfare* (Amsterdam: Rudopi, 1999) pp. 2–5.
22 Fraser, 'The Rise of Specialism and the Special Hospitals', p. 181; Newman, 'The Rise of Specialism and Postgraduate Education', pp. 173–6.

23 Joan Austoker and Linda Bryder (eds), *Historical Perspectives on the Role of the MRC* (Oxford, New York, and Tokyo: Oxford University Press, 1989), pp. 23–33; also see A. Landsborough Thomson, *Half a Century of Medical Research, Vols 1 and 2* (London: Medical Research Council, 1987).

24 On Lewis, see Arthur Hollman, *Sir Thomas Lewis: Pioneer Cardiologist and Clinical Scientist* (London and New York: Spring, 1996).

25 Cushing Papers, Microfilm Series II, Box 25, 469, Microfilm Reel 22, Letter from T. R. Elliott to Harvey Cushing, 14 November 1932; Letter from Harvey Cushing to T. R. Elliott, 25 November 1932.

26 Thomas Lewis, 'Research in Medicine: Its Position and its Needs', *British Medical Journal* (1930), 481; also see Thomas Lewis, 'Research Physicians', *British Medical Journal* (1930), 503–4; on Lewis, see Anon., 'Thomas Lewis, KT, CBE, MD Lond., DSc Wales. LL.D, FRCP, FRS', *Lancet* (1945), 419–20.

27 Lewis, 'Research in Medicine', 483.

28 Walter Fletcher, 'The National Organization of Medical Research in Peace after War', in *Contributions to Medical and Biological Research*, p. 469.

29 RSMA, K73, Council Minutes, 18 December 1919, p. 160; and 28 October 1920, p. 172.

30 Cf. Weisz, *Divide and Conquer*, pp. xx–xxx, 40–6, 163–9.

31 Cf. Douglas J Lanska, 'The Role of Technology in Neurologic Specialization in America', *Neurology* 48:6 (1997), 1722–7.

32 Anon., 'Sir Geoffrey Jefferson: A Great Neuro-Surgeon', *The Times* (30 January 1961), 12; Harold Himsworth, 'Sir Geoffrey Jefferson', *The Times* (1 February 1961), 15.

33 Fraenkel, *Hugh Cairns*, ch. 7.

34 AABN, Holmes to Weisenburg, 9 October 1925.

35 RSMA, K73, Council Minutes, 9 June 1926, p. 226.

36 Ibid.

37 AABN, James Purves Stewart, Anthony Feiling, and William Adie to Weisenburg, 22 June 1926.

38 Rockefeller Archive Center, Sleepy Hollow, NY (hereafter RAC), Record Group (hereafter R.G.) 1.1, Box 20, Folder 265, Series 401, A National Hospital for Nervous Diseases, 1930–1933; List of Americans Registered for Work in Neurology at the National Hospital Queen Square, 30 October 1930.

39 RSMA, K73, Council Minutes, 9 June 1926, p. 226; also see AABN, Programme of British-American Neurological Meeting, July 1927.

40 Benjamin White, *Stanley Cobb: A Builder of the Modern Neurosciences* (Boston, MA: Francis Countway Library of Medicine, 1984), pp. 100–24.

41 AABN, Adie to Weisenburg, 17 December 1926.
42 AABN, Holmes to Weisenburg, 25 January 1927.
43 AABN, Holmes to Weisenburg, 1 February 1927.
44 Purves Stewart to Bramwell, 26 September 1927.
45 For a similar story, see Daniela Barberis, 'Changing Practices of Commemoration in Neurology: Comparing Charcot's 1925 and 1993 Centennials', *Osiris* 14 (1999), 102–17.
46 Anon., 'British and American Neurologists: Meeting in London', *Lancet* (1927), 258–9; Anon., 'British and American Neurologists: Meeting in London', *Lancet* 6 (1927), 301–4. Also see, Archives World Federation of Neurology, London, Henry A Riley, 'Bernard Sachs: The Founder of the International Neurological Congresses', p. 249, attached with letter from Yahr to Toole, 13 November 2000.
47 AABN, Programme of British–American Neurological Meeting, July 1927.
48 AMCMA, Adolf Meyer Papers, Banquet Card: British–American Neurological Meeting, 28 July 1927, II/135/2 Meyer; Anon., 'A Meeting of Neurologists', *Lancet* (1927), 243; AABN, Programme of British–American Neurological Meeting, July 1927.
49 Anonymous article in *Science* 66 (2003), 149–50.
50 AMCMA, Adolf Meyer Papers, James Purves Stewart, *Mount Athos: A Survival of the Middle Ages. An Address at a Social Evening of the Royal Society of Medicine, July 15, 1927* (London: John Bale, Sons and Danielsson, 1927), pp. 83–91; AMCMA, Adolf Meyer Papers, British–American Neurological Meeting, 28 July 1927, II/135/2 Meyer.
51 AMCMA, Adolf Meyer Papers, Letter from Meyer to Bramwell, 23 April 1927; British–American Neurological Meeting, 28 July 1927, II/135/2 Meyer; also see in the same collection: Letter from Bramwell to Meyer, 21 June 1927; and Letter from Robertson to Meyer, 11 May 1927.
52 Archives of the World Federation of Neurology, Enclosure in Yahr to Toole, 13 November 2000: Henry A Riley, 'Bernard Sachs: The Founder of the International Neurological Congresses', pp. 249–55, 249.
53 NA, FD1/2747, Chevassut II, Memorandum of Meeting Held at 38 Old Queen Street on Friday 19 December 1930.
54 Anon., 'Bernard Halley Stewart', *British Medical Journal* (1931), 474. Also see the notice, 'Halley Stewart', *Lancet* (1937), 336.
55 Ibid.
56 See all of the letters in NA, FD 1/2750, Chevassut IV.
57 NA, FD 1/2750, Chevassut IV, Walshe to Halley Stewart, Jr, 30 March 1931.

58 See, Bernard Halley Stewart, *British Medical Journal*, 14 March 1931, p. 474.
59 NA, FD 1/2750 Chevassut IV, Fletcher to Frederick Chevassut, 24 June 1931.
60 See various letters in NA, FD 1/2750, Chevassut V.
61 NA, FD 1/2751, Chesterford Gardens, Fletcher to Walshe, 23 January 1932.
62 NA, FD 1/2751, Chesterford Gardens, Walshe to Fletcher, 25 January 1932.
63 NA, FD 1/2751, Chesterford Gardens, Edward Carmichael [co-authored with Francis Walshe – see the letter cited below], 'Proposal for Research Scheme Chesterford Gardens', received 1 February 1932, pp. 1–3, 1; Walshe to Fletcher, 30 January 1932.
64 Ibid., p. 2.
65 John C. Green, 'The Origins of Neurological Institutes', in Barrow Neurological Institute (ed.), *Horizons in Neurological Education and Research* (Springfield, Illinois: Charles C. Thomas, 1965), pp. 125–199, pp. 127, 147, 159, 176.
66 RAC, RG 1.1, Box 20, Folder 265, Daniel P. O'Brien, Diary excerpt 12 March 1932.
67 NA, FD 1/2751, Chesterford Gardens, Thompson to Carmichael and to Halley Stewart, 24 March 1932.
68 NA, FD 1/2751, Chesterford Gardens, Walshe to Fletcher, 11 May 1932.
69 NA, FD 1/2751, Chesterford Gardens, Halley Stewart to Fletcher, 16 June 1932.
70 NA, FD 1/2751, Chesterford Gardens, Fletcher to Walshe, 28 June 1932.
71 NA, FD 1/2751, Chesterford Gardens, Fletcher to Halley Stewart, 12 July 1932.
72 NA, FD 1/2413, Queen Square Neurology, Collier to Fletcher 14 July 1932.
73 RAC, RG 1.1, Box 20, Folder 265, Series 401, A National Hospital for Nervous Diseases, 1930–1933, Daniel P. O'Brien, Diary excerpt 11 March 1932.
74 NA, FD 1/2751, Chesterford Gardens, Walshe to Fletcher, 11 May 1932.
75 NA, FD 1/2413, Queen Square Neurology, Collier to Fletcher 14 July 1932.
76 See, for example, NA, FD 1/2413, Queen Square Neurology, Enclosure from Collier to Fletcher, 21 July 1932, 'Proposal for a Unit of the Medical Research Council at the National Hospital', pp. 1–2.
77 NA, FD 1/2751, Chesterford Gardens, Personal Note, Phone Transcript, 23 August 1932.

78 NA, FD 1/2751, Chesterford Gardens, Halley Stewart Sr to Fletcher, 23 August 1932; Fletcher to Halley Stewart, 31 August 1932; Halley Stewart to Fletcher, 3 September 1932.
79 NA, FD 1/2751, Chesterford Gardens, Fletcher to Halley Stewart, 22 September 1932.
80 Anon.,'University News,' *The Times* (20 April 1933), 8.
81 NA, FD 1/2413, Queen Square Neurology, Proposal for a Research Unit at the National Hospital, Queen Square, 17 October 1932, pp. 1–3.
82 NA, FD 1/2413, Queen Square Neurology, Fletcher to Halley Stewart Sr, 1 November 1932.
83 NA, FD 1/2413, Queen Square Neurology, Proposal for a Research Unit at the National Hospital, Queen Square, 17 October 1932, pp. 1–3.
84 NA, FD 1/2413, Queen Square Neurology, Collier to Fletcher, 31 October 1932; Hamilton to Fletcher, 9 November 1932.
85 NA, FD 1/2413, Queen Square Neurology, Halley Stewart to Fletcher, 3 November 1932.
86 NA, FD 1/2413, Queen Square Neurology, Fletcher to Halley Stewart, 10 November 1932.
87 NA, FD 1/2413, Queen Square Neurology, Fletcher to Halley Stewart, 14 December 1932.
88 NA, FD1/2415, Neurological Unit, Queen Square; also see, for example, RAC, RG 1.1, Box 20, Folder 267, Letter from Alan Gregg to William Lennox, 13 May 1935; O'Brien to Gregg, 3 September 1935; Gregg to O'Brien, 18 September 1935; Daniel O'Brien to J. G. Greenfield, 18 June 1936.
89 RAC, RG 1.1, Series 401, Box 20, Folder 265, O'Brien's Diary, 9 December 1933.
90 On Lennox, see White, *Stanley Cobb*, p. 90.
91 RAC, RG 1.1, Series 401, Box 20, Folder 267, Letter from William Lennox to Alan Gregg.
92 For example, RAC, RG 1.1, Series 401, Box 20, Folder 267, Letter from William Lennox to Alan Gregg, 2 June 1935; and in the same folder, Carmichael to O'Brien, 14 June 1937.
93 For example, fifty-four American postgraduates had studied at Queen Square from 1920 to 1940. RAC, RG 1.1, Series 401, Box 20, Folder 267, List of Americans.
94 A similar story is recounted in: Joel A. Vilensky, Sid Gilman, and Pandy Sinish, 'Denny-Brown, Boston City Hospital, and the History of American Neurology', *Perspectives in Biology and Medicine* 47:4 (2004), 505–18.
95 The correspondence is thick on this point, see for example UCL,

Francis Walshe Papers, Warfield Longcope to Francis Walshe, 24 June 1924; and AMCMA, Lewis H. Weed Collection, Henry Thomas to Francis Walshe, 17 October 1924, and attached letters. Also see RAC, RG 1.1, Series 401, Box 20, Folder 265, Lambert to O'Brien, 1 May 1930; Weed to Lambert, 5 Nov. 1930; Weed to Robert A. Lambert, 12 November 1930.

96 This was information Gordon Holmes provided when he came to America in 1930. RAC, RG 1.1, Box 20, Folder 265, Letter from Lewis Weed to Robert A. Lambert, 12 November 1930; RAC, RG 1.1, Box 20, Folder 265, Series 401, A National Hospital for Nervous Diseases, 1930–1933, List of Americans Registered for Work in Neurology at the National Hospital Queen Square, 30 October 1930.

97 This proved to be true later. RAC, RG 1.1, Series 401, Box 20, Folder 268, Carmichael to Gregg, 2 October 1936; enclosure, Carmichael to Gregg, 2 October 1936; also see correspondence RAC, RG 1.1, Series 401, Box 20, Folder 269, Letter from Lambert to Alan Gregg, 2 February 1937.

98 RAC, RG 1.1, Series 401A, Box 15, Folder 214, Letter from Pearce to Gregg, 13 February 1929; RAC, RF 1.1, Series 401, Box 20, Folder 265, Letter from O'Brien to Gregg, 6 April 1932; On Rockefeller Foundation funding generally in this period see William Schneider, 'The Men who Followed Flexner: Richard Pearce, Alan Gregg, and the Rockefeller Foundation Medical Divisions, 1919–1951', in William Schneider (ed.), *Rockefeller Philanthropy and Modern Biomedicine: International Initiatives from World War I to the Cold War* (Bloomington: Indiana University Press, 2002), pp. 7–60, for neurology specifically see pp. 43–7.

99 RAC, RG 1.1, Series 401, Box 20, Folder 273, O'Brien, Diary excerpt 12 March 1932; in the same folder, see: 'An Appeal to the Rockefeller Foundation by the National Hospital for Diseases of the Nervous System Queen Square for Aid in Research and Teaching in Neurology', p. 8.

100 See, for instance, RAC, RG 1.1, Series 401, Box 20, Folder 265, Francis Fraser to Alan Gregg, 6 June 1932, A National Hospital for Nervous Diseases, 1930–1933.

101 On the distribution of neurological institutes see Ingrid Farreras, Caroline Hannaway, and Victoria Harden (eds), *Mind, Brain, Body, and Behavior: Foundations of Neuroscience and Behavioral Research at the National Institutes of Health* (Amsterdam: OUS Press, 2004); DeJong, *A History of American Neurology*.

102 Pressman, *Last Resort*, pp. 30–5.

103 Bliss, *Harvey Cushing*, p. 496; E. W. Archibald (ed.), *Neurological Biographies and Addresses; Foundation Volume; Published for the*

Staff, to Commemorate the Opening of the Montreal Neurological Institute of McGill University (Oxford: Oxford University Press, 1936), pp. 7–12.

104 From the British point of view this was a controversial policy. The MRC especially disliked it. See Edward Mellanby's comments: NA, FD 1/2820, Personal Note 1581 1A-1B, 9 November 1937.

105 Developments at the National Hospital were thus not obstructed by their own local values. It seems that by the 1930s the foundation was more willing to not interfere with local customs, unlike it had been in Edinburgh in the 1920s. Cf. the foundation's programme in Edinburgh in the 1920s. Christopher Lawrence, *Rockefeller Money, the Laboratory and Medicine in Edinburgh, 1919–1930: New Culture in an Old Country* (Rochester, NY: University of Rochester Press, 2005).

106 RAC, RG 1.1, Series 401, Box 20, Folder 265, Gregg to Frederick Macmillan, 17 April 1935.

107 RAC, RG 1.1, Series 401, Box 20, Folder 265, Alan Gregg to Daniel O'Brien, 29 April 1932.

108 Indeed, this complaint had been lodged against the National Hospital and the organisation of British medicine generally by 1918. See J. G. Adami's comments in 'On the Problem of Graduate Medical Study in London', in *Contributions to Medical and Biological Research*, pp. 10–15.

109 The problem was one readily identified by younger neurologists. 'He [Derek Denny Brown] feels there is much need for a more closely knit structure in teaching and research. An important factor, he says, for the younger men – and this certainly would be the case for Carmichael – is the need for professorial or other University status. On this point, unfortunately, the older men are not especially interested, but the issue is most vital for the younger people.' RAC, RG 1.1, Series 401, Box 20, Folder 267, O'Brien to Gregg, 17 October 1936.

110 RAC, RG 1.1, Series 401, Box 20, Folder 265, National Hospital for Diseases of the Nervous System – London, 10 April 1935; RAC, RG 1.1, Series 401, Box 20, Folder 267, Letter from Gregg to Macmillan.

111 NA, FD 1/2415, Neurological Unit, Queen Square, Carmichael to Thompson, 8 July 1935.

112 NA, FD,1/2415, Neurological Unit, Queen Square, Carmichael to Green, 6 July 1934.

113 AABN, Minute Book, Association of British Neurologists (hereafter AABN, ABN Minutes), vol. 1, analysis of meetings on pp. 2–91.

114 In other words, 9 per cent of the participants were producing 16 per cent of the total work.

115 Ibid.

116 Anon., 'International Neurological Congress, Berne', *Journal of Neurology and Psychopathology* 12:45 (1931), 66–8, 67.
117 Ibid., 67–8.
118 Ibid., 68.
119 AABN, ABN Minutes, vol. 1, p. 2.
120 AABN, ABN Minutes, vol. 1, p. 3.
121 Edwin Bramwell Papers, Mackintosh to Bramwell, 12 May 1934.

Chapter 4

1 Stephen Casper and L. Stephen Jacyna (eds), *The Neurological Patient in History* (Rochester, NY: University of Rochester Press, 2012).
2 See, for instance, Philippon and Poirier, *Joseph Babinski*.
3 The best full-length discussion can be found throughout Bliss, *Harvey Cushing*, but also see all of Fraenkel, *Hugh Cairns*.
4 This fact has exercised enormous cultural commentary. For a review of the debates, see Matthew B. Crawford, 'The Limits of Neuro-Talk', *New Atlantis* (2008), 65–77.
5 Again the literature is huge, but the following works give some sense of those developments which influenced neurology and by extension medicine: David M. Oshinsky, *Polio: An American Story* (Oxford: Oxford University Press, 2006); Michael Bliss, *The Discovery of Insulin* (Edinburgh: Harris, 1983); Susan M. Reverby, *Examining Tuskegee: The Infamous Syphilis Study and its Implications* (Chapel Hill: University of North Carolina Press, 2009).
6 For an example, see Jesse F. Ballenger, 'Disappearing in Plain Sight: Public Roles of People with Dementia in the Meaning and Politics of Alzheimer's Disease', in Casper and Jacyna (eds), *The Neurological Patient in History*.
7 Rowland, *The Legacy of Tracy J. Putnam and H. Houston Merritt*.
8 An exemplary discussion of this problem is Shepherd, *Creating Modern Neuroscience*, pp. 176–92.
9 J. Wayne Lazar, 'Acceptance of the Neuron Theory by Clinical Neurologists of the Late-Nineteenth Century', *Journal of the History of Neurosciences* 19 (2010), 349–64, 362.
10 Shepherd, *Creating Modern Neuroscience*, pp. 39–55 and 206–17.
11 Cornelius Borck, *Hirnströme: eine Kulturgeschichte der Elektroenzephalographie* (Göttingen: Wallstein, 2005).
12 Rowland, *The Legacy of Tracy J. Putnam and H. Houston Merritt*, pp. 101–16; Jonas Salk, 'The Virus of Poliomyelitis: From Discovery to Extinction', *Journal of the American Medical Association* 250 (1983), 808–10.

13 The founding documents and associated records can be found throughout NA, FD 1/1422-1426. NA, FD 1/426, Minutes of the Burden Neurological Clinic is especially important and describes the foundation of the institute. Also see Ray Cooper and Jonathan Bird, *The Burden*.

14 See the reports from the unit for 1938–45 in NA, FD 1/5380, Neurological Unit, Queen Square, Annual Reports. An important discussion of research can be found in Rhodri Hayward, 'Germany and the Making of "English" Psychiatry: The Maudsley Hospital, 1908–1939), in Volker Roelcke, Paul J. Weindling, and Louise Westwood (eds), *International Relations in Psychiatry* (Rochester, NY; University of Rochester Press, 2010, pp. 67–81).

15 Gavrus, 'Men of Dreams and Men of Action'.

16 AABN, Macdonald Critchley, undated address [c. 1985].

17 Anon., 'Hughlings Jackson Centenary: A Commemorative Dinner', *British Medical Journal* (1935), 769–70.

18 AABN, ABN Minutes, vol. 1, p. 2.

19 AABN, Association of British Neurologists: List of Members, 1974, pp. 1–21, 3. A copy from 1974, for example, has the secretary's (Peter Robinson) pencilled revisions in the margins and texts: Anthony Feiling, an honorary member, had the word 'Dec'd' annotated next to a scratched-out mailing address.

20 AABN, ABN Minutes, vol. 1, p. 28. Members did not always attend: 'Attention was drawn to the failure of two members, D. K. Henderson and H. M. Traquiar to attend the last two meetings.'

21 AABN, Macdonald Critchley, undated address [c. 1985].

22 Robinson, *The History of the Association at the 50th Anniversary Meeting, 4th November 1983*, p. 5.

23 AABN, Association of British Neurologists, Rules, p. 1, undated. The rules changed very little between 1933 and 1960. When they did change, it was noted in the minutes, and thus the date of this source is not required.

24 AABN, ABN Minutes, vol. 1, p. 3.

25 Christopher Goetz, Teresa Chmura, and Douglas Lanska 'Part 1. The History of 19th Century Neurology and the American Neurological Association', *Annals of Neurology* 53:suppl. 4 (2003), s20.

26 Robinson, *The History of the Association at the 50th Anniversary Meeting, 4th November 1983*.

27 Ibid., p. 7.

28 Papers were delivered extemporaneously. AABN, Association of British Neurologists, Rules, p. 5; John Walton, *The Spice of Life* (London: Royal Society of Medicine Services, 1993), p. 341.

29 'John David Spillane', in *Lives of the Fellow (Munk's Roll)* (London: Royal College of Physicians, 1985), vol. 8, p. 479.
30 WL, PP/CPS/3, ABN Dinner.
31 AABN, ABN Minutes, vol. 1, pp. 100–1; Walton, *The Spice of Life*, p. 341.
32 Robinson, *The History of the Association at the 50th Anniversary Meeting, 4th November 1983*, p. 7.
33 AABN, ABN Minutes, vol. 1, p. 23.
34 Ibid., vol. 1, p. 27.
35 Ibid., vol. 1, pp. 28–9.
36 Ibid., vol. 1, pp. 31–2, Adrian on p. 31.
37 Ibid., vol. 2, p. 2.
38 It was the Neurological Society of Amsterdam. AABN, ABN Minutes, vol. 1, pp. 38–40.
39 Ibid., vol. 1, p. 40; this was probably done so that Derek Denny Brown could continue holding his membership despite an appointment in the United States. Edward G. Robinson had returned to Australia. He was the first overseas member to be admitted. He also played an important role in founding the Australian Association of Neurology.
40 AABN, ABN Minutes, vol. 1, pp. 55, 64–6.
41 Ibid., pp. 55–6.
42 Edwin Bramwell Papers, Edwin Bramwell, Diary entry, 5 May 1939, vol. 6, pp. 99–100.
43 Ibid., p. 100.
44 Description of the proceedings hereafter is taken from general observations from AABN, ABN Minutes, vol. 1, pp. 1–92 unless otherwise indicated.
45 AMCMA, Adolf Meyer Papers, Third International Neurological Congress, 11/290/2 International Neurological Congress.
46 Alan S. Milward, *War, Economy, and Society, 1939–1945* (Harmondsworth: Penguin Books, 1987), p. 111.
47 AABN, ABN Minutes, vol. 1, p. 54.
48 There is little work on the Second World War and British neurology. Relevant sources include: Bailey, 'The Present State of American Neurology', pp. 111–17; Wilder Penfield, 'Clinical Notes from a Trip to Great Britain', *Archives of Neurology and Psychiatry* 47 (1942), 1030–6; Wilder Penfield, 'Some Problems of Wartime Neurology', *Archives of Neurology and Psychiatry*, 47 (1942), 839–40; J. Clifford Richardson, 'Clinical Experiences with a R.C.A.M.C. Neuropsychiatric Division in England 1940 to 1944', *Proceedings of the Royal Society of Medicine* 2 (1944), 373–6.
49 Edgar Jones, Robin Woolven, Bill Durodie, and Simon Wessely,

'Civilian Morale during the Second World War: Responses to Air Raids Re-examined,' *Social History of Medicine* 17:3 (2004), 463–79.

50 Anon., 'Hospitals in War-Time: Advisers to Minister of Health,' *The Times* (8 March 1939), 8.

51 Stevens, *Medical Practice*, pp. 67–80.

52 Lovell, *Churchill's Doctor*, pp. 140–1.

53 Stevens, *Medical Practice*, p. 68.

54 Charles Webster, *The Health Services Since the War. Vol. 1: Problems of Health Care: The National Health Service before 1957* (London: HMSO, 1988), pp. 37–198.

55 Stevens, *Medical Practice*, p. 68.

56 Silver, *History of the Treatment of Spinal Injuries*, pp. 52–81; Susan Goodman, *Spirit of Stoke Mandeville: The Story of Sir Ludwig Guttman* (London: Collins, 1986), pp. 83–117; For the general context of these centres, see Hardy, *Health and Medicine in Britain since 1860*, pp. 126–32.

57 See NA, MH 76/159, Memorandum (June 1941), Peripheral Nerve Injuries Committee of the Medical Research Council, pp. 1–9.

58 NA, MH 76/159, Ministry of Health Emergency Hospital Scheme: Suggestions in regard to the Treatment of Peripheral Nerve Injuries of Service Cases in the E.M.S., 5 September 1940.

59 NA, MH 76/159, Committee on Peripheral Nerves – A Description, 27 September 1940.

60 NA, MH 76/159, Letter from Francis Fraser to Edward Mellanby, 27 September 1940; Letter from Fraser to George Riddoch, 7 October 1940; see also Riddoch to Fraser, 5 November 1941.

61 NA, MH 76/159, E.M.S.I. 231, Ministry of Health. Emergency Medical Services: Service Cases of Peripheral Nerve Injury, 30 September 1940.

62 NA, MH 76/159, Report E.M.S.I./495, Ministry of Health Emergency Medical Services: Special Units for Peripheral Nerve Injuries, August 1944.

63 NA, MH 76/159, Memorandum, Emergency Health Scheme: Follow-up of Certain Cases from Special Centres, 2 February 1942.

64 Ibid.

65 One professor wrote to the Ministry of Health angrily: 'these patients are not experimental animals; they cannot be caged up until the end of the investigation and we must allow them to return to a useful existence while providing for the re-examinations that are necessary for the fulfilment of our duty to our patients and the completion of a most important research.' NA, MH 76/159, Letter from H. J. Seddon to Francis Fraser, 12 May 1941.

66 NA, MH 76/159, After-Treatment of Service Cases of Peripheral Nerve Injury, 3 July 1941.

67 NA, MH 76/159, Memorandum (June 1941), Peripheral Nerve Injuries Committee of the Medical Research Council, especially pp. 8–9.

68 Silver, *History of the Treatment of Spinal Injuries*, pp. 52–81; Goodman, *Spirit of Stoke Mandeville*, pp. 83–117.

69 One socially significant impact of these centres was that they introduced the idea of athletic games for the disabled. This in turn led to the Special Olympics and now the Paralympics. In this Ludwig Guttmann at the Stoke Mandeville Treatment Centre for Spinal Injuries was particular important. Goodman, *Spirit of Stoke Mandeville*, pp. 118–46.

70 A typical complaint for neurology around the globe, see Lothar Kalinowsky and H. Houston Merritt, 'The Status of Neurology as a Specialty in Various Countries', *Neurology* 4 (1954), pp. 668–73.

71 Macdonald Critchley, 'George Riddoch (1889–1947)', in Critchley (ed.), *The Ventricle of Memory*, pp. 155–64.

72 Anon., 'George Riddoch, M.D., F.R.C.P.', *British Medical Journal* (1947), 711–12.

73 Anon., 'George Riddoch, M.D., Aberd., F.R.C.P.', *Lancet* (1947), 672–3.

74 Walter Russell Brain Private Papers Collection, private collection, Calgary, Canada (hereafter Brain Papers – Private), Letter from George Riddoch to W. Russell Brain, 25 September 1944.

75 A touching letter from this period is a reply by Riddoch's wife to Russell Brain's message of condolence. 'I appreciated your letter which was written immediately after George's operation more than I can tell, but it was not to be the he should recover from it though I know that everything was done that could possibly be done.' Brain Papers – Private, Letter from May Riddoch to W. Russell Brain, 28 October 1947.

76 Anon., 'Dr George Riddoch, Authority on Nervous Diseases', *The Times* (31 October 1947), 7.

77 E. D. Adrian, 'Dr George Riddoch', *The Times* (1 November 1947), 6.

78 NA, MH 76/159, Letter from Riddoch to Fraser, 4 August 1941.

79 Ibid.

80 NA, MH 76/159, Letter from Murchie to Riddoch, 12 August 1941.

81 NA, MH 76/159, Letter from Murchie to de Wesselow, 22 August 1941; Murchie to Patrick, 22 August 1941; de Wesslow to Murchie, 6 September 1941.

82 NA, MH 76/159, Letter from Murchie to Holmes, 13 September 1941.

83 NA, MH 76/159, Letter from Holmes to Murchie, 16 September 1941.

84 ARCP, Brain Papers, MS 3226/99, 'The Organization of Neurology in London After the War', [undated – c1945-1952].

85 ARCP, Brain Papers, MS 3226/99.5 and MS 3226/99.6 'The

Organization of Neurology in London after the War,' [undated, c. 1945–52].

86 Brain obviously knew a great deal about these centres. See his description of them in his obituary of Riddoch: 'George Riddoch, M.D., F.R.C.P.,' *British Medical Journal* (1947), 711–12.

87 Brain Papers – Private, George Riddoch Testimonial, 23 January 1927.

88 'George Riddoch arranged for me to become the first second HP at Maida Vale Hospital and so began an association which lasted all my professional life,' ARCP, Brain Papers, MS 3174.10, Autobiographical Notes by Lord Brain; also see Pickering, 'Walter Russell Brain, First Baron Brain of Eynsham,' 61–82.

89 AABN, ABN Minutes, vol. 1, p. 55.

90 Ibid.

91 Viscount Dawson, *Annual Address Delivered to the Royal College of Physicians by the President* (London: Royal College of Physicians, 1933), pp. 2–3.

92 Stevens, *Medical Practice*, p. 63.

93 Webster, *The Health Services since the War*, pp. 123 and 188.

94 AABN, ABN Minutes, vol. 1, p. 55.

95 Ibid. This was a fairly standard procedure for many specialties. See Stevens, *Medical Practice*, p. 370–5. It is noteworthy that the Diploma in Psychological Medicine was available by 1928.

96 Ibid.

97 AABN, ABN Minutes, vol. 1, p. 56.

98 Ibid., vol. 1, p. 57; see also p. 58: 'The draft of a letter to the Royal College of Physicians requesting the appointment of a Committee to deal with training and recognition of specialists in Neurology was considered and the Hon. Secretary was directed to forward it to the President of the College.'

99 Although the ABN requested this committee be formed, the Royal College of Physicians was also involved in forming such committees for medical specialties. See A. M. Cooke, *A History of the Royal College of Physicians of London* (Oxford: Clarendon Press, 1972), vol. 3, p. 1079.

100 AABN, ABN Minutes, vol. 1, for example, see pp. 58, 60, 68, 73–4.

101 Ibid., vol. 1, p. 80.

102 Ministry of Health, *Report of the Inter-Departmental Committee on the Remuneration of Consultants and Specialists* (London: HMSO, 1948), for neurologists see p. 6. For the conflation of general medicine with neurology see the tables on pp. 20–30.

103 In many ways this was rather strange. In 1949 neurology received the greatest number of distinction awards 'with 71.4% of the incumbents receiving awards.' That individuals' status in the field should have

been so well recognised by their peers, while at the same time the field should remain so marginal in its services, is very hard to explain, unless it is admitted that this had simply always been the status quo. Webster, *The Health Services since the War*, pp. 315–17; also see Lovell, *Churchill's Doctor*, pp. 324–5.

104 Ministry of Health, *Report of the Inter-Departmental Committee on Medical Schools* (London: HMSO, 1944).

105 ARCP, Royal College of Physicians London, Committee on Neurology, (hereafter Committee on Neurology), Royal College of Physicians Committee on Neurology Document M.1, 19 December 1944, 13C Minutes of the Committee of Neurology, vol. 1 (1944–66), Minutes; also see AABN, ABN Minutes, vol. 1, p. 57.

106 ARCP, Committee on Neurology, Royal College of Physicians Committee on Neurology Document M.1, 19 December 1944, 13C Minutes of the Committee of Neurology, vol. 1 (1944–66).

107 Ibid.

108 Ibid.

109 ARCP, Committee on Neurology, Royal College of Physicians Committee on Neurology Document M.2, 19 December 1944, 13C Minutes of the Committee of Neurology, vol. 1 (1944–66).

110 ARCP, Committee on Neurology, Royal College of Physicians, *Report of the Committee on Neurology* (London: Harrison & Sons, 1945).

111 Ibid., p. 15.

112 See, for example: ibid., p. 16.

113 Ibid., p. 4.

114 Ibid., p. 6.

115 Ibid., p. 7.

116 Eric J. Engstrom notes that a similar conversation occurred in the 1860s in Germany: Engstrom, *Clinical Psychiatry in Imperial Germany*, pp. 41–2.

117 Ministry of Health, *National Health Service: The Development of Consultant Services* (London: HMSO, 1950).

118 Ibid., p. 11.

119 Ibid., p. 12.

120 Ibid., p. 27.

121 Ibid.

122 Ibid.

123 This problem represented the general crisis within the National Health Service. Lovell, *Churchill's Doctor*, pp. 291–311.

124 ARCP, Committee on Neurology, Royal College of Physicians Committee on Neurology, 23 February 1953, 13C Minutes of the Committee of Neurology, vol. 1 (1944–66).

125 AABN, ABN Minutes, vol. 1, pp. 144–5.

126 ARCP, Committee on Neurology, Royal College of Physicians Committee on Neurology, 23 February 1953, 13C Minutes of the Committee of Neurology, vol. 1 (1944–66).

127 Royal College of Physicians, *Interim Report of the Committee on Neurology* (London: Harrison & Sons, 1954).

128 My emphasis. Ibid., p. 4.

129 Ibid., p. 8.

130 Ibid., quote on p. 5, see pp. 5–8.

131 Ibid., p. 8.

132 Ibid., p. 9.

133 Ibid., p. 9.

134 ARCP, Committee on Neurology, Document 11, Discussion of the Interim Report of the Committee on Neurology by the Council, April 1954, 1–7, 13C Minutes of the Committee of Neurology, vol. 1 (1944–66).

135 Ibid., p. 3.

136 Ibid., p. 6.

137 In fact the problem was one generally common within the health service during this period. See Webster, *The Health Services since the War*, pp. 1–30, especially 5–11.

138 AABN, ABN Minutes, vol. 1, p. 172.

139 Stevens, *Medical Practice*, p. 94, see also 148–50.

140 AABN, ABN Minutes, vol. 1, p. 187.

141 Ibid.

142 Ibid. pp. 214–15.

143 Ibid., p. 230.

144 Ibid., p. 234. In 1960 written confirmation of this status was also sent by the Neurological Section of the Royal Society of Medicine. The ABN effectively represented neurology in all of its political aspects in the United Kingdom. See ibid., p. 244.

145 Shepherd, *Creating Modern Neuroscience*, pp. 176–92.

146 Anon., 'E. A. Carmichael', *British Medical Journal* 1 (1978), 513–15.

147 F. M. R. Walshe, 'Training of the Neurologist', *Archives of Neurology and Psychiatry*, 29 (1933), 381.

148 Ibid.

149 For instance, see Charles Symonds, 'Reorientations in Neurology', *Lancet* (1949), 677–80; Derek Denny Brown, 'The Shattuck Lecture: The Changing Pattern of Neurologic Medicine', *New England Journal of Medicine*, 246:22 (1952), 846. Also see, Anon., 'Neurology Advances', *Lancet* (1952), 325; Anon., 'Neurology: A Weak Position', *Lancet* (1954), 1021; Francis Walshe, 'The Future of Neurology', *Proceedings of the Royal Society of Medicine* 48 (1955), 120–4; Brinton, 'Presidential Address, 263–4.

150 NA, FD 23/172, Minutes on Discussion on Neurological Research, 7 July 1960, pp. 1–2.
151 Ibid.
152 See NA, FD 23/173, Expenditures on Neurological Research, 1960.
153 NA, FD 23/174, Harold Himsworth to Russell Brain, 13 February 1961, Discussion on Neurological Research.
154 ARCP, Committee on Neurology, Minutes of the Committee of Neurology, 23 February 1953
155 ARCP, N. S. Alcock to John St Claire Elkington, 25 November 1952, Correspondence Neurological Committee, 26 November 1952–16 April 1953.
156 ARCP, Philip Buckley to J. St C. Elkington, 22 November 1952, Correspondence Neurological Committee, 26 November 1952–16 April 1953.
157 ARCP, David Kendal to Elkington, 24 November 1952; E. C. O. Jewerbury to Elkington, 1 December 1952; G. S. Graveson to J. St C. Elkington, 2 December 1952, Correspondence Neurological Committee, 26 November 1952–16 April 1953.
158 ARCP, A. M. Stewart Wallace to Elkington, 26 January 1953, Correspondence Neurological Committee, 26 November 1952–16 April 1953.
159 ARCP, John Penman to Elkington, 28 November 1952, Correspondence Neurological Committee 26 November 1952–16 April 1953.
160 Royal College of Physicians Committee on Neurology, *The Neurological Services in Great Britain* (London: Harrison & Sons, 1965), p. 5.

Chapter 5

1 Brinton 'President's Address', 263–5; Denis Brinton, 'The Neurological Services of England and Wales', *Lancet* (1963), 663.
2 Association of British Neurologists, *Neurology in the United Kingdom: Towards 2000 and Beyond* (London: Association of British Neurologists, 1997); David L. Stevens, *Neurology in the United Kingdom: Numbers of Clinical Neurologists and Trainees* (London: Association of British Neurologists, 1996).
3 C. B. Carroll, D. S. Tengah, C. Lawthorn, and G. Venables, 'The Feminisation of British Neurology: Implications for Workforce Planning', *Clinical Medicine* 7:4 (2007), 339–42.
4 R. Langton Hewer and V. A. Wood, 'Neurology in the United Kingdom. I: Historical Development', *Journal of Neurology, Neurosurgery, and Psychiatry* 55 (1992), 2–7.

5 Henry Miller, 'The Organization of Neurological Services and Neurological Training', *Proceedings of the Royal Society of Medicine* 61 (1968), 1004–10; Henry Miller, 'Neurology in a General Hospital', *British Medical Journal* 1 (1958), 477–80.
6 Goodman, *Spirit of Stoke Mandeville*, pp. 118–46.
7 ARCP, Committee on Neurology, Royal College of Physicians Committee on Neurology, 13C Minutes of the Committee of Neurology, Minutes from a Meeting of the Neurology Committee Held at the Royal College of Physicians on Thursday 14 June, 1962.
8 Christopher Pallis, *ABC of Brainstem Death: Articles Published in the British Medical Journal* (London: British Medical Journal, 1983).
9 Ballenger, *Self, Senility, and Alzheimer's Disease in Modern America*, pp. 81–112.
10 George Canguilhem, *The Normal and the Pathological* (New York: Zone Books, 1991), in particular pp. 233–87.
11 Jon Turney and Brian Balmer, 'The Genetic Body', in Roger Cooter and John Pickstone (eds), *Companion to Medicine in the Twentieth Century* (London and New York: Routledge, 2003), pp. 411–12; Alice Wexler, *The Woman who Walked into the Sea: Huntington's and the Making of Genetic Disease*, (New Haven and London: Yale University Press, 2008), pp. 94–122.
12 Bonnie Evans, 'Mental Defectives, Childhood Psychotics and the Origins of Autism Research at the Maudsley Hospital, 1913–1983' (PhD dissertation, University of Cambridge, 2010).
13 Daniel R. Wilson and Gerald A. Cory, Jr, *The Evolutionary Epidemiology of Mania and Depression: A Theoretical and Empirical Interpretation of Mood Disorders* (Lampeter, Edwin Mellen Press, 2007).
14 For a review, see Peter Conrad and Kristin K. Barker, 'The Social Construction of Illness: Key Insights and Policy Implications', *Journal of Health and Social Behavior* 51:S (2010), S67–79.
15 WL, PP/DOL/A/1/22, Letter from Brian Matthews to Richard Doll, 13 September 1970; on prions, see Anderson, *The Collectors of Lost Souls*; Kiheung Kim, *The Social Construction of Disease: From Scrapie to Prion* (London and New York: Routledge, 2007).
16 Karl Friston, 'A Short History of SPM', in Karl J. Friston, John T. Ashburner, Stefan J. Kiebel, Thomas E. Nichols, and William D. Penny (eds), *Statistical Parametric Mapping: The Analysis of Functional Brain Images* (London and New York: Elsevier, 2007), pp. 1–9.
17 WL, PP/DOL/A/1/22, Letter from Brian Matthews to Richard Doll, 3 May 1974.

18 WL, PP/DOL/A/1/22, Letter from Richard Doll to Brian Matthews, 6 May 1974.
19 John Krige, *American Hegemony and the Postwar Reconstruction of Science in Europe* (Cambridge, MA: MIT Press, 2006).
20 Vilensky, Gilman, and Sinish, 'Denny-Brown, Boston City Hospital, and the History of American Neurology', 505–18.
21 WL, PP/DOL/A/1/22, Letter from Paul B. Beeson to Professor Richard Doll, 14 November 1969.
22 Anthony Hopkins, 'Different Types of Neurologist', *British Medical Journal* 288 (1984), 1736.
23 Weisz, *Divide and Conquer*, pp. 191–225.
24 See, as one example, Beard 'Editorial'.
25 John Walton (Lord Walton of Detchant), '50 Years in Neurology, A Retrospect', *Practical Neurology* 3 (2003), 55.
26 Paul Forman, 'The Primacy of Science in Modernity, of Technology in Postmodernity, and of Ideology in the History of Technology', *History and Technology* 23:1/2 (2007), 1–152; Paul Forman, '(Re)cognizing Postmodernity: Help for Historians – of Science Especially', *Berichte zur Wissenschaftsgeschichte* 33:2 (2010), 157–75.
27 It is remarkable that Engstrom's excellent *Clinical Psychiatry in Imperial Germany* frames much of its analysis of jurisdiction disputes in terms of the rhetoric and achievements of few individuals. Implicitly such a frame suggests that reforms and conflicts among groups were restricted and atypical. See pp. 199–203.
28 Cf. Shepherd, *A War of Nerves*, pp. 21–168.
29 Anon., 'International Neurological Congress, Berne', *Journal of Neurology and Psychopathology*, 12:45 (1931), 66–8.
30 The decline was actually experienced across the world but British neurologists, confronting so many changes in the practice of medicine with the advent of the National Health Service, were particularly affected. See K. J. Zülch, 'The Place of Neurology in Medicine and Its Future', in P. J. Vinker and G. W. Bruyn (eds), *Handbook of Neurology* (Amsterdam: North-Holland Publishing Co., 1968), pp. 1–44.
31 On this ambiguity see RCPA, *Report of the Committee on Neurology*, Royal College of Physicians, July 1945, pp. 1–17; RCPA, *Future Needs of Neurological Staffing*; Royal College of Physicians Committee on Neurology, 13C Minutes of the Committee of Neurology, vol. 1 (1944–1966); also see Stevens, *Medical Practice*, pp. 42–3; Webster, *The Health Services since the War*, vol. 1, p. 310, Table VII, Consultant Numbers.
32 Lawrence, 'Still Incommunicable', p. 96.
33 Anon., 'Francis Carmichael Purser, M.D.Dub.', *Lancet* (1934), 545.

34 Anon., 'Ronald Grey Gordon, M.D., D.Sc., Edin., F.R.C.P.E.', *Lancet* (1950), 932.

35 Anon., 'R. G. Gordon, M.D., F.R.C.P.Ed.', *British Medical Journal* (1950), 1080–2, especially 1081.

36 Anon., 'Conrad Meredyth Hinds Howell, M.A., D.M., Oxon., F.R.C.P.', *Lancet* (1960), 1136.

37 The total number of individuals in this study was 200. Here the obituaries of 100 members of the ABN were used, the number of obituaries available for those neurologists totalling 294. Further details for the statistical portion of this study were supplemented by *Munk's Roll* and other biographical sources, including student records. When I could find them, I used sources from personal papers collections, the MRC archives, and the Ministry of Health.

38 Anon., 'Donald Elms Core, M.D. Manch., F.R.C.P. Lond.', *Lancet* (1934), 377.

39 His textbook offers few hints of such behaviour. His chapter 'X-Ray's and the Nervous System', for example, makes no reference to it as a tool to be used only after the history has failed to turn up the problem: Donald Core, *The Examination of the Central Nervous System* (Edinburgh, E. & S. Livingstone, 1928), pp. 209–17.

40 Anon., 'Edwin Bramwell, M.D., LL.D. Edin., M.D., Melb., F.R.C.P., F.R.C.P.E.', *Lancet* (1952), 726–7; for a discussion of Bramwell's patrician ethos, see Lawrence, *Rockefeller Money, the Laboratory and Medicine in Edinburgh*.

41 See, for instance, Private Collection, Edwin Bramwell, Diary; 6 February 1935, p. 222.

42 Anon., 'Eric Alfred Blake Pritchard, M.A., M.D.Cantab., F.R.C.P.', *Lancet* (1962), 1361; Anon., 'Frederick Lucien Golla, O.B.E., B.M.Oxon., F.R.C.P.', *Lancet* (1968), 367; Anon., 'Helen Dimsdale, M.D.Cantab., F.R.C.P', *Lancet* (1977), 1018; Anon., 'Charles Putnam Symonds', *Lancet* (1978), 1389–90; Anon., 'Richard Sydney Allison', *Lancet* (1978), 1108–9. See Casper, 'The Idioms of Practice', Appendix C for career information.

43 The archives for this exhibit are held in the Neuroscience Archives, University of California, Los Angeles, Webb Haymaker Collection, '1953 *Founders of Neurology*'.

44 Otis Historical Archives, National Museum of Health and Medicine Armed Forces Institute of Pathology, Silver Spring, Maryland (hereafter AFIP), Series 1, Box 2, Enclosure ,'Publicity for *The Founders of Neurology*', Founders of Neurology (Omissions).

45 Webb Haymaker, *The Founders of Neurology: One-Hundred and Thirty-Three Biographical Sketches* (Springfield, IL: Charles C. Thomas, 1953), p. xi.

46 Webb Haymaker and Francis Schiller, *The Founders of Neurology: One-Hundred Forty-Six Biographical Sketches by Eighty-Nine Authors* (Springfield, IL: Charles C. Thomas, 1970), p. vi.
47 For example, AFIP, Series 1, Box 2, Francis Schiller to Webb Haymaker, 13 November 1967; Francis Schiller to Webb Haymaker, 28 December 1967; Francis Schiller to Webb Haymaker, 6 July 1968, Francis Schiller to Webb Haymaker, 9 September 1968.
48 AFIP, Series 1, Box 2, Francis Schiller to Webb Haymaker, 11 September 1968.
49 AFIP, Series 1, Box 2, William McMenemy to Webb Haymaker, 15 October 1968.
50 AFIP, Series 1, Box 2, Francis Schiller to Webb Haymaker, 13 June 1967.
51 AFIP, Series 1, Box 2, Francis Schiller to Webb Haymaker, 22 August 1968.
52 AFIP, Series 1, Box 2, David Bodian to Webb Haymaker, 20 September 1968.
53 Haymaker and Schiller, *The Founders of Neurology*, pp. vi–vii.
54 AFIP, Series 1, Box 2, Francis Schiller to Webb Haymaker, 13 November 1967.
55 Haymaker, *The Founders of Neurology*, p. 206.
56 Ibid., p. 304.
57 On George Riddoch's contributions to British Neurology, see Casper, 'The Idioms of Practice', ch. 7.
58 Personal correspondence with Royalty Division of Charles C. Thomas, 2 May 2007.
59 Anon., 'Editorial: The Future of Neurology', 792.
60 Brain, 'Neurology: Past, Present, and Future', *British Medical Journal* (1958), 355.
61 Ibid.
62 Abbott, *The System of the Professions*, pp. 59–62.
63 Abbott, noting this feature generally in professions, writes: 'Today... when the vast majority of professionals are in organizational practice, and indeed when only about 50 percent of even doctors and lawyers are in independent practice, the public continues to think of professional life in terms of solo, independent practice. Similarly, the ideas that lawyers spend large amounts of time in court, or doctors in hospitals, or that architects spend most of their time actually designing buildings persist long after the realities they imply disappeared. To some extent, of course, this archaism is self-consciously maintained since it provides the older professions with a legitimating link to a romanticized past.' Abbott, *System of the Professions*, p. 61.

64 This was a view that was reproduced. Remember that in 1945 the neurologist was to be a consultant not a specialist. Anon., 'Neurological Training of the Future', *British Medical Journal* (1945), 292.

65 For a similar argument, see Gadi Algazi, 'Food for Though: Hieronymus Wolf Grapples with the Scholarly Habitus', in Rudolf Dekker (ed.), *Egodocuments and History: Autobiographical Writings in its Social Context since the Middle Ages* (Hilversum: Verloren, 2002), pp. 21–5. See also how Steven Shapin and Christopher Lawrence contest this positivist tradition, 'Introduction: The Body of Knowledge', in Christopher Lawrence and Steven Shapin (eds), *Science Incarnate: Historical Embodiments of Natural Knowledge* (Chicago: University of Chicago Press, 1998), pp. 13–16.

66 This had been the case for their instructors, teachers, advisors, and mentors.

67 In part the movement of clinical neurology away from functional subjects may serve as an explanation for why in the early 1970s clinical neurology and neuroscience returned to (and in some sense reinvented) memory via biomechanistic synaptic explanations, epitomised, for example, by hypotheses like long-term potentiation (LTP) and long-term depression (LTD) of cerebral neurons.

68 Aldous Huxley, *Brave New World* (New York: HarperPerennial Modern Classics, 2006), p. 166.

69 Head, 'Presidential Address', 6.

70 Canguilhem, *The Normal and the Pathological*, pp. 233–87.

71 Forman, 'The Primacy of Science in Modernity'; Forman, '(Re) cognizing Postmodernity'.

72 Shepherd, *Creating Modern Neuroscience*, pp. 136–236; Robert L. Grubb, *Neurosurgery at Washington University: A Century of Excellence* (St Louis: The Washington University, 2010), pp. 199–322; Roger Smith, *Being Human: Historical Knowledge and the Creation of Human Nature* (New York: Columbia University, 2007).

73 *Report of the Committee on Teaching/Research Manpower and Needs in Basic Neurologic and Communicative Sciences. Manpower in Basic Neurologic and Communicative Sciences: Present Status and Future Needs* (Washington, DC: National Academy of Sciences, 1977), p. 132.

74 Vidal, 'Brainhood, Anthropological Figure of Modernity', 15–36; Rose, 'Neurochemical Selves'.

75 Foucault, *The Birth of the Clinic*, p. 185.

Select bibliography

Archives

Alan Mason Chesney Medical Archives of Johns Hopkins Medical Institutions, Baltimore, Adolf Meyer Papers (Adolf Meyer Papers)

Archives of the Association of British Neurologists, London (AABN)

Archives and Special Collections A. C. Long Health Sciences Library, Columbia University, New York City, New York, Henry A. Riley Papers.

Archives of the Royal College of Physicians London (ARCP)

- Association of Physicians of Great Britain and Ireland (AP)
- Committee on Neurology Papers, Royal College of Physicians, London
- Walter Russell Brain Papers (Brain Papers)

Archives of the World Federation of Neurology, London

Bakken Library and Museum, Minneapolis, MN (Bakken Library)

British Library (BL)

London Hospital Archives

London Metropolitan Archives

National Archives, London (NA)

National Archives Scotland (NAS)

Edwin Bramwell Papers, Carnoustie, Scotland, Private Collection (Bramwell Papers)

Neuroscience Archives, University of California, Los Angeles, Webb Haymaker Collection

Otis Historical Archives, National Museum of Health and Medicine Armed Forces Institute of Pathology, Silver Spring, MD

Rockefeller Archive Center, Sleepy Hollow, NY (RAC)

Rockefeller Medical Library, Institute of Neurology, National Hospital, Queen Square, London

Red Cross Archives

Royal Holloway University Library, London (RHUL)

Royal Society of Medicine Archives, London (RSMA)

- Neurological Section of the Royal Society of Medicine
- Neurological Society of the United Kingdom

Special Collections, Brotherton Library, University of Leeds
University College London Special Archives and Collections (UCL)
Francis Walshe Papers (Francis Walshe Papers)
University of Birmingham, Special Collections
University of Minnesota, Biomedical Library, Minneapolis, Minnesota
Walter Russell Brain Papers Private Collection, Calgary, Canada, Private Collection (Brain Papers – Private)
Wellcome Library, London (WL)
Yale University Library, Manuscripts and Archives, Harvey Cushing Papers (Cushing Papers)

Periodicals and newspapers consulted

Archives of Neurology from the Pathological Laboratory of the London County Asylums
Archives of Neurology
Archives of Neurology and Psychiatry
Brain: A Journal of Neurology
British Medical Journal
Bulletin of the History of Medicine
Guy's Hospital Gazette
Guy's Hospital Reports
Journal of the History of Medicine and Allied Sciences
Journal of Neurology and Psychopathology
Journal of Neurology and Psychiatry
Journal of Neurology, Neurosurgery, and Psychiatry
Lancet
Medical History
Practitioner
Proceedings of the Royal Society of Medicine (PRSM)
Quarterly Journal of Medicine
Review of Neurology and Psychiatry
Science
St Mary's Gazette
St Bartholomew's Hospital Reports
The Times (London)
Transactions of the Ophthalmological Society of the United Kingdom (*Trans.*)

Books and journal articles

Abbott, Andrew, *The System of the Professions: An Essay on the Division of Expert Labor* (Chicago: University of Chicago Press, 1988).

Abel-Smith, Brian, *The Hospitals, 1800–1948: A Study in Social Administration in England and Wales* (London: Heinemann, 1964).

Ackernecht, Erwin H., *Medicine at the Paris Hospital* (Baltimore: Johns Hopkins University Press, 1967).

Adams, Raymond D., 'The Clinical Method of Neurology: Comments and Suggestions', *Medical Clinics of North America* 36:5 (1952), 1393–408.

Adrian, E. D., 'Croonian Lecture: The Messages in Sensory Nerve Fibres and their Interpretation', *Proceedings of the Royal Society of London* 109:760 (1931), 1–18.

—— *'The Electrical Reactions of Muscles Before and After Nerve Injury'*, *Brain* 39 (1916), 1–31.

—— 'The Nervous System', *Science* 84 (1936), 275–8.

Allen, David, 'Arcana ex multitudine: Prosopography as a Research Technique', *Archives of Natural History* 17 (1990), 349–59.

Althaus, Julius, *The Functions of the Brain: A Popular Essay* (London: Longmans and Co., 1880).

Anderson, Benedict, *Imagined Communities: Reflections on the Origin and Spread of Nationalism* (London and New York: Verso, 1991).

Anderson, Warwick, *The Collector of Lost Souls: Turning Kuru Scientists into Whitemen* (Baltimore: Johns Hopkins University Press, 2008).

Anning, S. T., *The General Infirmary at Leeds. Vol.. 2: The Second Hundred Years, 1869–1965* (Edinburgh and London: E. & S. Livingston, 1966).

Anon., 'British Postgraduate Medical Federation: New Specialist Institutes', *British Medical Journal* (1946), 581.

Anon., 'The Clinical Method in Neurology and Psychiatry', *Archives of Neurology and Psychopathology* 13 (1933), 359–62.

Anon., 'Discussion of the Mental and Physical Symptoms of the Presenile Dementias', *Proceedings of the Royal Society of Medicine* 26 (1933), 1077–91.

Anon., 'Discussion on Penicllin Neurology', *Proceedings of the Royal Society of Medicine* 40 (1947), 681–6.

Anon., 'Editorial: International Neurological Congress, Berne', *Journal of Neurology and Psychopathology* 21:45 (1931), 66–8.

Anon., 'Editorial: Neurological Training of the Future', *British Medical Journal* (1945), 292.

Anon., 'Editorial: The Future of Neurology', *Lancet* (1923), 792–3.

Anon., 'Limits to S. H. M. O. Grade', *British Medical Journal* (1950), 876.

Anon., 'Medical Auxiliaries in National Health Service', *British Medical Journal* (1951), 877–9.

Anon., 'The Medical Staff and the Management of the National Hospital for the Paralyzed and Epileptic, Queen Square', *Lancet* (1900), 351–2.

Anon., 'National Hospital for the Paralysed and Epileptic: The Electrical Room', *Lancet* (1866), 576–7.

Anon., 'The National Hospital for the Paralysed and Epileptic: Extraordinary Meeting Held at the Hospital, Queen Square, W. C', *Lancet* (1900), 551–8.

Anon., 'National Hospital for the Paralysed and Epileptic, Queen Square: Report on the Committee of Inquiry', *Lancet* (1901), 1855.

Anon., 'Needed Reforms in Psychiatry and Neurology', *Archives of Neurology and Psychopathology* 17 (1937), 176–80.

Anon., 'Neurological Problems of To-Day', *British Medical Journal* (1928), 803.

Anon., 'Neurological Therapeutics', *Archives of Neurology and Psychopathology* 16 (1936), 369–73.

Anon., 'Neurology Advances', *Lancet* (1952), 325–7.

Anon., 'Neurology in Great Britain', *Lancet* (1960), 1394.

Anon., 'Post-graduate Teaching in Neurology', *British Medical Journal* (1918), 597.

Anon., *Proceedings of the First International Neurological Congress, Berne (Switzerland), August 31 to September 4, 1931* (Berne: Stämpfli, 1932).

Anon., 'Recent Researches on the Condition of the Cerebro-Spinal Fluid in Nervous Disease', *Lancet* (1914), 1130.

Anon., 'Society of British Neurological Surgeons', *British Medical Journal* (1947), 650.

Anon., 'The Story of "Brain": Complimentary Dinner to Dr Head', *British Medical Journal* 2 (1924), 880–1.

Anon., 'Student's Guide, 1938–39: Neurology', *Lancet* (1938), 538.

Anon., 'The Scope of Neurology in Hospital Practice', *Journal of Neurology and Psychopathology* 3:10 (1922), 168.

Anon., 'Thirty-Five Years of Neurology', *Lancet* (1956), 828–9.

Anon., 'The Undergraduate Training in Neurology', *Archives of Neurology and Psychopathology* 10 (1929), 328–31.

Association of British Neurologists, *Neurology in the United Kingdom: Towards 2000 and Beyond* (London: Association of British Neurologists, 1997).

Austoker, Joan, and Linda Bryder, *Historical Perspectives on the Role of the MRC* (Oxford, New York, and Tokyo: Oxford University Press, 1989).

Bagnold, Enid, *A Diary without Dates* (London: Virago, 1978).

Bailey, Percival, 'The Present State of American Neurology', *Journal of Neuropathology and Experimental Neurology* 1 (1942), 111–13.

Ballenger, Jesse F., *Self, Senility, and Alzheimer's Disease in Modern America: A History* (Baltimore: Johns Hopkins University Press, 2006).

Barberis, Daniela, 'Changing Practices of Commemoration in Neurology: Comparing Charcot's 1925 and 1993 Centennials', *Osiris* 14 (1999), 102–17.

Barton, Ruth, '"An Influential Set of Chaps": The X-Club and Royal Society Politics, 1864–85', *British Journal for the History of Science* 23 (1990), 53–4.

Beach, Thomas G., 'The History of Alzheimer's Disease: Three Debates', *Journal of the History of Medicine and Allied Sciences* 42 (1987), 327–49.

Beard, George, 'Editorial', *Archives of Electrology and Neurology: A Journal of Electro-Therapeutics and Nervous Diseases* 1 (1874), 116–21.

Bell, Charles, 'Reprint of the "Idea of a New Anatomy of the Brain"', *Journal of Anatomy and Physiology* 3:1 (1868), 147–82.

Berg, Marc, 'Turning a Practice into a Science: Reconceptualizing Postwar Medical Practice' *Social Studies of Science* 25:3 (1995), 437–76.

Berkowitz, Carin, 'Medical Science as Pedagogy in Early Nineteenth-Century Britain: Charles Bell and the Politics of London Medical Reform' (PhD dissertation, Cornel University, 2010).

Bichat, Xavier, *Physiological Researches on Life and Death*, trans. F. Gold (London: Longman, Hurst, Rees, Orme and Brown, n.d.).

Bliss, Michael, *Harvey Cushing: A Life in Surgery* (New York: Oxford University Press, 2005).

—— *The Discovery of Insulin* (Edinburgh: Harris, 1983).

Blustein, Bonnie Ellen, 'Medicine as Biology: Neuropsychiatry at the University of Chicago, 1928–1939', *Perspectives on Science: Historical, Philosophical, Social* 1:3 (1993), 416–44.

—— 'New York Neurologists and the Specialization of American Medicine', *Bulletin of the History of Medicine* 53 (1979), 170–83.

—— 'Percival Bailey and Neurology at the University of Chicago, 1928–1939', *Bulleting of the History of Medicine* 66:1 (1992), 90–113.

—— *Preserve your Love for Science: Life of William A. Hammond, American Neurologist* (Cambridge: Cambridge University Press, 1991).

Blythe, Ronald, *The Age of Illusion: England in the Twenties and Thirties, 1919–40* (Middlesex: Penguin, 1963).

Bogacz, Ted, 'War Neurosis and Cultural Change in England, 1914–22: The Work of the War Office Committee of Enquiry into "Shell Shock"', *Journal of Contemporary History* 24:2 (1989), 227–56.

Bonner, Thomas Neville, *Medical Education in Britain, France, Germany, and the United States, 1750–1945* (Baltimore and London: Johns Hopkins University Press, 1995).

Borck, Cornelius, 'Electrifying the Brain in the 1920s: Electrical Technology as a Mediator in Brain Research', in Paolo Bertucci and Giuliano Pancaldi (eds), *Electric Bodies: Episodes in the History of Medical Electricity* (Centro Internazionale per la Storia delle Universita e della Scenza, 2001).

Bourdieu, Pierre, *Homo Academicus* (Oxford: Blackwell, 1990).

—— *The Logic of Practice* (Oxford: Blackwell, 2003).

Brain, W. Russell, *Diseases of the Nervous System* (London, New York, and Toronto: Oxford University Press, 1951).

Brand, Jeanne L., 'Neurology and Psychiatry', in Ronald L. Numbers (ed.), *The Education of American Physicians: Historical Essays* (Berkeley, Los Angeles and London: University of California Press, 1980).

Brinton, Denis, 'President's Address: The Development of Neurological Services under the NHS', *Proceedings of the Royal Society of Medicine* 53:261 (1960), 261–3.

—— 'The Neurological Services of England and Wales', *Lancet* (1963), 663.

Bristowe, J. S., 'On the Nature and Relations of Mind and Brain', *Brain* 14 (1891), 18–34.

Broadbent, M. E. (ed.), *The Life of Sir William Broadbent* (London: John Murray, 1909).

Brown, Derek Denny, 'The Shattuck Lecture: The Changing Pattern of Neurologic Medicine', *New England Journal of Medicine* 246:22 (1952), 839–46.

Brown, Edward M., 'Neurology and Spiritualism in the 1870s', *Bulletin of the History of Medicine* 57 (1983), 562–77.

Brown, Michael, *Performing Medicine: Medical Culture and Identity in Provincial England, c. 1760–1850* (Manchester : Manchester University Press, 2011).

Bruce, Alexander, 'Preliminary Statement', *Review of Neurology and Psychiatry* 1 (1903), 1–2.

Brumberg, Joan Jacobs, *Fasting Girls: The History of Anorexia Nervosa* (New York: Vintage Books, 2000).

Bulkley, L. Duncan, 'The Relations of the Nervous System to Diseases of the Skin', *Archives of Electricity and Neurology* 1 (1874), 242–68.

Burnham, John C., 'The Founding of the Archives of Neurology and Psychiatry; or, What Was Wrong with the Journal of Nervous and Mental Disease', *Journal of the History of Medicine and Allied Sciences* 34 (1981), 310–24.

—— *How the Idea of Profession Changed the Writing of Medical History* (London: Wellcome Institute for the History of Medicine, 1998).

—— (ed.), *After Freud Left: A Century of Psychoanalysis in America* (Chicago: University of Chicago Press, 2012).

Burr, Charles W., *The S. Weir Mitchell Oration: S. Weir Mitchell: Physician, Man of Science, Man of Letters, Man of Affairs* (Philadelphia: The College, 1920).

Bury, Judson S., *Diseases of the Nervous System* (Manchester: The University Press, 1912).

Butterfield, Herbert, *The Origins of Modern Science* (New York: Free Press, 1957).

Butterfield, Isabel Kennedy (ed.), *The Making of a Neurologist. The Letters of Foster Kennedy M.D. F.R.S.Edin. 1884–1952 to his Wife* (Hatfield: Stellar Press, 1981).

Buzzard, E. Farquhar. 'The Evolution of Neurology and its Bearing on Medical Education', *British Medical Journal* (1922), 718.

—— 'Hughlings Jackson and his Influence on Neurology', *Lancet* (1934), 909–13.

—— 'Lettsomian Lecture on the Principles of Treatment in Relation to Diseases of the Nervous System', *Lancet* (1926), 484–9.

Buzzard, Thomas. 'On the Simulation of Hysteria By Organic Disease of the Nervous System', *Brain* 13 (1890), 1–44.

Bynum, W. F. *Science and the Practice of Medicine in the Nineteenth Century*. New York: Cambridge University Press, 1994.

Bynum, William F., 'The Nervous Patient in 18th- and 19th-century Britain: The Psychiatric Origins of British Neurology', in William Bynum, Roy Porter, and Michael Shepard (eds), *The Anatomy of Madness: Essays in the History of Psychiatry* (London: Tavistock Publications, 1985).

Cameron, H. C., *Mr Guy's Hospital, 1726–1948* (London, New York, and Toronto: Longmans, Green and Co., 1954).

Canguilhem, Georges, *The Normal and the Pathological* (New York: Zone Books, 1991).

Carney, T. F., 'Prosopography: Payoffs and Pitfalls', *Phoenix* 27 (1973), 159–79.

Carroll, C. B., D. S. Tengah, C. Lawthorn, and G. Venables, 'The Feminisation of British Neurology: Implications for Workforce Planning', *Clinical Medicine* 7:4 (2007), 339–42.

Casper, Stephen T., 'Atlantic Conjunctures in Anglo-American Neurology: Lewis H. Weed and Johns Hopkins Neurology, 1917–1942', *Bulletin of the History of Medicine* 82 (2008), 646–71.

—— 'The Idioms of Practice: British Neurology, 1880–1960' (PhD dissertation, University College London, 2006).

—— '"Then Why Not an Association of British Neurologists?" British Neurologists and the Founding of an Elite Medical Society', *Annals of Clinical Neuroscience and Rehabilitation* 7 (2007), 16–17.

—— 'Trust, Protocol, Gender, and Power in Interwar British Biomedical Research: Kathleen Chevassut and the "Germ" of Multiple Sclerosis', *Journal of the History of Medicine and Allied Sciences* 66:2 (2011), 180–215.

—— and L. Stephen Jacyna (eds), *The Neurological Patient in History* (Rochester, NY: University of Rochester Press, 2012).

Charcot, Jean M., *Lectures on the Diseases of the Nervous System* (New York: Hafner Publishing Co., 1962).

Cheyne, George, *The English Malady or a Treatise of Nervous Diseases of all Kinds as Spleen, Vapours, Lowness of Spirits, Hypochondriacal, and Hysterical Distempers, etc.* (London: Strathan, 1733).

Cho Kim, Ock-Joo, 'The Integration of Science with the Healing Art: Harvey Cushing's Development of Neurosurgery, 1896–1912 (PhD dissertation, University of Minnesota, 1998).

Clarke, Edwin, and L. Stephen Jacyna, *Nineteenth-Century Origins of Neuroscientific Concepts* (Berkley: University of California Press, 1992).

—— and C. D. O'Malley, *The Human Brain and Spinal Cord: A Historical Study Illustrated by Writings from Antiquity to the Twentieth Century* (San Francisco: Norman Publishers, 1996).

Cohen, H. Floris, *The Scientific Revolution: An Historiographical Inquiry* (Chicago: University of Chicago Press, 1994).

Cohen, Henry, 'Fifty Years of Medical Research and Practice', *British Medical Journal* (1950), 16–21.

Collier, James, 'Inventions and the Outlook in Neurology', *Lancet* (1934), 855–9.

Committee on Teaching/Research Manpower and Needs in Basic Neurologic and Communicative Sciences, *Manpower in Basic Neurologic and Communicative Sciences: Present Status and Future Needs* (Washington, DC: National Academy of Sciences, 1977).

Conrad, Peter, and Kristin K. Barker, 'The Social Construction of Illness: Key Insights and Policy Implications', *Journal of Health and Social Behavior* 51:S (2010), S67–79.

Cook, A. M., *A History of the Royal College of Physicians of London, Vol. 3* (Oxford: Clarendon Press, 1972).

—— *Sir E. Farquhar Buzzard, Bt., K.C.V.O., D.M., F.R.C.P.: An Appreciation* (London: Royal Society of Medicine, 1975).

Cooper, Ray, and Jonathan Bird, *The Burden: Fifty Years of Clinical and Experimental Neuroscience at the Burden Neurological Institute* (Bristol: White Tree Books, 1989).

Cooter, Roger, *The Cultural Meaning of Popular Science: Phrenology and the Organisation of Consent in Nineteenth Century Britain* (Cambridge: Cambridge University Press, 1985).

—— *Surgery and Society in Peace and War: Orthopaedics and the Organisation of Modern Medicine, 1880–1948* (Houndmills: Macmillan, 1993).

—— and John Pickstone, *Companion to Medicine in the Twentieth Century* (London and New York: Routledge, 2003).

—— and Steve Sturdy, 'Science, Scientific Management, and the Transformation of Medicine in Britain c. 1870–1950', *History of Science* 36 (1998), 421–66.

——, Mark Harrison, and Steve Sturdy, *War, Medicine, and Modernity* (Stroud: Sutton, 1998).

Core, Donald, *The Examination of the Central Nervous System* (Edinburgh: E. & S. Livingstone, 1928).

Crawford, Matthew B., 'The Limits of Neuro-Talk', *New Atlantis* (2008), 65–77.

Crenner, Christopher, *Private Practice: In the Early Twentieth-Century Medical Office of Dr Richard Cabot* (Baltimore: Johns Hopkins University Press, 2005).

Crichton-Browne, James, *Victorian Jottings, from an Old Commonplace Book* (London: Etchells & Macdonald, 1926).

Critchley, Macdonald, *The Ventricle of Memory: Personal Recollections of Some Neurologists* (New York: Raven Press, 1990).

—— (ed.), *The Divine Banquet of the Brain and Other Essays* (New York: Raven Press, 1979).

—— and Eileen A Critchley, *John Hughlings Jackson: Father of English Neurology* (New York: Oxford University Press, 1998).

Cubitt, Geoffrey, and Allen Warren, *Heroic Reputations and Exemplary Lives* (Manchester and New York: Manchester University Press, 2000).

Cushing, Harvey, *From A Surgeon's Journal, 1915–1918* (Boston, MA: Little, Brown and Co., 1936).

—— *The Life of William Osler, Vol. 1* (Oxford: Clarendon Press, 1925).

Dale, Henry, 'Scientific Method in Medical Research', *British Medical Journal* (1950), 1185–90.

Dandy, Walter, 'Ventriculography Following the Injection of Air in the Cerebral Ventricles', *Annals of Surgery* 68 (1918), 5–11.

Danziger, Kurt, *Constructing the Subject: Historical Origins of Psychological Research* (New York: Cambridge University Press, 1990).

Davis, Dona L., and Setha M. Low, *Gender, Health, and Illness: The Case of Nerves* (New York: Hemisphere, 1989).

de Sio, Fabio, 'Leviathan and the Soft Animal: Medical Humanism and the Invertebrate Models for Higher Nervous Functions, 1950s–90s', *Medical History* 55:3 (2011), 369–74.

DeJong, Russell N., *A History of American Neurology* (New York: Raven Press, 1982).

Dekker, Rudolf (ed.), *Egodocuments and History: Autobiographical Writings in its Social Context since the Middle Ages* (Hilversum: Verloren, 2002).

Denison, Charles, 'The Influence of the Climate of Colorado on the Nervous System', *Archives of Electricity and Neurology* 1 (1874), 179–93.

Denning, Michael, *The Cultural Front: The Laboring of American Culture the Twentieth Century* (London and New York : Verso, 1996).

Denny-Brown, Derek, 'On Inhibition as a Reflex Accompaniment of the Tendon Jerk and of other Forms of Active Muscular Response', *Proceedings of the Royal Society of London* 103:725 (1928), 321–36.

Digby, Anne, *The Evolution of British General Practice, 1850–1948* (New York: Oxford University Press, 1999).

—— *Making a Medical Living: Doctors and Patients in the English Market for Medicine, 1720–1911* (Cambridge: Cambridge University Press, 1994).

Duffin, Jacalyn, *History of Medicine: A Scandalously Short Introduction* (Toronto and London: University of Toronto Press, 1999).

Dwyer, Ellen, 'Toward New Narratives of Twentieth Century Medicine', *Bulletin of the History of Medicine* 74 (2000), 786–93.

Dyhouse, Carol, 'Driving Ambitions: Women in Pursuit of a Medical Education, 1890–1939', *Women's Historical Review* 7 (1998), 321–43.

—— 'Women Students and the London Medical Schools, 1914–39: The Anatomy of a Masculine Culture', *Gender History* 10 (1998), 110–32.

Eadie, Mervyn, *The Flowering of a Waratah: The History of the Australian Neurology and of the Australian Association of Neurologists* (Eastleig : John Libby, 2000).

Eastwood, Martin, and Anne Jenkinson, *A History of the Western General Hospital: Craigleith Poorhouse, Military Hospital, and Modern Teaching Hospital* (Edinburgh: John Donald Publishers, 1995).

Eksteins, Modris, *Rites of Spring: The Great War and the Birth of the Modern Age* (London: Bantam Press, 1989).

Engstrom, Eric J., *Clinical Psychiatry in Imperial Germany: A History of Psychiatric Practice* (Ithaca, NY, and London: Cornell University Press, 2003).

Eulner, Hans-Heinz, *Die Entwicklung der medizinischen Specizlfächer an den Universitäten des deutschen Sprachgebietes* (Stuttgart: Ferdinand Enke Verlag, 1970).

Evans, Bonnie, 'Mental Defectives, Childhood Psychotics and the Origins of Autism Research at the Maudsley Hospital, 1913–1983' (PhD thesis, University of Cambridge, 2010).

Farreras, Ingrid, Caroline Hannaway, and Victoria Harden, *Mind, Brain, Body, and Behavior: Foundations of Neuroscience and Behavioral Research at the National Institutes of Health* (Amsterdam: OUS Press, 2004).

Feiling, Anthony, *A History of the Maida Vale Hospital for Nervous Diseases* (London: Butterworth & Co., 1958).

Feindel, William, 'The Beginning of Neurology: Thomas Willis and his Circle of Friends', in F. Clifford Rose (ed.), *A Short History of British*

Neurology: The British Contribution: 1660–1910 (Oxford: Butterworth Heinemann, 1999).
—— 'Thomas Willis...The Founder of Neurology', *Canadian Medical Association Journal* 87 (1962), 289–96.
Ferrier, David, 'The Croonian Lecture: Experiments on the Brain of Monkeys – Second Series', *Transactions of the Royal Society of London* 165 (1875), 433–88.
—— 'Experiments on the Brain of Monkeys – First Series', *Proceedings of the Royal Society* 23 (1875), 409–32.
—— *The Functions of the Brain* (London: Smith, 1876).
—— 'Localisation of Function in the Brain', *Proceedings of the Royal Society* 22 (1874), 229–32.
Finger, Stanley, *Origins of Neuroscience: A History of Explorations into Brain Function.* New York: Oxford University Press, 2001.
Finger, Stanley, Francois Boller, and Kenneth L. Tyler, *History of Neurology* (Edinburgh and New York: Elsevier, 2010).
Forman, Paul, 'The Primacy of Science in Modernity, of Technology in Postmodernity, and of Ideology in the History of Technology', *History and Technology* 23:1 (2007), 1–152.
Forman, Paul, '(Re)cognizing Postmodernity: Help for Historians – of Science Especially', *Berichte zur Wissenschaftsgeschichte* 33:2 (2010), 157–75.
Foucault, Michael, *The Birth of the Clinic* (London: Routledge, 2000).
Fraenkel, G. J., *Hugh Cairns: First Nuffield Professor of Surgery University of Oxford* (Oxford: Oxford University Press, 2003).
Frank, Robert G., 'Instruments, Nerve Action, and the All-or-None Principle', *Osiris* 9 (1994), 208–35.
Fraser, Francis, 'Postgraduate Education and the National Health Service', *British Medical Journal* (1946), 353–7.
—— 'The Rise of Specialism and the Special Hospitals', in F. N. L. Poynter (ed.), *The Evolution of Hospitals in Britain* (London: Pitman Medical Publishing, 1964).
French, John D. (ed.), *Frontiers in Brain Research* (New York and London: Columbia University Press 1962).
Friston, Karl, 'A Short History of SPM', in Karl J. Friston, John T. Ashburner, Stefan J. Kiebel, Thomas E. Nichols, and William D. Penny (eds), *Statistical Parametric Mapping: The Analysis of Functional Brain Images* (London; New York: Elsevier, 2007).
Fulton, John F., 'Arnold Klebs and Harvey Cushing at the 1st International Neurological Congress at Berne in 1931', *Bulletin of the History of Medicine* 8 (1940), 332–54.
Fye, W. Bruce., *American Cardiology: The History of a Specialty and Its College* (Baltimore: Johns Hopkins University Press, 1996).

Galison, Peter, *Image and Logic: A Material Culture of Microphysics* (Chicago: University of Chicago Press, 1997).

Garrison, Fielding H., 'History of Neurology', in Charles L. Dana (ed.), *Text-Book of Nervous Diseases: For the Use of Students and Practitioners of Medicine* (New York: William Wood and Co., 1925).

Gavrus, Delia, 'Men of Dreams and Men of Action: Neurologists, Neurosurgeons, and the Performance of Professional Identity, 1920–1950', *Bulletin of the History of Medicine* 85 (2011), 57–92.

Geddes, J. F., 'The Doctors' Dilemma: Medical Women and the British Suffrage Movement', *Women's Historical Review* 18 (2009), 203–18.

Geison, Gerald L., '"Divided We Stand": Physiologists and Clinicians in the American Context,' in Martha Vogel and Charles E. Rosenberg (eds), *The Therapeutic Revolution: Essays in the Social History of Medicine* (Philadelphia: University of Pennsylvania Press, 1979).

—— *Michael Foster and the Cambridge School of Physiology: The Scientific Enterprise in Late Victorian Society* (Princeton: Princeton University Press, 1978).

Gelfand, Toby, *Professionalizing Modern Medicine: Paris Surgeons and Medical Science and Institutions in the 18th Century* (Westport, CT: Greenwood Press, 1980).

Gijswijt-Hofstra, Marijke, and Roy Porter, *Cultures of Neurasthenia: From Beard to the First World War* (Amsterdam and New York: Rodopi, 2001).

Goetz, Christopher, Michel Bonduelle, and Toby Gelfand, *Charcot: Constructing Neurology* (New York and London: Oxford University Press, 1995).

Goldstein, Jan E., *Console and Classify: The French Psychiatric Profession in the Nineteenth Century* (New York: Cambridge University Press, 1987).

Golla, F. L., 'The Nervous System and the Organic Whole', *Proceedings of the Royal Society of Medicine* 29 (1935), 109–18.

Gooddy, William, P. C. Gautier-Smith, and E. W. Dunkley, 'Neurological Practice in a Mental Observation Unit', *Lancet* (1960), 1290–2.

Gowers, William, 'The Designation of Musical Notes in Science and Medicine', *Review of Neurology and Psychiatry* 1 (1903), 228–33.

—— *Diseases of the Nervous System* (Philadelphia: B. Plackston Son and Co., 1899).

—— *A Manual and Atlas of Medical Ophthalmoscopy* (London: J. & A. Churchill, 1879).

—— 'Reports: Pathological', *Mind* 1:4 (1876), 552–4.

Granit, Ragnar, *Charles Scott Sherrington: An Appraisal* (London: Thomas Nelson, 1966).

Greenblatt, Samuel, 'Harvey Cushing's Paradigmatic Contribution to Neurosurgery and the Evolution of his Thoughts about Specialisation', *Bulletin of the History of Medicine* 77:4 (2003), 789–822.

—— 'The Major Influences on the Early Life and Works of John Hughlings Jackson', *Bulletin of the History of Medicine* 39:4 (1965), 346–76.

Gritzer, Glenn, and Arnold Arluke, *The Making of Rehabilitation: A Political Economy of Medical Specialization* (Berkeley: University of California Press, 1985).

Grob, Gerald A., *From Asylum to Community: Mental Health Policy in Modern America* (Princeton: Princeton University Press, 1991).

—— *Mental Illness and American Society, 1875–1940* (Princeton: Princeton University Press, 1983).

Grubb, Robert L., *Neurosurgery at Washington University: A Century of Excellence* (St Louis: Washington University, 2010).

Guillain, Georges, *J.-M. Charcot, 1825–1893: His Life - His Work*, ed. Pearce Bailey (New York: Paul B. Hoeber, 1959).

Guthrie, Leonard George, *Contributions to the Study of Precocity in Children: The History of Neurology. The Fitzpatrick Lectures on the History of Medicine, Delivered at the Royal College of Physicians in the Years 1907 and 1908* (London: E. G. Millar, 1921).

Hale, Nathan G., *The Rise and Crisis of Psychoanalysis in the United States: Freud and the Americans, 1917–1985* (New York: Oxford University Press, 1995).

Hale-White, William, *Great Doctors of the Nineteenth Century* (London: Edward Arnold, 1935).

Halpern, L., 'Neurology at the Crossroads', *Confinia Neurologica* 13 (1953), 124–6.

Hardy, Anne, *Health and Medicine in Britain since 1860* (New York: Palgrave, 2001).

—— 'Poliomyelitis and the Neurologists: The View from England, 1896–1966', *Bulletin of the History of Medicine* 71:2 (1997), 249–72.

Harrington, Anne, *Medicine, Mind, and the Double Brain: A Study in Nineteenth-Century Thought* (Princeton: Princeton University Press, 1987).

Harris, Henry, *The Birth of the Cell* (New Haven: Yale University Press, 1999).

Haymaker, Webb (ed.), *The Founders of Neurology: One-Hundred and Thirty-Three Biographical Sketches* (Springfield, IL: Charles C. Thomas, 1953).

—— and Francis Schiller, *The Founders of Neurology: One-Hundred Forty-Six Biographical Sketches by Eighty-Nine Authors* (Springfield, IL: Charles C. Thomas, 1970).

Hayward, Rhodri, 'Demonology, Neurology, and Medicine in Edwardian Britain', *Bulletin of the History of Medicine* 78:1 (2004), 37–58.

—— 'The Tortoise and the Love-Machine: Grey Walter and the Politics of Electroencephalography', *Science in Context* 14:4 (2001), 615–41.

Head, Henry, 'Presidential Address: Some Principles of Neurology', *Proceedings of the Royal Society of Medicine* 12 (1918), 1–12.

Heaman, E. A., *St Mary's: The History of a London Teaching Hospital* (Montreal, Kingston, London, and Ithaca, NY: Liverpool University Press and McGill Queen's University Press, 2003).

Herrick, C. Judson, 'A Neurologist Makes up his Mind', *Scientific Monthly* 49:2 (1939), 99–110.

Hewer, R. Langton, and V. A. Wood, 'Neurology in the United Kingdom. I: Historical development', *Journal of Neurology, Neurosurgery, and Psychiatry* 55 (1992), 2–7.

Hobsbawm, Eric, *Age of Extremes: The Short Twentieth Century, 1914–1991* (London: Michael Joseph, 1994).

Hodgkin, Alan, 'Edgar Douglas Adrian, Baron Adrian of Cambridge. 30 November 1889–4 August 1977', *Biographical Memoirs of Fellows of the Royal Society* 25 (1979), 1–73.

Hodgson, Shadworth H., 'The Philosophical Relations of Neurology', *Brain* 14 (1891), 1–17.

Hollman, Arthur, *Sir Thomas Lewis: Pioneer Cardiologist and Clinical Scientist* (London and New York: Spring, 1996).

Holmes, Gordon, 'Disturbances of Spatial Orientation and Visual Attention, with Loss of Stereoscopic Vision', *Archives of Neurology and Psychiatry* 1:4 (1919), 385–407.

—— *The National Hospital, Queen Square, 1860–1948* (Edinburgh: Livingstone, 1954).

—— 'The Symptoms of Acute Cerebellar Injuries from Gunshot Wounds', *Brain* 40 (1917), 461–535.

—— and W. Lister, 'Disturbances of Vision from Cerebral Lesions with Special Reference to the Cortical Representation of the Macula', *Brain* 39 (1917), 34–73.

Hopkins, Anthony, 'Different Types of Neurologist', *British Medical Journal* (1984), 1736.

Howell, Joel, '"Soldier's Heart": The Redefinition of Heart Disease and Specialty Formation in Early Twentieth-Century Great Britain', in William F. Bynum, Christopher Lawrence and Vivian Nutton (eds), *The Emergence of Modern Cardiology* (London: Wellcome Institute Press, 1985).

Hunting, Penelope, *The History of the Royal Society of Medicine* (London: Royal Society of Medicine Press, 2001).

Hurst, Arthur, 'Psycho-analysis and War Neuroses', *Guy's Hospital Gazette* 31 (1917), 308–9.

Hutchinson, Herbert (ed.), *Jonathan Hutchinson, Life and Letters* (London: W. Heinemann, 1946).

Isler, Hansruedi, *Thomas Willis, 1621–1675: Doctor and Scientist* (New York and London: Hafner, 1968).

Jackson, J. Hughlings, 'Case Illustrating the Value of the Ophthalmoscope in the Investigation and Treatment of Diseases of the Brain', *Lancet* (1880), 906.

—— 'Ophthalmology and Diseases of the Nervous System', *Transactions of the Opthalmological Society of the United Kingdom* 6 (1886), 1–22.

—— 'Value of the Ophthalmoscope in the Investigation and Treatment of Diseases of the Brain', *Lancet* (1880), 906.

Jacyna, L. Stephen, 'Galvanic Influences: Themes in the Early History of British Animal Electricity', in Marco Bresadola and Giuliano Pancaldi (eds), *Luigi Galvani: International Workshop Proceedings* (Bologna: Centro Internazionale per la Storia della Universita, 1999).

—— *Lost Words: Narratives of Language and the Brain, 1825–1926* (Princeton: Princeton University Press, 2000).

—— *Medicine and Modernism: A Biography of Henry Head* (London and Brookfield, VT: Pickering & Chatto, 2008).

—— 'Somatic Theories of Mind and the Interest of Medicine in Britain, 1850–1879', *Medical History* 26:3 (1982), 233–58.

James, Frederick Ernest, 'The Life and Work of Thomas Laycock, 1812–1876' (PhD dissertation, University College London, 1995).

Jenkinson, Jacqueline. 'The Role of Medical Societies in the Rise of the Scottish Medical Profession, 1730–1939', *Social History of Medicine* 4 (1991), 253–75.

Jenner, Mark S. R., and Patrick Wallis, *Medicine and the Market in England and its Colonies, c. 1450–c. 1850* (Basingstoke: Palgrave Macmillan, 2007).

Jewson, N. D., 'The Disappearance of the Sick Man from Medical Cosmology, 1770–1870', *Sociology* 10 (1976), 225–44.

——, 'Medical Knowledge and the Patronage System in 18th-Century England', *Sociology* 8 (1974), 369–85.

Jones, Carolyn, and Peter Galison, *Picturing Science, Producing Art* (New York: Routledge, 1998).

Jones, Edgar, Robin Woolven, Bill Durodie, and Simon Wessely, 'Civilian Morale During the Second World War: Responses to Air Raids Re-examined', *Social History of Medicine* 17:3 (2004), 463–79.

Jones, Helen, *Health and Society in Twentieth Century Britain* (London and New York: Longman, 1994).

Jordanova, Ludmilla, *Defining Features: Scientific and Medical Portraits, 1660–2000* (London: Reaktion Books, 2000).

Kalinowskyp, Lothar, and H. Houston Merritt, 'The Status of Neurology as a Specialty in Various Countries', *Neurology* 4 (1954), 668–73.

Kennaway, James, *Bad Vibrations: The History of the Idea of Music as a Cause of Disease* (Farnham and Burlington, VT: Ashgate, 2012).

Kevles, Daniel, and Gerald Geison, 'The Experimental Life Sciences in the Twentieth Century' *Osiris* 10 (1995), 97–121.

Kidd, Leonard J., 'Lachrymal Reflexes: Pressure-Sensibility of Head and Neck: And the Squeezed-Tongue Sensation', *Review of Neurology and Psychiatry* 7 (1909), 167–80.

Kim, Kiheung, *The Social Construction of Disease: From Scrapie to Prion* (London and New York: Routledge, 2007).

Kragh, Helge, 'Problems and Challenges in the Historical Study of the Neurosciences', *Journal of the History of Neurosciences* 11 (2002), 55–62.

Krige, John, *American Hegemony and the Postwar Reconstruction of Science in Europe* (Cambridge, MA: MIT Press, 2006).

Kroker, Kenton, 'Epidemic Encephalitis and American Neurology, 1919–1940', *Bulletin of the History of Medicine* 78:1 (2004), 18–147.

Kushner, Howard, *A Cursing Brain: The Histories of Tourette's Syndrome* (Cambridge, MA, and London: Harvard University Press, 1999).

Lanska, Douglas J., 'The Role of Technology in Neurologic Specialization in America', *Neurology* 48:6 (1997), 1722–7.

——, T. A. Chumura, and Christopher Goetz.,'Part 1: The History of 19th-Century Neurology and the American Neurological Association', *Annals of Neurology* 53 (2003), S2–26.

Laureno, Robert, *Raymond Adams: A Life of Mind and Muscle* (New York: Oxford University Press, 2009).

Lawrence, Christopher, 'Incommunicable Knowledge: Science, Technology and the Clinical Art in Britain, 1850–1914', *Journal of Contemporary History* 20:4 (1985), 503–20.

—— 'The Nervous System and Society in the Scottish Enlightenment', in Barry Barnes and Steven Shapin (eds), *Natural Order: Historical Studies of Scientific Culture* (London: Sage, 1979).

—— *Rockefeller Money, the Laboratory and Medicine in Edinburgh, 1919–1930: New Culture in an Old Country* (Rochester, NY: University of Rochester Press, 2005).

—— 'Still Incommunicable: Clinical Holists and Medical Knowledge in Interwar Britain', in Christopher Lawrence and George Weisz (eds), *Greater than the Parts, Holism in Biomedicine, 1920–1950* (Oxford and New York: Oxford University Press, 1998).

Laycock, Thomas, *Mind and Brain: Or, The Correlations of Consciousness and Organization; Systemically Investigated and Applied to Philosophy, Mental Science, and Practice.* New York: Appleton, 1869.

—— 'On the Reflex Function of the Brain: A Correction of Dates', *British Medical Journal* (1874), 705–6.

Lazar, J. Wayne, 'Acceptance of the Neuron Theory by Clinical Neurologists of the Late-Nineteenth Century', *Journal of the History of Neurosciences* 19 (2010), 349–64.

Leese, Peter, *Shell Shock: Traumatic Neurosis and the British Soldiers of the First World War* (Basingstoke: Palgrave Macmillan, 2002).

Leneman, Leah, 'Medical Women at War, 1914–1918', *Medical History* 38 (1994), 160–77.

Lepore, F. E., 'Harvey Cushing, Gordon Holmes, and the Neurological Lessons of World War I', *Archives of Neurology* 51 (1994), 711–22.

Levack, Iain, and Hugh Dudley, *Aberdeen Royal Infirmary: The People's Hospital of the North-East* (London, Philadelphia, Toronto Sydney, and Tokyo: Bailliere Tindall, 1992).

Lewis, Thomas, 'Research in Medicine: Its Position and its Needs', *British Medical Journal* (1930), 481.

—— 'Research Physicians', *British Medical Journal* (1930), 503–4.

Lhermitte, Jean, 'Training of the Neurologist', *Archives of Neurology and Psychiatry* 30 (1933), 405–12.

Liddell, Edward George Tandy, *The Discovery of Reflexes* (Oxford: Clarendon Press, 1960).

Lindsey, Almont, *Socialised Medicine in England and Wales, The National Health Service, 1948–1961* (Chapel Hill: University of North Carolina Press, 1962).

Link, Arthur S. (ed.), *Fifty Years of American Neurology: An Historical Perspective* (Winston-Salem, NC: Stratford Books, 1998).

Loudon, Irvine, *Medical Care and the General Practitioner, 1750–1850* (Oxford: Clarendon Press, 1986).

Lovell, Richard, *Churchill's Doctor: A Biography of Lord Moran* (London: Royal Society of Medicine, 1992).

Lyotard, Jean-François, *The Postmodern Condition: A Report on Knowledge*, trans. Geoff Bennington and Brian Massumi (Minneapolis: University of Minnesota Press, 1999).

McConica, James K., 'The Prosopography of the Tudor University', *Journal of Interdisciplinary History* 3 (1973), 543–54.

MacCormac, William, and George Henry Makins, 'Discussion on the Localization of Function in the Cortex Cerebri', in *Transactions of the International Medical Congress* (London: J. W. Klockman, 1881).

McMenemey, W. H., 'The History of Neurology: Neurological Investigation in Britain from 1800 to the Founding of the National Hospital', *Proceedings of the Royal Society of Medicine* 53 (1960), 33–40.

McMurray, T. P., 'The Teaching of Anatomy to the Medical Student', *British Medical Journal* (1949), 510–12.

MacPherson, W. G., W. P. Herringham, T. R. Elliot, and A. Balfour, *History of the Great War, Based on Official Documents: Medical Services, Diseases of the War. Vol. 2* (London: HMSO, 1923).

MacQueen, Loudon, and Archibald B. Kerr, *The Western Infirmary, 1874–1974: A Century of Service to Glasgow* (Glasgow and London: John Horn, 1974).

Marchildon, John, *The Wasserman Reaction: Its Technic and Practical Application in the Diagnosis of Syphilis* (London: Henry Kimpton, 1912).

Marks, Harry M., *The Progress of Experiment: Science and Therapeutic Reform in the United States, 1900–1990* (Cambridge: Cambridge University Press, 1997).

—— '"Until the Sun of Science...the True Apollo of Medicine Has Risen": Collective Investigation in Britain and America, 1880–1910', *Medical History* 50 (2006), 154–6.

Martensen, Robert L., *The Brain Takes Shape: An Early History* (Oxford and New York : Oxford University Press, 2004).

Marwick, Arthur, *The Deluge: British Society and the First World War* (Basingstoke: Palgrave Macmillan, 2006).

—— *A History of the Modern British Isles, 1914–1999* (London: Blackwell, 2000).

Matthews, W. B., *Practical Neurology* (Oxford: Blackwell Scientific Publications, 1963).

Mayr, Ernst, 'When is Historiography Whiggish', *Journal of the History of Ideas* 51:2 (1990), 301–9.

Micale, Mark, *Approaching Hysteria: Disease and its Interpretations* (Princeton: Princeton University Press, 1995).

Miller, Henry, 'Neurology in a General Hospital', *British Medical Journal* (1958), 477–80.

—— 'The Organization of Neurological Services and Neurological Training', *Proceedings of the Royal Society of Medicine* 61 (1968), 1004–10.

Miller, Samuel, *A Brief Retrospect of the Eighteenth Century. Vol. 1: A Sketch of the Revolutions and Improvements in Science, Arts, and Literature during that Period* (London: Ellllerton and Byworth, 1805).

Millett, David, 'Illustrating a Revolution: An Unrecognized Contribution to the "Golden Era" of Cerebral Localisation', *Notes and Records of the Royal Society* 5 (1998), 292–3.

—— 'Wiring the Brain: From the Excitable Cortex to the EEG, 1870–1940' (PhD dissertation, University of Chicago, 1998).

Milward, Alan S., *War, Economy, and Society, 1939–1945* (Harmondsworth: Penguin Books, 1987).

Ministry of Health, *National Health Service: The Development of Consultant Services* (London: HMSO, 1950).

—— *Report of the Inter-Departmental Committee on the Remuneration of Consultants and Specialists* (London: HMSO, 1948).

—— *Report of the Inter-Departmental Committee on Medical Schools* (London: HMSO, 1944).

Minney, R. J., *The Two Pillars of Charing Cross: The Story of a Famous Hospital* (London : Cassell, 1967).

Mitchell, S. Weir, *A Comedy of Conscience* (New York: Century Co., 1903).

—— *The Complete Poems* (New York: Century, 1914).

—— *Constance Trescot: A Novel* (New York: Century Co., 1905).

Mitchell, T. J., and G. M. Smith, *History of the Great War, Based on Official Documents: Medical Services, Casualties and Medical Statistics of the Great War* (London: HMSO, 1931).

Monrad-Krone, G. H., 'Diagnostic Errors in Neurology', *Acta Medica Scandinavica* 142 (1952), 733–42.

Montreal Neurological Institute, *Neurological Biographies and Addresses: Foundation Volume Published for the Staff, to Commemorate the Opening of the Montreal Neurological Institute of McGill University* (London: Oxford University Press, 1936).

Morris, R. J., *Clubs, Societies, and Associations. Vol. 3: Social Agencies and Institutions*, in F. M. L. Thompson (ed.), *The Cambridge Social History of Britain, 1750–1950* (Cambridge: Cambridge University Press, 1990).

Mott, Frederick, 'Presidential Address: The Inborn Factors of Nervous and Mental Disease', *Proceedings of the Royal Society of Medicine* 5 (1911), 1–30.

Murray, Ian, *The Victoria Infirmary of Glasgow: History of a Voluntary Hospital, 1890–1948* (Glasgow: C. L. Wright, 1967).

Musselman, Elizabeth Green, *Nervous Conditions: Science and the Body Politic in Early Industrial Britain* (Albany, NY: State University of New York Press, 2006).

Neuburger, M., *Die historische Entwicklung der experimentellen Gehern und Rüchenmarks-physiologie vor Flourens* (Stuttgart: Ferdinand Enke, 1897).

Neve, Michael, and Trevor Turner, 'What the Doctor Thought and Did: Sir James Crichton-Browne (1840–1938)', *Medical History* 39 (1995), 399–432.

Newman, Charles, 'The Rise of Specialism and Postgraduate Education', in F. N. L. Poynter (ed.), *The Evolution of Medical Education in Britain* (London: Pitman Medical Publishing, 1966).

Nieman, Eric, 'Wilfred Harris (1869–1960), Pioneer of Neurology at St. Mary's Hospital', *St Mary's Gazette* 104:2 (1998), 733.

Nightingale, Florence, *Notes on Nursing* (New York: Dover Publications, 1969).

Oldroyd, David, *Darwinian Impacts: An Introduction to the Darwinian Revolution* (Milton Keynes: Open University Press, 1983).

Oliff, Andrew, 'History and Development of Neurology as a Distinct Specialty in America', *Journal of Civil War Medicine* 3 (1999), 33–41.

Oppenheim, Janet, *Shattered Nerves: Doctors, Patients, and Depression in Victorian England* (Oxford: Oxford University Press, 1991).

Oshinsky, David M., *Polio: An American Story* (Oxford: Oxford University Press, 2006).

Pallis, Christopher, *ABC of Brainstem Death: Articles Published in the British Medical Journal* (London: British Medical Journal, 1983).

Penfield, Wilder, 'Clinical Notes from a Trip to Great Britain', *Archives of Neurology and Psychiatry* 47 (1942), 1030–6.

—— 'Psychical Seizures', *British Medical Journal* (1946), 639–41.

—— 'Some Problems of Wartime Neurology', *Archives of Neurology and Psychiatry* 47 (1942), 839–40.

—— 'The Training of a Neurologist', *Archives of Neurology and Psychiatry* 31 (1934), 842–4.

Pera, Marchello, *The Ambiguous Frog: The Galvani-Volta Controversy on Animal Electricity* (Princeton: Princeton University Press, 1992).

Peterson, M. Jeanne, *The Medical Profession in Mid-Victorian London* (Berkley, Los Angeles, and London: University of California Press, 1978).

Philippon, Jacques, and Jacques Poirier, *Joseph Babinski: A Biography* (New York and Oxford: Oxford University Press, 2008).

Pick, Daniel, *Faces of Degeneration: A European Disorder, c. 1848–c. 1918* (Cambridge: Cambridge University Press, 1989).

Pickering, George W., 'Walter Russell Brain, First Baron Brain of Eynsham, 1895–1966', *Biographical Memoirs of Fellows of the Royal Society* 14 (1968), 61–82.

Pickstone, John, *Medicine and Industrial Society: A History of Hospital Development in Manchester and its Region, 1752–1946* (Manchester: Manchester University Press, 1985).

Pinel, Philippe, *A Treatise on Insanity in which are Contained the Principles of a New and More Practical Nosology of Maniacal Disorders than Has Yet Been Offered to the Public*, trans. D. D. Davis (Sheffield: W. Todd, 1806).

Porter, Roy, *Flesh in the Age of Reason* (New York and London: W. W. Norton and Co., 2003).

—— *The Greatest Benefit to Mankind: A Medical History of Humanity* (New York and London: W. W. Norton, 1997).

Porter, Theodore M., *The Rise of Statistical Thinking, 1820–1900* (Princeton: Princeton University Press, 1986).

Poser, Charles M., 'The World Federation of Neurology: The Formative Period, 1955–1961', *Journal of Neurological Sciences* 120 (1993), 218–27.

Power, D'Arcy (ed.), *British Medical Societies* (London: Medical Press, 1939).

Pressman, Jack, *Last Resort: Psychosurgery and the Limits of Medicine* (Cambridge: Cambridge University Press, 1998).

Purves Stewart, James Morgan, *The Diagnoses of Nervous Diseases* (London: Edward Arnold, 1906).

—— *Mount Athos: A Survival of the Middle Ages. An Address at a Social Evening of the Royal Society Medicine* (London: John Bale, Sons and Danielsson, 1927).

—— *Sands of Time, Recollections of a Physician in Peace and War* (London: Hutchinson & Co, 1939).

Pyenson, Lewis, '"Who the Guy's Were": Prosopography in the History of Science', *History of Science* 15 (1977), 155–88.

Raj, Kapil, *Relocating Modern Science: Circulation and the Construction of Knowledge in South Asia and Europe, 1650–1900* (Basingstoke: Palgrave Macmillan, 2007).

Rapport, Richard, *Nerve Endings: The Discovery of the Synapse. The Quest to Find How Brain Cells Communicate* (New York and London: St Edmundsbury Press, 2005).

Report of the War Office Committee of Inquiry into 'Shell-Shock' (London: HSMO, 1922).

Reverby, Susan M., *Examining Tuskegee: The Infamous Syphilis Study and its Implications* (Chapel Hill: University of North Carolina Press, 2009).

Richardson, Alan, *British Romanticism and the Science of the Mind* (Cambridge: Cambridge University Press, 2001).

Richardson, J. Clifford, 'Clinical Experiences with a R.C.A.M.C. Neuropsychiatric Division in England 1940 to 1944', *Proceedings of the Royal Society of Medicine* 37 (1944), 373–6.

Richter, Jochen, 'The Brain Commission of the International Association of Academies', *Brain Research Bulletin* 52:6 (2000), 445–57.

Riese, Walther, 'An Outline of a History of Ideas in Neurology', *Bulletin of the History of Medicine* 23:2 (1949), 111–36.

Robinson, Peter, *The History of the Association at the 50th Anniversary Meeting, 4th November 1983* (Winchester: Peter Robinson, 1985).

Roelcke, Volker, Paul J. Weindling, and Louise Westwood (eds), *International Relations in Psychiatry* (Rochester, NY: University of Rochester Press, 2010).

Rolleston, Humphrey, *Life of Sir Clifford Allbutt* (London: Macmillan and Co., 1929).

Romano, Terrie, *Making Medicine Scientific: John Burdon Sanderson and the Culture of Victorian Science* (Baltimore: Johns Hopkins University Press, 2002).

Rose, F. Clifford, 'Historiography: An Introduction', *Journal of the History of Neurosciences* 11 (2002), 35–7.

—— (ed.), *A Short History of British Neurology: The British Contribution, 1660–1910* (Oxford and Boston, MA: Butterworth-Heinemann, 1999).

—— (ed.), *Twentieth-Century Neurology: The British Contribution* (London and River Edge, NJ: World Scientific Publishing Co., 2002).

Rose, Nikolas S., 'Neurochemical Selves', *Society* (2003), 46–59.

—— *The Psychological Complex: Psychology, Politics and Society in England, 1869–1939* (London: Routledge, 1985).

Rosen, George, *The Specialization of Medicine with Particular Reference to Ophthalmology* (New York: Froben Press, 1944).

Rosenberg, Charles E., and Janet Golden (eds), *Framing Disease: Studies in Cultural History* (New Brunswick, NJ: Rutgers University Press, 1992).

Ross, Dorothy (ed.), *Modernist Impulses in the Human Sciences, 1870–1930* (Baltimore and London: Johns Hopkins University Press, 1994).

Roudebush, Marc, 'A Battle of Nerves: Hysteria and its Treatment in France during World War I', in Mark S Micale and Paul Lerner (eds), *Traumatic Pasts: History, Psychiatry, and Trauma in the Modern Age, 1870–1930* (Cambridge: Cambridge University Press, 2001).

Rousseau, George S., *Nervous Acts: Essays on Literature and Sensibility* (Houndmills and Basingstoke: Palgrave Macmillan, 2005).

—— '"The Torpedo-Act": Prosopography as Biography', *Annals of Science* 42 (1985), 431–5.

Rousseau, Jean-Jacques, *The Social Contract* (Ware: Wordsworth Editions, 1998).

Rowland, Lewis P., *The Legacy of Tracy J. Putnam and H. Houston Meritt: Modern Neurology in the United States* (New York: Oxford University Press, 2008).

Royal College of Physicians, *Interim Report of the Committee on Neurology* (London: Harrison & Sons, 1954).

—— *Report of the Committee on Neurology* (London: Harrison & Sons, 1945).

Royal College of Physicians Committee on Neurology, *The Neurological Services in Great Britain* (London: Harrison &Sons, 1965).

Saliba, George, *Islamic Science and the Making of the European Renaissance* (Cambridge, MA, and London: MIT Press, 2011).

Salisbury, Laura, and Andrew Shail, *Neurology and Modernity: A Cultural History of Nervous Systems, 1800–1950* (Basingstoke: Palgrave Macmillan, 2010).

Schneider, William (ed.), *Rockefeller Philanthropy and Modern Biomedicine: International Initiatives from World War I to the Cold War* (Bloomington: Indiana University Press, 2002).

Schwab, Sidney 'The Neurologic Dilemma', *Archives of Neurology and Psychiatry* 6:3 (1921), 255–62.

Scott, Anne, Mervyn Eadie, and Andrew Lees, *William Richard Gowers, 1845–1915* (Oxford: Oxford University Press, 2012).

Scull, Andrew, *Social Order/Mental Disorder: Anglo-American Psychiatry in Historical Perspective* (Berkeley: University of California Press, 1989).

Senior, John E., 'Meteorological Awakenings', in Eileen Magnello and Anne Hardy (eds), *The Road to Medical Statistics* (Amsterdam and New York: Rodopi, 2002).

—— 'Rationalising Electrotherapy in Neurology, 1860–1920' (PhD dissertation, Oxford University, 1994).

Shapin, Steven, 'History of Science and its Sociological Reconstructions', *History of Science* 198:20 (1982), 157–211.

—— 'The Royal Society of Edinburgh: A Study of the Social Context of Hanoverian Science' (PhD. dissertation, University of Pennsylvania, 1971).

—— and Arnold Thackray, 'Prosopography as a Research Tool in History of Science: The British Scientific Community, 1700–1900', *History of Science* 12 (1974), 1–28.

Sharpey-Shäfer, E. A., 'The Nerve Cell Considered as the Basis of Neurology', *Brain* 16 (1893), 134–69.

Shephard, Ben, *A War of Nerves: Soldiers and Psychiatrists, 1914–1994* (London: 2002).

Shepherd, Gordon M., *Creating Modern Neuroscience: The Revolutionary 1950s* (New York and Oxford: Oxford University Press, 2010).

Sherrington, Charles, *The Endeavour of Jean Fernel: With a List of the Editions of his Writings* (Cambridge: Cambridge University Press, 1946).

—— *The Integrative Action of the Nervous System* (London: Oxford University Press, 1906).

—— *Man on his Nature* (Cambridge: Cambridge University Press, 1951).

Shorter, Edward, 'The Borderland between Neurology and History', *Neurologic Clinics* 13:2 (1995), 229–37.

—— *A History of Psychiatry: From the Era of the Asylum to the Age of Prozac* (New York: John Wiley, 1997).

Showalter, Elaine, *The Female Malady: Women, Madness, and English Culture, 1830–1980* (New York: Pantheon Books, 1985).

Silver, John Russell, *History of the Treatment of Spinal Injuries* (New York: Kluwer Academic/Plenum Publishers, 2003).

Slobodin, Richard, *W. H. R. Rivers* (New York: Columbia University Press, 1978).

Smith, Roger, *Being Human: Historical Knowledge and the Creation of Human Nature* (New York: Columbia University, 2007).

—— *Inhibition: History and Meaning in the Sciences of the Brain and Mind* (London: Free Association Books, 1992).

Söderqvist, Thomas, 'Neurobiographies: Writing Lives in the History of Neurology and the Neurosciences', *Journal of the History of Neurosciences* 11:1 (2002), 38–48.

Solomon, Susan Gross (ed.), *Doing Medicine Together: Germany and Russia between the Wars* (Toronto and London: University of Toronto Press, 2006).

Soury, Jules, *Le système nerveux central, structure et fonctions, histoire critique des théories et des doctrines* (Paris: Georges Carré et C. Naud, 1889).

Star, Susan Leigh, *Regions of the Mind: Brain Research and the Quest for Scientific Certainty* (Stanford: Stanford University Press , 1989).

Starr, Paul, *The Social Transformation of American Medicine* (New York: Basic Books, 1982).

Stevens, David L., *Neurology in the United Kingdom: Numbers of Clinical Neurologists and Trainees* (London: Association of British Neurologists, 1996).

Stevens, Rosemary, *American Medicine and the Public Interest: A History of Specialization* (London: University of California Press, 1998).

—— *Medical Practice in Modern England: The Impact of Specialization and State Medicine* (New Haven: Yale University Press, 1966).

Sturdy, Steve, 'The Political Economy of Scientific Medicine: Science, Education and the Transformation of Medical Practice in Sheffield, 1890–1922', *Medical History* 36 (1992), 125–59.

Suckling, C. W., *On the Diagnosis of Diseases of the Brain, Spinal Cord, and Nerves* (London: H. K. Lewis, 1887).

Sully, James, 'Dr Hughlings Jackson on Morbid Affections of Speech', *Mind* 5:17 (1880), 105–11.

Symonds, Charles, 'Reorientations in Neurology', *Lancet* (1949), 677–80.

Taylor, James, 'The Ophthalmological Observations of Hughlings Jackson and their Bearing on Nervous and Other Diseases', *Brain* 38 (1915), 391–417.

Temkin, Owsei. *The Double Face of Janus and Other Essays in the History of Medicine* (Baltimore: Johns Hopkins University Press, 1977).

—— *The Falling Sickness: A History of Epilepsy: From the Greeks to the Beginnings of Modern Neurology* (Baltimore: Johns Hopkins University Press, 1971).

Thomson, A. Landsborough, *Half a Century of Medical Research. Vol. 1* (London: Medical Research Council, 1987).

Thomson, H. Campbell, *The Story of the Middlesex Hospital Medical School* (London: John Murray, 1935).

Todd, Robert Bentley, and William Bowman, *The Physiological Anatomy and Physiology of Man* (Philadelphia: Blanchard and Lea, 1857).

Tuchman, Arleen Marcia, *Science, Medicine, and the State in Germany: The Case of Baden, 1815–1971* (Oxford : Oxford University Press , 1993).

Tuke, Daniel Hack, *Illustrations of the Influence of the Mind upon the Body in Health and Disease to Elucidate the Action of the Imagination* (London: J. & A. Chuchill, 1884).

Tuke, John Batty, 'The Relation of the Lunacy Laws to the Treatment of Insanity', *Brain* 28 (1905), 1–12.

Turner, W. Aldren, 'Presidential Address: The Influence of Psychogenic Factors in Nervous Disorders', *Proceedings of the Royal Society of Medicine* 13 (1919), 1–16.

Vess, David M., *Medical Revolution in France, 1789–1796* (Gainesville: University Presses of Florida, 1975).

Vidal, Fernando, 'Brainhood, Anthropological Figure of Modernity', *History of the Human Sciences* 22:1 (2009), 15–36.

—— *The Sciences of the Soul: The Early Modern Origins of Psychology*, trans. Saskia Brown (Chicago and London: University of Chicago Press, 2011).

Vilensky, Joel A., Sid Gilman, and Pandy Sinish, 'Denny-Brown, Boston City Hospital, and the History of American Neurology', *Perspectives in Biology and Medicine* 47:4 (2004), 505–18.

Walshe, F. M. R., 'The Evolution of the Teaching-Hospital Physician in our Time', *Proceedings of the Royal Society of Medicine* 54 (1961), 525–32.

—— 'The Future of Neurology', *Proceedings of the Royal Society of Medicine* 48 (1955), 120–4.

—— 'Physiology of the Cerebral Motor Cortex: The Contribution of Clinical Study', *British Medical Journal* (1947), 830–2.

—— 'Training of the Neurologist', *Archives of Neurology and Psychiatry* 29 (1933), 368–81.

Walshe, Stephen, *Stravinsky: A Creative Spring Russia and France: 1882–1934* (London: Pimlico, 2002).

Walton, John, '50 Years in Neurology: A Retrospect', *Practical Neurology* 3 (2003), 55.

—— *The Spice of Life* (London: Royal Society of Medicine Services, 1993).

Wear, Andrew, *Knowledge and Practice in English Medicine, 1550–1680* (Cambridge: Cambridge University Press, 2000).

—— (ed.), *Medicine in Society: Historical Essays* (Cambridge: Cambridge University Press, 1992).

Webster, Charles, *The Health Services Since the War. Vol. 1: Problems of Health Care: The National Health Service Before 1957* (London: HMSO, 1988).

Weisenburg, Theodore H., 'The Military History of the American Neurological Association', *Archives of Neurology and Psychiatry* 1 (1919), 1–13.

Weiss, Sheila Faith, *The Nazi Symbiosis: Human Genetics and Politics in the Third Reich* (Chicago and London: University of Chicago, 2010).

Weisz, George, *Divide and Conquer: A Comparative History of Specialization* (Oxford: Oxford University Press, 2006).

Wexler, Alice, *The Woman who Walked into the Sea: Huntington's and the Making of Genetic Disease* (New Haven; London: Yale University Press, 2008).

Whitaker, Harry, C. U. M. Smith, and Stanley Finger, *Brain, Mind and Medicine: Essays in Eighteenth-Century Neuroscience* (New York: Springer, 2007).

White, Benjamin, *Stanley Cobb: A Builder of the Modern Neurosciences* (Boston, MA: Francis Countway Library of Medicine, 1984).

Wilks, Samuel, *A Memoir: On the New Discoveries or New Observations Made during the Time he Was a Teacher at Guy's Hospital* (London: Adlard and Son, 1911).

Williams, David, 'RSM 1907: The Acceptance of Specialization', *Journal of the Royal Society of Medicine* 93 (2000), 642–5.

Williams, Denis, 'Advances in Neurology', *Practitioner* 173 (1954), 395–402.

Wilson, Daniel R., and Gerald A. Cory, *The Evolutionary Epidemiology of Mania and Depression: A Theoretical and Empirical Interpretation of Mood Disorders* (Lampeter: Edwin Mellen Press, 2007).

Wilson, S. A. Kinnier, *Neurology. Vol. 1* (Baltimore: Williams and Wilkins Co., 1955).

Winter, Alison, *Mesmerized: Powers of Mind in Victorian Britain* (Chicago and London: University of Chicago Press, 1998).

Worster-Drought, C., 'Penicillin in Neurosyphilis', *British Medical Journal* (1947), 559–64.

——, H. J. B. Fry, and G. Roche Lynch, 'Observations on the Colloidal Gold Reaction in Neurosyphilis and other Diseases of the Central Nervous System', *Lancet* (1922), 1063–4.

York, George K., and David A. Steinberg, *An Introduction to the Life and Work of John Hughlings Jackson* (London: Wellcome Trust Centre for the History of Medicine at UCL, 2006).

Young, Robert M., 'The Functions of the Brain: Gall to Ferrier (1808–1886)', *Isis* 59:3 (1968), 250–68.

—— *Mind, Brain, and Adaptation in the Nineteenth Century* (New York: Oxford University Press, 1990).

Zülch, K. J., 'The Place of Neurology in Medicine and its Future', in by P. J. Vinker and G. W. Bruyn (eds), *Handbook of Neurology* (Amsterdam: North-Holland Publishing Co., 1968).

Index

Adie, William John 76, 82, 107, 121, 168
Adrian, Edgar Douglas 126–7, 129–30, 135
Aldren Turner, William 50, 89
American Neurological Association 22, 106–9, 202n.6
ancient tradition of medicine 4, 6–8
animal electricity 9, 15
animal spirits 9
Apothecaries Act (1815) 7
Association of British Neurologists (*also* ABN) 26, 57, 99, 113, 120–1, 124–31, 143, 145–6
  advice on remuneration 139
  Advisor on Neurology 145
  Committee on Neurology 140
  eclectic membership of 126
  meeting in Edinburgh 127
  membership lists 125
  official body representing British neurology 137, 143
  origins of 118–19
  overseas membership in 128
  physiology and neurology 129
  Second World War and 128
  teaching and practice 137
  women members 129
Association of Physicians of Great Britain and Ireland 52, 64, 66–8, 74, 84, 89, 95, 105, 120, 162
asylums 7, 11, 21, 50, 117

bacteriology 11, 97, 124, 170
Barlow, Thomas 53, 55
Barnes, Arthur Stanley 93, 126, 128, 140
Bastian, Henry Charlton 37, 48–50
Beard, George 6
Bell, Charles 9–10, 46
Bernard, Claude 12
Beveridge Committee 138
Bichat, Marie François Xavier 7
biochemistry 113, 123–4, 148–9, 170
borders between specialties *see* jurisdictions
Bowman, William 32, 45, 47
Bradford, John Rose 53, 55, 66
Brain: A Journal of Neurology 12, 39, 107, 170
Brain, Walter Russell 59–60, 69–74, 76–7, 84, 140, 143, 148, 169–71
  career of 74
  educational background 69–70
  pacifism of 70–3
  Report on Neurological Services 90–1, 136–7
  views of malingering 73–4
  x-ray technician 69–75
brain death criteria 155
brainhood 28, 177
Bramwell, Byrom 1, 46, 63, 108
Bramwell, Edwin 1, 5, 23, 60, 89–90, 108, 121, 126–9, 164–5
Broadbent, William 22, 37, 45
Brown-Séquard, Charles Édouard 48
Bucknill, John 37, 39, 50
Burden Neurological Institute and Clinic 93, 123, 224n.13
Burdon-Sanderson, John 30, 48–9
Buzzard, Edward Farquhar, 61, 89, 126, 128

Buzzard, Thomas 36–8, 48

Cairns, Hugh 106
Cajal, Santiago Ramón y 167
cardiology 14, 142
Carmichael, Edward Arnold 97–9, 103, 112–15, 123, 146–7
  Director of MRC Clinical Neurological Research Unit 115–18
Carpenter, William 48
cell theory 10
  see also neuron theory
Chair of Clinical Neurology at Oxford University 213–14n.189
Charcot, Jean-Martin 18, 22–3
Chevassut, Kathleen 97–9, 103, 106, 110–13
  see also Halley Stewart Trust
Cloake, Philip 93, 130, 140
club culture 26, 41, 48, 63–4, 126–7, 130
Cohen, Henry 121, 126
Committee on Neurology at Royal College of Physicians *see* Royal College of Physicians London
conscientious objectors 69
Core, Donald 121, 164
Cornwall 150
cortical localisation 11, 29, 40, 45, 50, 57, 156
Crichton-Browne, James 29, 37, 39, 46
Critchley, Macdonald 61, 91, 125–6
Cushing, Harvey 1, 5, 79, 89, 94, 106

Dale, Henry 47, 167
Decade of the Brain 157
Denny Brown, Derek 116, 157, 220n.109
Devon 150
diagnosis 23, 43, 123, 139, 159
  controversy in shell shock 96
  diagnostic medicine 122
  diagnostic practices 95
  diagnostic technologies 105
  eyes in diagnostics 36
  hysteria 81
  method of 87
  semiology 122
  uncertainty of 42
Diploma in Neurology 138, 141
distinction awards in neurology 228–9n.103
division of labour xv, 14, 34–5, 103
Dott, Norman 94, 106
Douglas Powell, Richard 66
drugs 122–3

economics 95, 158, 177
electroencephalography 122–3
electrology 6, 11, 160
electron microscope 149
Elkington, John 140
Emergency Medical Services 135
evolution 33–5, 87, 156, 176–8
eyes 19, 32, 36
  diseases of the eyes 8

Feiling, Anthony 93, 121, 140
Ferrier, David 29, 37, 46, 48, 50
First World War 25, 68–84, 96, 99, 109, 153, 172, 174
  demography of wounded 75
  functional nervous disorders 75
  head wounds in 76
  nerve patients 79
    see also shell shock
  neurological injuries 75
  research on war injuries 89
  specialisation 25
  specialised bodies 74
  wounded soldiers 69–73
Fletcher, Walter Morley 104, 111–15
Foster, Michael 30, 47
Founders of Neurology 166–9
France 7, 74–9, 82, 92, 117, 157, 159
Freud, Sigmund 81
Freudianism 78–9, 82, 84
functional nerve disorders 22, 40, 74–5, 78–80, 87, 175
  see also nervous diseases

Galton, Francis 37
Galvani, Luigi 9
Garrod, Archibald 66, 102, 104
general hospitals 18
  fiscal crisis of 19–20
  neurological departments in 91–4
general medicine 165
  career in 20
  commonalities with neurology 139
  and specialism 103
general physicians
  remuneration 139
  with an interest in neurology 25, 94, 145, 150–1
general practice
  importance of training medical students 20
general practitioners 150, 153
generalism *see* medical generalism
generalist
  advantages to being 17
  antipathy to specialism 93
  monopoly power 95
  with special interests 24
generations 6, 11, 15, 17, 23, 25, 59, 68–9, 72, 74, 76, 79, 86, 88, 95, 121, 123–5, 147, 164–5, 172
  conflicts between 86–8, 125, 139
  definition of neurology 6, 95, 121, 164–5, 209n.126
  and founding specialties 15
  specialist mentalities 17, 25, 76
  war experience 68–9, 74, 76
genetics 123–5, 149
Germany 23, 55, 69, 73, 117, 131, 159
Godber, George Edward 150
Goodenough Report 140
Gordon, Ronald Grey 121, 164
Gowers, William 1, 12, 33, 36
Greenfield, James Godwin 121, 130, 140
Guttman, Ludwig 155

habitus 27, 173
Haldane Commission 85, 103
Hale-White, William 19, 53, 66
Hall, Marshall 10, 46–7
Halley Stewart Jr., Barnard 110
Halley Stewart Sr., Barnard 111–12
Halley Stewart Trust 98, 111–15, 130
  Chesterford Gardens 111–15
  research fellowships 25, 115, 118
Harris, Wilfred 43, 91, 121
Haymaker, Webb 166
Head, Henry 47, 56, 59–60, 66, 77, 84–8, 104, 152, 176
  medical unit at the London Hospital 8, 56
  presidential address to Neurological Section or RSM 86–8
head wounds 76
Himsworth, Harold 148
Hinds Howell, Conrad Meredyth 164
histology 11, 123
historiography of neurology 166
Hitzig, Eduard 29, 45
Holmes, Gordon 43, 76–80, 82, 121, 132, 136
  anti-Freudianism 78–9
  functional neuroses and 78
  job offer at Johns Hopkins 100–1, 116
  military commission of 78
  Red Cross work in First World War 77
  on shell shock 82
  spinal injuries and 78
Horsley, Victor 40, 44–5
Hughlings Jackson Lectureship 45, 87
Hurst, Arthur 83, 89, 92
Hutchinson, Jonathan 37, 46, 66, 196n.12
Huxley, Thomas Henry 30, 47–8

imaging science 122, 156
imaging technologies 149, 157, 176
immunology 155
integration and neurology 33–5, 158–62

International Neurological Congresses 109, 119, 143
1931 Congress in Berne 110
1935 Congress in London 105, 125
1939 Congress in Copenhagen 131
internationalism
League of Nations 104
meetings 25, 107
and neurology 99
and specialism 100, 105, 109
invented tradition 101, 108, 235n.63
commemoration and memory 105
of neurology 2

Jackson, John Hughlings 19, 21, 23, 29, 32, 37, 45–7, 50, 86–7, 105, 152
and Herbert Spencer 33–5, 196n.21
justifications for specialisation 35
Jefferson, Geoffrey 106
Johns Hopkins Hospital and Medical School 100–1
Johnson, William 79, 82, 92, 121
Journal of Neurology and Psychopathology 119
jurisdictions 54–5, 142, 161, 207n.97
alienists and neurologists 34
internal medicine and neurology 56
neurology and general medicine 140–2, 144
neurology and psychiatry 140, 142, 144
neurosurgery and neurology 105
ophthalmologists and physicians with interests in nervous diseases 32
ophthalmology and neurology 32, 32–7
orthopaedic surgeons and neurologists 135–6
physicians of nervous diseases and neurologists 92–4
physiology and neurology 47
psychoanalysis and neurology 81–2

Kennedy, Foster 78, 81
Kerr Anderson, Hugh 47, 50
Kinnier Wilson, S. A. 91, 93, 121, 172

La Salpêtrière 23
laboratory medicine 102, 116
Laycock, Thomas 10, 19, 46
Lennox, William 116, 118–19
Lewis, Thomas 103–4, 114
London teaching hospitals 21
Lord, John Robert 50–1

McAlpine, Douglas 91–2
Maida Vale Hospital for Nervous Diseases 21, 79
malingering 73–4, 80
Mapother, Edward 91
Medical Act (1858) 7, 18–19
medical generalism 2, 15–17, 52, 54–5, 95, 101–2
decline of 106
generalism to specialism 60
generalist societies 66
influence of general medicine on specialisation 3, 13, 92–3
patrician tastes 67
specialist medical societies and 31
Medical Research Council (MRC) 25, 97, 103–4, 112–15, 147
Medico-Psychological Association 50
mesmerism 9, 15
metaphors 10–11, 33, 35, 160, 176
specialisation and the body medical 33
Meyer, Adolf 40, 108–9
Mind 12
mind and brain 11, 156
Ministry of Health 80, 131, 135–6, 136, 143, 145, 150
collaboration with MRC on nerve injuries 132
lack of recognition of neurologists 134

Ministry of Pensions 80, 90, 133, 135
Montreal Neurological Institute 1
Mott, Frederick 50, 168
MRC *see* Medical Research Council

National Health Service 94, 124, 131, 142, 144–5, 149–50, 157
National Hospital for Nervous Diseases, Queen Square 19–21, 25, 40, 48, 50, 100–1, 112–15, 129
  Medical Research Council Clinical Neurological Research Unit 116–18, 123, 146
  postgraduates from America 116, 220n.93
National Union of Neurologists 89, 104
nerve injuries 131–6
nervous diseases 4, 80, 149
  Alzheimer's disease 149, 156
  chronic disorders 149
  chronic epileptics 145
  chronic patients 90, 110, 122, 149
  Creutzfeld-Jakob's disease 156
  cultural construction of 8
  differentiating nerve patients 22
  inability to treat 145
  multiple sclerosis 97–9, 109–10
  Parkinson's disease 149
nervous system 149, 174
  anatomy of the brain and nerves 9–10
  autonomic responses of 146
  cultural construction of 95
  masculinity and the 10
  physiology of 11, 12
networks in Victorian science 46–52
neuro-culture 2, 27–8, 176, 178
neurochemical self 177
Neurological Society of the United Kingdom 24, 30, 36–58, 173
  Brain: A Journal of Neurology and 39
  Darwinians in 48
  demography of 40, 51
  Fellows of Royal Society in 46–8
  formation of 36
  integration in 38
  patients in 42–4
  training young members 41–4
  women in 39
neurology and evolution 34, 176
neuron theory 44, 123, 167, 236n.67
neuropsychiatry 93, 117, 161
neurosciences 27, 123, 146
neuroscientists 149
neurosurgery 105
neurosurgical centre 144
Nevin, Samuel 118, 127, 140
Newcastle neurology 155
number of neurologists 151, 154

O'Brien, Daniel P. 114
obituaries 163–5, 234n.37
Ophthalmological Society of the United Kingdom 24, 30-7, 52, 120
  John Hughlings Jackson's Bowman Lecture 33–6
  and Royal Society of Medicine 57
opposition to specialisation 13, 14, 17, 20, 22, 24–5, 102, 157–9
  internal medicine and 56
  regional hospital boards 143–5
Osler, William 55–6, 66, 68, 84

Pallis, Christopher 155
Paralympics 155
pathology 10–11
patients 22, 43–4, 122, 142
patrician mentality 3, 67, 153, 162
pharmacology 149, 155
phrenology 5, 9, 11, 15–16
Physiological Society of the United Kingdom 50
physiology 123–4, 149
Proceedings of the Royal Society of Medicine 44
professional designation of 'neurologist' 54, 121
  retrospective reconstruction of identity xv, 58, 165–9

self-described neurologists 25, 209–10n.126
professional identity xv, 21, 23, 94–5, 135–6, 162–5, 169–71
crisis of 26
declinism in neurology 125, 147
defining neurology 147–8
fluidity of 54, 139
integrative identity of neurologists 27, 154, 158, 169–72
membership lists of societies 46, 51, 163
networks 46–52
neurologists lack of recognition in Ministry of Health 134
professors of neurology 1–2, 155
see also specialist departments
psychiatry 5, 11–13, 17, 54, 81, 124, 140–4, 148, 161, 164, 169–70, 175, 177
see also jurisdictions
psychology 9–12, 15, 17, 38, 54, 124, 148, 161, 175
see also jurisdictions
Purves-Stewart, James Morgan 75, 97–9, 101, 106–10 119, 215n.8

Queen Square *see* National Hospital

regional hospital boards 149
see also opposition to specialisation
Review of Neurology and Psychiatry 12
Riddoch, George 89, 130, 134–7, 140, 168
Risien Russell, James Samuel 50
Rockefeller Foundation 100, 107, 113, 116
endowment of research at National Hospital 116–18
motivations for supporting neurology 117
Romanes, George John 37
Royal College of Physicians, London 19, 145
Comitia of 144–5
Committee on Neurology 124, 138, 140–5, 149, 151
Royal Medico-Psychological Association 138
Royal Society 30, 46–52
Royal Society of Medicine (*also* RSM) 24, 65–8, 86–90, 120, 159, 162
amalgamation of medical societies 24, 56
formation of 61–2
growing evidence of specialisation 67
Russell, Dorothy 129

Sargent, Percy 78, 89
Schiller, Francis 166–7
Scotland 93
Second World War 124, 157, 175
nerve injuries in *see* nerve injuries
Section of Neurology, Royal Society of Medicine 104–8, 145, 173–4
see also Royal Society of Medicine
Sharpey-Schafer, Edward Albert 37, 40–2, 44
shell shock 80–4
Gordon Holmes and 82
hereditary nature 80
morale 83
political debates about 82
Report of the War Office Committee on Shell Shock 82–4
Sherrington, Charles 47, 50, 87, 168, 172
Society of British Neurological Surgeons 106, 120, 127, 129
specialist departments 8, 18, 91–5, 151
Cardiff Royal Infirmary 94
Edinburgh University 94
General Infirmary, Leeds 93
Guy's Hospital 92–3
King's College Hospital 93
lack of neurological departments in regional centres 142
London Hospital 59, 85–6, 88
Middlesex Hospital 91

specialist departments (*continued*)
- Royal Victorian Infirmary, Newcastle 93
- St Bartholomew's Hospital 216n.20
- St George's Hospital 93
- St Mary's Hospital, 22, 91
- Scotland 93–4
- Swansea General Hospital 94
- University College Hospital 93
- Victoria Infirmary, Glasgow 93–4
- Wales 94
- Western Infirmary, Glasgow 94
- Wrexham Emergency Hospital 94

specialist hospitals 8, 11, 18, 20–2, 90–1, 159
Spencer, Herbert xv, 33–5, 37, 57, 196n.21, 196n.29
Spillane, John David 127
Standing Joint Committee 137–8
Symonds, Charles 61–2, 74, 138
- appointment as Assistant Physician in Nervous Diseases 92–3

technology 105–6, 155, 176
- and generalism 105
- and neurosurgery 105
- role in specialism 13, 36

therapeutics 122
- electric therapy 40

training
- importance of training medical students in general practice 20, 92–3
- of neurologists and psychiatrists 138, 140
- neurology training for general practitioners after First World War 207n.92
- training of specialists in neurology 143

Transactions of the Ophthalmological Society of the United Kingdom 31–2

unification of medicine 24
Union of Medical Societies 62, 66
United States of America 100, 116–17, 154, 157
- American Civil War 22
- patronage of science 157
- specialisation in 22

universal suffrage 96, 101

vaccines 16, 97–9, 110, 123
Vesalius, Andreas 5
Volta, Alessandro 9

Wales 94
Walshe, Francis Martin Rouse 62, 81, 89, 91, 98, 112–14, 127, 146–7
- Catholicism of 111
- denial of wartime specialist status 75

Walton, John 161
War Office
- number of specialists in nervous diseases 75
- *Report of the War Office Committee on Shell Shock* 82–4
  - *see also* shell shock

Weir Mitchell, Silas 18
welfare state 16
West End Hospital for Nervous Diseases 21, 134
- number of beds 90

West Riding Lunatic Asylum 29
Willis, Thomas 5, 168
Wilson, Charles 140
women and neurology 39, 97–8, 154, 185n.51
work in neurology 149–52
- holiday and sick leave 150
- long distances 151

World Federation of Neurology 145
Worster-Drought, Cecil 91, 121

X-club 48, 200n.97
x-ray 69–75
- bismuth meal techniques 70

CPSIA information can be obtained
at www.ICGtesting.com
Printed in the USA
FFOW03n0229270116
20701FF

9 780719 099816